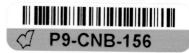

MIRACLES FROM
THE VAULT
ANTHOLOGY OF UNDERGROUND CURES

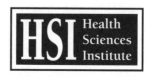

HSI Health Sciences Institute

Miracles from the Vault: Anthology of Underground Cures

610B000196

Table of Contents

Part III: Heart

Part IV: Asthma and COPD

Part V: Anti-Aging, Energy, and Weight Loss

Part VI: Osteoporosis

Part VII: Diabetes

Part VIII: Memory

Part IX: Immune System

Part X: Vital Health Secrets

Part I

Pain

CHAPTER ONE

Ancient herb meets modern science to slash rheumatoid arthritis symptoms in half

There's an interesting debate heating up among supporters of Cat's Claw. On the one hand, its track record providing centuries of relief speaks for itself. On the other, a group of scientists has, for lack of a better term, dissected it—and their findings are what's causing the controversy.

In the 1970s, scientists began to investigate this herb, used for centuries in South and Central America to treat disorders from asthma to ulcers. They identified several components that may contribute to its power. They cataloged at least six types of alkaloids, called oxindole alkaloids, which they found to have immune-boosting properties.

In dozens of clinical studies since then, Cat's Claw's oxindole alkaloids have demonstrated their ability to stimulate the immune response and increase white blood cell production, as well as decrease inflammation.[1-4] In fact, based on this research, Cat's Claw became a popular complementary treatment for fighting cancer and AIDS.

Scientists isolate alkaloids responsible for the power of Cat's Claw

Then a few years ago, a group of Austrian scientists probed a little deeper. They classified Cat's Claw's oxindole alkaloids into two distinct groups: pentacyclic oxindole alkaloids (POAs) and tetracyclic oxindole alkaloids (TOAs). Their research showed that the POAs alone were responsible for Cat's Claw's immune-enhancing effects—and that the TOAs actually inhibited the positive effects of the POAs.[1,2] In one study, the author went so far as to say: "Recent studies have shown that the tetracyclic alkaloids exert antagonistic effects on the action of the pentacyclic alkaloids. Mixtures of these two types of drugs are therefore unsuitable for medicinal uses."[3]

But the idea that one of the constituents "does all the work" doesn't sit well with a lot of people. It reminds me of the old commercial for peanut butter cups—is it the chocolate or the peanut butter that's responsible for the taste? Obviously, it's both.

HSI panelist Leslie Taylor is among those herbal researchers that's skeptical about the validity of the findings against TOA. They point to decades of Cat's Claw research that demonstrates the plant's power without specifying TOA and POA content, and to the synergistic effects of the many other active phytochemicals in Cat's Claw.

In fact, in a report titled, "The Cat's Claw TOA/POA Controversy," Taylor wrote: "I've seen too many times where nature has provided us with a great beneficial and biologically-active medicinal plant—and a rich indigenous history of effective use—but some have a compelling need to alter its chemical composition. The number of compounds present in such plants is staggering, and their interactions are subtle; science can only hope to understand most of them. I don't believe that science can state, at this point, that Cat's Claw's 'active constituents' are its alkaloids (or just one group of alkaloids), extract them, and expect them to work as efficiently as the natural form."

Could one herb slash tender joint pain in half?

The jury may still be out on TOA-free Cat's Claw. And I have to wonder if the researchers behind it don't want it that way. Just recently, a study at Austria's Innsbruck University Hospital demonstrated the effectiveness of TOA-free Cat's Claw against rheumatoid arthritis. In this clinical trial, doctors recruited 40 patients who fulfilled the American College of Rheumatology's criteria for RA. All of the patients were taking sulfasalazine (Azulfidine) or hydroxyxhloroquine (Plaquenil) for their condition, as well as small doses of NSAIDs and/or prednisolone as needed, but still suffered with painful, swollen joints and morning stiffness. On average, the participants had been dealing with RA symptoms for seven years.

In the first phase of the study, participants were divided into two groups and received either a capsule containing 60 mg of TOA-free Cat's Claw extract or a placebo three times a day. In the second phase, all participants received the Cat's Claw extract capsules. Phase one lasted 24 weeks; phase two continued another 28 weeks after that.

This is where my curiosity gets aroused. If they are so confident that TOA-free Cat's Claw is superior, wouldn't it have made sense to have a three-way trial—one that tested standard Cat's Claw vs. the TOA-free variety vs. a placebo? That would have allowed them to measure any true impact the TOA was having—negative or positive.

But back to the study they did do. At the beginning of phase one, all the RA patients' symptoms were assessed in a number of ways: by number of tender and swollen joints; by the Ritchie index, a widely accepted tool for assessing RA symptoms; and by duration of stiffness each morning. Participants were also asked to use a visual analog scale (VAS), which is essentially a long line they mark to reflect the severity of their pain. At the end of the first 24 weeks, the Cat's Claw-treated patients' scores had been cut in half in several significant areas. Their number of tender joints fell from 7.7 to 3.8, and their Ritchie index scores declined from 5.5 to 2.9. (In comparison, the placebo group went from 8.3 to 6.3 respectively, and their Ritchie Index scores moved from 4.8 to 4.2.) During phase two, the phase one placebo group began taking Cat's Claw, and soon they began reaping the benefits as well. After beginning Cat's Claw therapy, the former placebo group lowered its number of tender joints to 2.7, and saw its Ritchie Index score plummet to 1.8. Even better, the original treated group continued to see additional gains in phase two; its number of tender joints was reduced to 2.5, and Ritchie Index fell to 2.4.[4] And during the entire study period, there were no adverse effects attributed to Cat's Claw treatment.

Ninety-eight percent of patients improved; more energy, better mental clarity, and more

Another recent study, published in the *British Naturopathic Journal*, supports these findings on RA and reports on TOA-free Cat's Claw's efficacy against a wide range of other health concerns.

In this clinical review, John Kule M.D. of the East Aiken Health Center in South Carolina discussed his treatment of 60 patients with the new formulation. Overall, Dr. Kule says that 98 percent of his patients have shown clinical improvement after treatment. Specifically, he highlights seven case studies showing that TOA-free Cat's Claw increases energy, improves mental clarity, decreases inflammation, lowers blood pressure, and reduces blood sugar.[5]

TOA-free formulas come at a premium

As the debate between the Cat's Claw camps continues, there's one thing everyone agrees on: TOA-free Cat's Claw doesn't come cheap. In fact, it costs about three times more than regular Cat's Claw. Its proponents justify the price jump as necessary to cover the additional expenses of harvesting and verifying the plant's alkaloid content.

Critics say the additional testing is unnecessary and consumers can obtain the same benefits with regular Cat's Claw. They point out that it's been used for at least 2,000 years to relieve pain and treat rheumatism, arthritis, swelling, and infections. And since the two have never been tested against each other, our advice would be to let your pain and your pocketbook decide.

On a related note, Taylor stresses the need to know your Cat's Claw source, and make sure you are getting Uncaria tomentosa and not one of the other varieties out there. As Cat's Claw has become more popular, Uncaria tomentosa has become harder to find, and some suppliers are now substituting another Cat's Claw species called Uncaria guianensis. Taylor recommends reading labels carefully to ensure that you are getting the real thing.

Whichever one you choose, the evidence is clear that Cat's Claw is safe and without side effects. For information on how to order both forms of Cat's Claw, see the Member Source Directory on page 529.

CHAPTER TWO

Breakthrough Chinese formula sends drug-resistant joint pain packing

"I couldn't wait to tell you."

That's how the letter began. What followed was one woman's incredible story of her recovery from crippling knee arthritis—in a matter of *hours*. So it's not surprising that Jim English (CEO of Tango Advanced Nutrition) made a point of passing the news along to me— adding that the brand-new product behind this story is without doubt one of the most promising formulas he's come across in years.

So, to borrow from the amazing testimonial English received mere days after sending his few samples out, I just couldn't wait to tell you— about ArthriPhase, that is. Like all of Tango's products, it's a carefully selected blend of potent Chinese herbs—but it's also the first arthritis product Tango has ever distributed.

I can tell you now: It's a perfect fit. Like every Tango product that's made the cut before it, this isn't just any old formula. And its benefits reach way beyond pain relief—meaning that finally, there's a *real* solution for your arthritis. And one that's completely safe, too.

But before I explain what makes ArthriPhase so unique, let me take a minute to expose some little-known truths about your arthritis pain—and to tell you why so many mainstream treatments just don't work.

Dissecting the "disease" of chronic pain

Researchers know more about chronic pain today than they ever have before. But unfortunately, the news isn't great. In fact, it appears that chronic pain isn't so much a symptom after all—and it might actually be better classified as a disease in and of itself.

This distinction has everything to do with the physiological differences that scientists have discovered between chronic pain and its shorter, more immediate counterpart (better known as acute pain). While the exact specifics of these differences are too complicated to get into here, let me take a minute to explain them as simply as I can.

Normal acute pain essentially acts as your body's natural alarm system. When tissue is injured, it prompts a cascade of inflammatory chemicals that trigger your brain to signal pain. These pain signals are then carried by your body's sensory pain receptors (called nociceptors), which communicate with nerves in your spinal cord.

From there, the signal is transmitted to the cerebral cortex—at which point you will feel the signal as pain, and be able to identify its location. And this sensation is critical to proper healing and to avoiding injurious situations in the future.

What you may not realize, though, is that this elaborate signaling system has a very important counterpart—and its purpose is to dull the very same pain, by means of natural painkilling chemicals like endorphins and norephinephrine.

Think about it: The sensation you experience from a simple cut or bruise subsides quickly relative to the amount of time these injuries take to completely heal. And it's a good thing, too—if every minor injury persisted with the same amount of pain you experienced when it initially happened, you'd barely be able to function. So it's easy to see how essential your natural painkilling mechanism is—and how many problems can arise if it somehow goes haywire.

Unfortunately, that's exactly what happens in cases of chronic pain like fibromyalgia or arthritis. You see, nociceptors use the neurotransmitter glutamate to relay their message to your spinal cord. In smaller amounts, glutamate only activates the receptors responsible for acute pain (called AMPA receptors)—but after repeated activation, or when glutamate is released in larger amounts, a different set of receptors (called NDMA receptors) is activated instead.

And it just so happens that this transition has some disastrous physical consequences.

Why mainstream "solutions" just don't work

When acute pain becomes chronic pain, the entire structure of your body's pain response is changed—and often, there's not much that can be done to help it. That's because pain receptors become more excitable and sensitive as a result of this switch—and require less input to receive a pain signal. Consequently, even greater amounts of input are required to dull this signal, and over time, your natural painkilling mechanism will exhaust itself trying to keep up with these oversensitive receptors.

This extreme transformation in chemical pathways means that your pain becomes estranged from the original injury that triggered it. Instead, it permanently remains as part of a vicious self-continuing cycle—in much the same way that a vivid memory of a traumatic event can continue to cause emotional distress years later.

The result is chronic pain and inflammation—often with no identifiable source, and with even more resistance to conventional attempts to relieve it. It's precisely this type of stubborn, debilitating pain that serves as the most common indicator of the two main types of arthritis: osteoarthritis (OA) and rheumatoid arthritis (RA). But it's still worth noting some of the major differences between the two conditions.

Unlike osteoarthritis—which is a condition attributed to age- or injury-related "wear and tear" in your joints—RA is an autoimmune disease. It sets in when your immune system turns on your body, and begins attacking healthy tissue—a phenomenon that leads to a state of near-perpetual inflammation in your body's joints (usually the smaller ones that are closer to your hands, like your knuckles).

Over time, this inflammation can destroy your joints completely—and sometimes in a matter of only a couple of years or less. Pain relievers (whether they're over-the-counter NSAIDs or that infamous class of drugs called COX-2 inhibitors) are powerless against this gradual degeneration—and while they may control some of the symptoms of your arthritis, the end result remains the same.

Not that you would want to rely on either of these so-called "solutions" anyway—you've already heard the warnings. The same COX-2 inhibitors that were once hailed as breakthroughs (think Vioxx and Celebrex) quickly revealed themselves to cause an increased risk of heart attacks. And the NSAIDs you're left with (like ibuprofen and naproxen) will tear up your insides over time.

For that same reason, the outlook isn't so much brighter if you're suffering with the more common condition of osteoarthritis. In fact, some research has shown that patients using anti-inflammatories to treat their OA pain might actually experience a *faster* progression in joint damage over time.[1] But whether or not that's true in all cases, the fact still remains that the pain, inflammation, and cartilage degradation involved in both types of arthritis will almost always surpass any treatment's ability to keep up with it.

Ask any doctor, and he'll probably tell you that when it comes to chronic forms of arthritis, there's not much more you can do beyond temporarily treating the pain with dangerous medicines—or subjecting yourself to side-effect laden immune-modulators like steroids and other marginally effective drugs.

The fact is, mainstream medicine's contributions to arthritis treatment have been fleeting at best—and deadly at worst. But you know as well as I do that the pain and physical limitations your arthritis imposes are downright impossible to ignore. And simply living with your symptoms is not an option.

10 years of pain erased in a single week

Chances are good that you've already made the switch to a safer natural arthritis treatment—like glucosamine, chondroitin, or MSM—one that promises pain relief and support in joint regeneration. If so, maybe you've seen improvements from these supplements already.

But if you haven't seen any improvements—or if you just haven't seen *enough*—then ArthriPhase is exactly what you've been looking for. The twelve herbs that comprise the formula work in tandem to help soothe inflammation, reduce swelling, and boost circulation—thereby assisting in new cartilage formation.

Most notable is that more than half of the herbs in the formula (among them, Gastrodia elata, Tang-kuei, Notopterygium, Cyathula, Angelica Pubescens, Aconite, and Scrophularia—for a complete list, see above) have been shown in animal studies to act on receptors that are specific to chronic pain and to calm overly excited nerves. And as I discussed earlier, this action helps to restore normal pain responses—thereby providing more effective, longer-term relief.

But these effects haven't been noted in animals alone—Chinese clinical studies show that this unique benefit applies to humans, too.

In one trial, 310 arthritis patients received ArthriPhase for 30 days. By the tenth day, a remarkable 70 percent had already reported noteworthy reductions in joint pain. At the end of the study, these reports were supported by the results of two diagnostic blood tests—one that measured the subjects' erythrocyte sedimentation rates (or ESR—a marker of inflammation), and one that measured for rheumatoid factor (RF—a marker of rheumatoid arthritis).

These tests revealed that 50 percent of the subjects had normal ESR values. But just as impressive was that 24 of the 38 subjects who began the study with rheumatoid arthritis tested *negative* for the marker at the end of the 30 days.

Similar results have been reported in Tango's dozens of rigorous evaluations: Every tester reported greater range of motion, less stiffness, and reduced pain—with some, as I mentioned earlier, reporting incredible improvements in mere hours. In fact, one subject—who was diagnosed with rheumatoid arthritis prior to beginning treatment with ArthriPhase—reported a complete absence of joint pain after the preliminary test period.

"Within one week," he reported, "my daily pain is gone"—adding that his joints only ache now from overuse or extreme cold. But it's his final remark that says it all: "Overall, I feel better than I have in 10 years."

You can find ordering information for ArthriPhase in the Member Source Directory.

ArthriPhase is a proprietary blend of the following time-tested and scientifically proven arthritis-fighting herbs:

Gastrodia Elata	Rehmannia (root)
Tang-kuei (root)	Notopterygium (root)
Eucommia (bark)	Chinese Ligusticum (root)
Cyathula (root)	Scrophularia (root)
Viscum (stem and leaf)	Angelica Pubescens (root)
Processed Aconite (root)	Typhonium (root)

CHAPTER THREE

Eliminate excruciating kidney pain for good with this all-in-one stone-crushing cure

I'll never forget it: finding my good friend collapsed in pain on his kitchen floor, clutching his side, unable to move, and only barely able to speak. After being ushered to the emergency room via ambulance and given a hefty dose of pain medication, the cause of his crippling condition finally came to light.

It was a kidney stone, they said. And though it was the first time I had ever seen the devastating side effects of a passage like this, you can believe that I know them when I see them now. And that goes a million times over for my friend who suffered through it. He said it was the most unimaginable pain he'd ever experienced.

You might already be familiar with this nightmarish pain first-hand—and if so, the product I'm about to share with you could literally change your life. A far cry from the mainstream's so-called "solution" of prescription painkillers, it turns out that there is a safe, natural—and very effective—cure.

It's called KGP Flush, and it's a brand-new formula from panelist

Jon Barron that I learned about just a few short weeks ago.

The single-herb answer to destroying dangerous kidney stones

If you've been a member for a while now, you might remember the first time we told you about a potent Peruvian herb called chanca piedra—literally, *stone breaker*. (It's also the main ingredient in Barron's new formula.) This herb can effectively destroy kidney stones by breaking them into smaller pieces and thereby making them easier to pass.[1]

I probably don't have to tell you that this will spare you a tremendous amount of agony—in both the short and the long term.

That's because the size of the kidney stone you're passing is what dictates the level of pain you'll experience. Believe it or not, these deposits (formed from calcium in the urine, mixed with a salt called oxalate, or alternatively, uric acid) are quite common. In fact, most of us will pass stones in our lifetimes—many of which go completely unnoticed.

If these stones are large enough, however—about the size of a grain of sand or bigger—you won't be so lucky. A dull, throbbing pain in your back and side will become a sharp stabbing pain as a stone moves from your kidney to your urethra to be passed. (Remember, however small these stones may appear, they are composed of jagged edges that tear through your flesh as they move.) This horrible process can take hours, even days.

To make matters worse, one incident of this kind usually portends another (if not many more) to come. And if later stones are any larger, the complications reach much further than excruciating pain. A stone that's too large to be passed can block urine flow in your kidneys—and ultimately lead to permanent (and potentially deadly) damage.

In cases like these, your only real options are surgery, or a procedure called extracorporeal shock- wave lithotripsy (ESWL for short, wherein shockwaves are sent through your tissue to crush the stones).

Either way, you're still looking at a lifetime of unpredictable attacks and a dizzying regimen of prescription pain management.

Fortunately, none of this has to happen—not if you keep your kidney stones under control from the start. And regular consumption of chanca piedra is the key.

Not only does it break down your stones, making them less painful as they move through your body (imagine the difference between the consistency of gravel and a consistency more like toothpaste, Barron suggested), but it also acts as an anti-inflammatory, an antibacterial, and a diuretic.

Even more impressive is the fact that chanca piedra can keep those stones from coming back, too. Although researchers are still investigating exactly how it works, the herb has been shown to have a "potent and effective" inhibitory effect on kidney stone formation—even at very high concentrations of calcium oxalate.[2]

By harnessing the power of chanca piedra, KGP Flush provides all of the herb's best benefits. But that's not all it does—not by a long shot.

7 steps to keeping your kidneys healthier than ever

In developing this formula, Barron demanded an approach that was thorough and comprehensive—one that, in his experience, isn't often assumed by your average kidney product. As he explained it, most kidney supplements focus solely on the antilithic (or stone-breaking) action—and for good reason, as that's probably the most important aspect of kidney stone relief.

But in focusing only on that one element, you are forgetting all of the essential actions that your kidneys perform. Your kidneys are responsible for the filtering your blood and eliminating waste, preserving the appropriate amounts of electrolytes and water in your body, and producing key blood-protective, bone-protective, and heart-protective hormones.

And if something goes awry in your kidneys, all of these functions can eventually be affected.

That's why Barron believes that any good kidney formula will perform six essential duties beyond simply being antilithic. To truly address the many sources of kidney stones and the pain that accompanies them, a formula would also have to be diuretic (water removing), antiseptic (infection killing), anti-hepatotoxic and anti-nephrotoxic (liver and kidney cleansing), soothing to urinary tract tissue, anti-inflammatory, and lastly, stimulating to renal tissue (so that damage can be repaired quickly and efficiently).

In addition to chanca piedra, KGP Flush boasts a long list of 13 other ingredients, each with manifold influences on the health of your kidneys—and on the relief of kidney stone-related pain.

- Hydrangea root is a potent diuretic (which lessens the likelihood of infection along the entire urinary tract, including the bladder and the prostate) in addition to being antilithic. (The Native Americans have used the herb in this capacity for generations.) Recent research has also shown that hydrangea root offers more antioxidant protection to your liver than milk thistle and turmeric combined.[3]

- Gravel root is also a potent diuretic and antilithic agent. In addition, it facilitates the excretion of excess uric acid (making it an ideal treatment for gout and rheumatism too).

- Marshmallow root soothes inflamed tissues in the kidneys and urinary tract—making stones easier (and less painful) to pass.

- Juniper berry is a strong antiseptic and a natural diuretic that fights and flushes out infection.

- Corn silk is another diuretic (often used to treat bladder and prostate infections as well).

- Uva ursi has strong antiseptic, antioxidant, and antilithic properties. It is especially useful in soothing, calming, and strengthening bladder walls, protecting you against chronic infection.

- Parsley root is another diuretic that also clears uric acid (thereby preventing stone formation) and also prevents histamine release (meaning it can help with allergies, too).

- Carrot tops help to clear infection and alkalize the blood (removing stress from the kidneys).

- Dandelion leaf is a traditional diuretic, antiseptic, and pain reliever. It's also rich in potassium—a mineral that's often lost by excessive urination.

- Horsetail is another popular diuretic.

- Orange peel is a natural antiseptic, antibacterial, and fungicidal agent.

- Peppermint soothes and relaxes the muscles in the urinary tract, reducing pain and spasms.

- Goldenrod flushes excess water from the body—without flushing out essential electrolytes (like salt and potassium), a common problem with many diuretics (prescription or natural).

Each of these ingredients taken in combination with the antilithic chanca piedra can safely and effectively wash out your existing kidney stones—without the telltale sharp, stabbing pain you've come to dread. But just as important is that it keeps those stones from returning, while healing, restoring, and regenerating damaged tissue in your kidneys—not to mention your entire urinary tract. (In fact, this formula can help to break down stones in your liver, pancreas, and gall bladder, too, while flushing and restoring all of those organs—and keeping them healthy for life.)

You may have noticed, however, that many of the above ingredients are diuretic in nature—meaning that they also have the potential to increase any toxic effects from certain medications you may already be taking. If you're currently on medications, you'll want to stay on the safe side and work with your doctor while using KGP Flush.

Now you might be wondering, as you've probably come to wonder with any formula that promises an end to otherwise untreatable chronic pain: What's the catch? And when I tell you that KGP Flush isn't a capsule, but a tincture (it was the only way to include all of the necessary ingredients without compromising quality, Barron explained) you might think that you've found the catch right there.

But let me also say this: As tinctures go, this particular blend is the exception to every unspoken rule. The taste (while still bitter) is not reminiscent of the usual overpowering foulness that assaults your tongue with many other products—and neither is the smell. In fact, as soon as you open your bottle of KGP Flush, you'll inevitably recognize the distinct woodsy aroma of gin—courtesy of the juniper berries, no doubt. (If martinis are your drink of choice, you might even find this tincture pleasant.)

20 years of unbearable pain reversed in just 3 days

Like I said before, this product is brand new—so new, in fact, that Baseline is still ironing out details as I write this. But already, reports are coming in about KGP Flush's incredible capabilities. And Patty, a woman who has suffered with "incurable" kidney sludge for 20 years, will be the first to volunteer her story. Before she began taking Barron's new product, her pain was so severe that, at one point, she had to receive liquid Morphine every hour (a treatment usually reserved for terminal cancer patients) just to make it bearable.

Because she was diagnosed with sludge (small sand-like particles with no larger stone as a source), neither surgery nor lithotripsy were an option. The doctors told her that there was nothing more they could do. Several other natural remedies had already failed her—KGP Flush was her last resort. Fortunately for Patty, it was also the most effective.

After just three days of taking the formula, all of her kidney symptoms began to disappear. The pressure in her back released, and she was able to urinate without any straining or burning. By the evening of the fourth day, her symptoms had reversed so much that she was able to completely eliminate her evening dose of pain medication—and stay pain-free for the first time in 10 years. A full week later, she is still pain-free—and overwhelmingly amazed at the way this new formula has transformed her life. She'll continue to flush with KGP Flush once a month—and still can't believe that her days of unbearable and disabling pain might finally be behind her.

Like Patty, you'll want to mix 4 ounces of KGP Flush with a quart of fresh apple juice (usually recommended for its taste—but any juice you prefer is fine) and a quart of water. You'll drink the entire mixture over a course of four days (that's about a pint a day). Your stones should soften enough for a painless passage in as little as two to eight days. And in most cases, according to Barron, flushing with KGP Flush only twice a year should be enough to keep them away for good.

CHAPTER FOUR

Your glucosamine supplement could be useless... Uncover the secret source of your joint discomfort

You just can't figure it out. You've been taking glucosamine faithfully, but your joints are still stiff and uncomfortable.

Turns out, you could actually be treating the <u>wrong source</u> of your joint discomfort.

Because cartilage is not the only mechanism of action in your joints.

Joints can start aching for a number of different reasons. We all know one reason—the cartilage that cushions the joints breaks down and bone surfaces become less protected. So things that put weight on your joints—even the simplest things like walking and standing—become almost unbearable.

But there's another cause of joint distress—one you might not have heard of until now. That's because, until now, the only way to treat this aspect of joint health was through injections. But new research has changed that—and now it's one of the targets of the three-pronged approach that could keep your joints moving smoothly.

It's all in an exclusive formula called SynerFlex—combining several joint-savers that were never before brought together.

Synovial fluid—the secret to smooth, flowing movement

You might not have heard of synovial fluid before now, but it turns out it's one of the biggest factors in joint comfort.

It's a thick, stringy fluid found in the cavities of joints. This fluid, made mostly of hyaluronic acid (HA), reduces friction between the cartilage and other tissues in joints, lubricating and cushioning them during movement.

Of course, like so many other things, synovial fluid breaks down as we age. Without the "gel pack" of synovial fluid protecting them, joints and cartilage are left bare. So they rub against one another, sometimes causing excruciating pain.

Think about that stiff feeling you get when you suddenly stand after sitting for a long time—the synovial fluid has stiffened up. It usually takes just a few moments to get flowing again. But what if it takes longer?

Glucosamine is great for helping rebuild the cartilage that's rubbing away, but it won't do anything for synovial fluid.

For that, you have to replenish the very thing it's made of.

HA is present in nearly all the tissues of your body, but it's particularly important to the makeup of your skin as well as to the synovial fluid that cushions your joints (where it's the primary force in keeping joints lubricated).

It may also stimulate collagen production and plays an important role in the tissue-repair process.

And by replacing the diminishing HA in synovial fluid, you could actually help keep "bare joints" comfortable.

For a long time, it was assumed that HA only worked when it was injected directly into the site where it was needed. Without getting too technical on you, it has to do with the size of the HA molecules—it was assumed that, taken orally, they would never be absorbed by the body. But new research—and a brand new approach to isolating HA— is changing all that. And it's starting to show that HA could do the job even when swallowed in a pill.

Most HA is produced by bacterial fermentation. And it's always done the job—if you don't mind getting poked with needles regularly.

Still, the team that created Hyal-Joint® figured they could do one better. So they created a revolutionary extraction process to create HA that could be taken orally and could give the same—or better—results as fermented HA.

It starts with rooster comb, which yields an end product with the same molecular weight as the HA naturally found in the human joint.

They found that their process, though it created a less "pure" form of HA, actually resulted in a more effective product. Usually, the fermentation process breaks things down until only HA is left. But with Hyal-Joint, the extraction process is stopped before all of the other great stuff in the rooster comb is taken out. The collagen and glycosaminglycans—essential to joint health—are left in. So you get the benefit of HA as a "whole food"—rather than just one isolated element.

When it was put up against fermented HA in an *in vitro* study of human synovial fluid, Hyal-Joint clearly came out on top. After 24 hours, the highest levels of HA were measured in cells stimulated with Hyal-Joint, and the lowest levels were in those stimulated with fermented HA. Researchers concluded that Hyal-Joint is more active in synovial fluid cells.[1]

Then it was time for human trials. One study in particular, conducted on 20 subjects taking 80 mg of Hyal-Joint, or a placebo, orally over the course of eight weeks, is quite promising. By the end of the study, the subjects who took HA felt they had experienced statistically significant improvement in comfort and physical function.

Researchers concluded that Hyal-Joint appeared to be effective for promoting joint comfort, improving physical function, and enhancing several aspects of quality of life.[2]

Earlier, I mentioned that this is a three-pronged approach. HA is only the beginning when it comes to supporting your joints.

A healthy response to inflammation

SynerFlex doesn't stop at helping to replenish the HA that makes up your synovial fluid. It also promotes a healthy inflammatory response. The ingredients in SynerFlex work together to help maintain smooth joint movement and flexibility.

The natural anti-inflammatory properties of SynerFlex come from boswellia, an extract of the Indian frankincense tree that has been used historically to promote joint health. It contains various boswellic acids, the most potent of which is acetyl-11-keto-boswelllic acid (AKBBA).

Any kind of boswellia will give you some kind of results. But it really shines when it's standardized to contain a high percentage of AKBBA. Then, it builds on the effects of HA—helping to maintain flexibility.

The boswellia included in SynerFlex has been standardized to an impressive 20 percent. You're just not going to see that in all other joint supplements.

There have been several trials on how boswellia aids in healthy inflammatory response.

In one experiment with rabbits, oral administration of boswellia significantly reduced the population of inflammatory leukocites in the knee. The effect appeared within 6-12 hours after treatment, and persisted for over a month.

While the number of human trials is small, they show that boswellia may help preserve the structural integrity of joint cartilage and support connective tissue by stopping the breakdown of glycosaminoglycans, which help lubricate the joints.

It may also help support the healthy activity of leukotrienes, enzymes that cause inflammation. This can help keep joints comfortable and moving smoothly. But it doesn't stop there—an *in vitro* study showed that boswellia can actually help regulate the production of osteoclasts, cells that are involved in bone health.

So we've taken care of maintaining healthy HA levels in the synovial fluid and promoting a healthy response to inflammation—how about joint comfort?

Soothe and comfort your joints safely and naturally

You might have heard of hops before—it shows up in various sleep formulas. But the hops extract in SynerFlex, which is a little different and doesn't cause drowsiness, serves a very different purpose. And that's helping keep joints comfortable.

One study showed that hops supported healthy COX-2 in an *in vitro* model of inflammation.

And in a human study, subjects took 500 mg of hops twice daily for six weeks. It supported knee joint comfort and range of motion. Furthermore, hops have been shown to have a much lower potential for GI risk as compared to NSAIDs.

The surprise nutrient you're just not getting enough of

Boswellia, hops, and HA make up a pretty impressive joint health formula on their own. But then there's the surprising addition—a nutrient that research suggests promotes bone strength and could help prevent many of the joint worries we think are just a normal part of aging.

It also could go a long way in combating the underlying cause of joint concerns.

Boron is found in fruits and vegetables—when the soil they're grown in is boron-rich, of course. And as early as 1963 it was suggested that boron deficiency in food and/or water might worsen joint health. Surgeons have observed that patients taking boron supplements have much harder bones, and that broken bones heal more quickly among those patients.

Boron was put to the test in a trial exploring its effects on bone density in vitamin-D-depleted rats. Over the course of eight weeks, rats treated with 35 mg of boron showed a significant trend toward higher bone density.[3]

In a pilot human trial on joint comfort, 50 percent of patients given 6 mg of boron per day improved, as compared with 10 percent of subjects given placebo. And it's generally recognized as an essential nutrient for bone and joint health.

In another trial, 20 subjects with joint health concerns took boron for eight weeks. After just four weeks, 62.5 percent of the participants were more comfortable, and 87.5 percent felt less stiffness or no stiffness. And, after eight weeks, 70.8 percent had more comfort, 87.5 percent felt less stiffness, and 77.77 percent had less movement restriction. No serious side effects were reported.[4]

The problem is that, until now, there just wasn't a *safe* way to get a potent daily intake of boron. Everything scientists came up with was rather toxic, so it looked as if this bone-building miracle would just fall by the wayside.

Until a natural form, actually present in the food chain for millennia, was discovered. NorthStar snapped up this safe, food-sourced form of boron, called FruiteX-B®, and it became one of the powerful elements of SynerFlex.

The first product of its kind changes the way we approach joint health

I asked the NorthStar development team what makes SynerFlex special. They told me it's the first formula they know of to combine these joint-protective ingredients. They also told me they'd first looked into HA more than six years ago, but had been patiently waiting for solid research to show that an oral form of it really works.

And now, thanks to the innovation, quality, and research behind the Hyal-Joint HA, they are thrilled to build a new solution for joint health around it and the other joint-saving powerhouses in the formula.

SynerFlex is rounded out with a bio-enhancer blend containing ginger, black pepper, and long pepper. Ginger adds another measure of anti-inflammatory power, and the two kinds of pepper may also enhance the bioavailability of a number of nutrients, including boswellia.

Ordering information for SynerFlex is in the Member Source Directory on page 529.

CHAPTER FIVE

One-time charge for long-time relief from chronic pain

I n the May 1998 issue of *Members Alert*, HSI wrote about the FDA ban on one of the products we had featured several years before— a pain relieving blanket made from a fabric called Farabloc™. That's right: It's not just vitamins, herbs, and other natural supplements the FDA wants to get rid of—it's all alternative therapies, even items as harmless as a blanket.

Although it demonstrated fantastic success for pain management and had proven itself in clinical studies, the FDA removed Farabloc from the American market. It declared that there was insufficient evidence to "adequately demonstrate the safety and effectiveness of Farabloc" technology.

In addition to the clinical trials supporting it, it had also earned enthusiastic endorsements from physicians, insurance agencies, and consumer groups. And the feedback we received from scores of HSI members related near-miraculous results—including the elimination of knee pain, stiff necks, stump pain, arthritis, hip pain, muscle sprains, menstrual cramps, and migraines. In fact, one of our own staff members swore that the Farabloc blanket was the best—and only—relief she ever found from constant lower back pain caused by a slipped disk.

But, again, sometimes when a product works—really works—and the market demands access to it, things have a way of re-emerging. And Farabloc happens to be one of those things that really, truly works.

A new way to weather your painful symptoms

For generations, anecdotal evidence has demonstrated that people can predict weather changes based on symptom flare-ups they feel in their bodies. Maybe you've noticed your own joints aching just before a rainstorm or when a cold front moves in. Well, in 1969, a German scientist named Frieder Kempe began researching those claims to determine if there was any hard evidence to back them up.

He theorized that the shifts in electromagnetic fields causing weather changes may also be behind the physical symptom changes people experience during these times. To test out his theory, he created his own version of something called a Faraday cage and used it on his father, a WWII veteran who had lost a limb in combat and suffered phantom limb pain during climate and other environmental changes.

A Faraday Cage is a physical shield that completely blocks external electrical fields from coming into contact with—or affecting in any way—the object beneath it.

Granted, it sounds rather difficult to employ in real-world applications, but it's actually used every day in nearly every hospital. MRI machines utilize the concept of the Faraday cage as a means to keep the room free from radiation. The actual "cage" used for MRIs is made of an iron-containing metal, arranged in a grid pattern, that blocks high level electromagnetic frequencies or radiation from escaping the tunnel.

The fabric Kempe developed for his Farabloc blanket is made in the same way, only with a much finer grid. Of course, Farabloc isn't protecting outside environments—it's actually doing the reverse: protecting you—and all your cells—from the impact of those electromagnetic fields that cause atmospheric and environmental fluctuations.

To create his first prototype, Kempe hired a Belgian-based firm to spin fine steel mesh onto nylon thread. He then hired a German firm to weave the fibers into cloth. The result was a thick, stiff, uncomfortable, itchy fabric. Not exactly ideal—but it worked. When his father tried it, he reported complete relief from his phantom limb pain.

So following his initial success, Kempe set out to create a thinner, softer, more comfortable fabric.

He tested cotton and linen versions, but found them both less durable than the nylon fabric he'd originally chosen. The final version available today, is made of microthin threads of stainless steel fibers woven with nylon. This lightweight fabric looks and feels like linen, and, with proper care, it can last for years.

Weaving the way to relief from phantom limb pain, muscle fatigue, and even fibromyalgia

Since our first report on Farabloc in July 1996, many studies have been done—perhaps as a vehement retort to the FDA's position that there was insufficient evidence to "adequately demonstrate the [product's] safety and effectiveness."

Most of the research has been devoted to phantom limb pain like the kind Kempe's father experienced. However, Farabloc is also holding its own in demonstrating relief for other conditions—from arthritis to fibromyalgia.

One award-winning double-blind, cross-over study published in January of 2000 examined the effects of Farabloc and a placebo fabric on a condition called delayed-onset muscle soreness (DOMS), which occurs following strenuous exercise.

The researchers concluded that Farabloc worked significantly better than the placebo at reducing post-exercise stiffness and soreness. It also reduced the subsequent build-up of lactic acid and free-radical damage.

And I recently got a sneak peak at two not-yet-published studies conducted by Gerhard L. Bach, M.D., professor of medicine/rheumatology at the University of Munich in Germany on the use of Farabloc to treat fibromyalgia. Although the studies were small, they concluded that Farabloc showed a strong positive effect on the pain and tenderness associated with this condition.

As I said, these studies are so recent they haven't even been published yet—so you're among the first people to hear about Farabloc's proven effects on fibromyalgia. There's so little available to help alleviate this debilitating condition that these studies, and the re-introduction of Farabloc to the U.S. market, may revolutionize the future of fibromyalgia therapy—and dramatically improve the lives of those people afflicted with it.

The faces peeking out from under this "miracle blanket"

When I spoke to Pat Winterton, president of ABC Health Solutions, Farabloc's former U.S. distributor, I wasn't at all surprised when she told me she had a personal motive for bringing Farabloc back into the U.S.—her husband. After a stroke, he was left partially paralyzed and suffering from terrible nerve pain. Although she admits that Farabloc does not help everyone and that each person's response time varies—due to environment, lifestyle, disease, etc.—she will tell you that it's the only thing that has truly brought her husband any relief. And Mr. Winterton isn't the only one getting a long-sought-after reprieve from pain. Check out what some other people have experienced:

Three years ago, Pauletta L. was diagnosed with peripheral neuropathy. She says her feet would get ice cold, lose feeling, and generally make it very hard for her to walk comfortably. Her doctor told her that there was really no treatment for the condition, but he did prescribe her a drug that he said would relieve her symptoms somewhat.

But then, Pauletta explained, a friend gave her a Farabloc blanket to try.

"I slept with this blanket around my feet that night," Pauletta told me, "and as soon as I woke up in the morning and stepped on my floor, I could feel a difference in my feet… My feet still occasionally get cold, but I simply wrap them in the blanket for a few moments and they are OK again."

"To keep my feet feeling good I sleep with the blanket over them two or three nights per week. I am eternally grateful to my friend for this gift that she gave me. I can now walk around and shop for hours without needing to sit and put my feet up. They are no longer swollen after a long day on them as they used to be."

"I was a skeptic. Even my doctor asked me if I had to put an aluminum foil antenna on my head to get the blanket to work. I am a believer now. Drug free. Pain free. Swelling free. And, most importantly, no longer freezing cold. This product worked a miracle for me."

An investment in relief

Since its creation, Farabloc fabric has taken on many forms. There are, of course, the original blanket versions, which range in size from 12 inches by 30 inches to 34 inches by 58 inches. But there are also unique variations like socks, mitts, cummerbunds, and even full short- or long-sleeved jackets. You can also have an item custom-made, if you have a particular need that the other Farabloc products don't address.

Prices range from $50 all the way up to over $550, depending on which specific product and size you choose. So Farabloc isn't necessarily a bargain. But considering that it's reusable (and even machine washable, provided you don't wring it out), it may very well be an investment that you can continue to collect returns from for years to come.

And there are no side effects to worry about unless you happen to be allergic to nylon or steel.

To be quite honest, we're not sure what changed the FDA's mind about Farabloc. They've refused to see the light on numerous other highly effective natural products.

But regardless of the reason or motive behind the decision, it's great news for people who have been without this powerful pain reliever for the past six years. And, who knows? Maybe this will pave the way for the re-introduction of other previously banned products that could be a godsend for you or someone you love. See the Member Source Directory on page 529 for complete ordering information.

CHAPTER SIX

Soothe your pain on contact

Backache... sore muscles... aching joints... sprains... strains. As we get older, it seems as if pain becomes a constant companion. Just getting out of a chair can become challenging, let alone enjoying simple pleasures like gardening and strolling through the park. Taking aspirin helps, but it can eventually tear up your stomach. And prescription drugs have side effects that only compound the underlying problem. About 50 percent of the population is suffering from occasional aches and pains.[1]

Most medical schools don't teach pain relief

Mainstream medicine is finally becoming aware of the need to relieve pain. Hospitals now have pain-management teams. Palliative care—a relatively new medical specialty—was developed to address pain relief. Pain centers are also opening across the country as more and more people look for relief. But they all concentrate on mainstream "cures"—drugs and surgery, which are rife with uncomfortable and even life-threatening side effects.

Unfortunately, doctors aren't receiving much training in medical school about pain intervention. According to a survey of oncology surgeons, 90 percent of respondents said they received 10 hours or less of medical-school education on palliative care and 79 percent said they received no more than 10 hours of instruction in palliative care during their surgical residency.[2]

Healed injuries can continue to flare up over time

Effective pain management is a complex issue, because your body responds with all its defenses to protect and heal an injury. When you injure yourself, your body sends protective fluids, such as histamine, bradykinin, prostaglandin, and substance P, to surround and heal the area. But they can also irritate the injury over time.

Another problem associated with pain is referred to as the "snowball effect." This is the result of pain caused by injury and inflammation, which in turn causes distress and, as a result, continued pain and inflammation. This cyclic pattern snowballs and results in discomfort even after the original injury has been healed.

While you may have done everything possible to heal an injury for good, that doesn't mean the hurt will leave once your injury has healed. Most people can relate to occasional flare ups from past injuries, or subsequent pulled muscles or aching backs that come from trying to compensate for the original injury.

Putting a stop to the pain cycle

Finding a way to stop the pain cycle has been a goal of Health Sciences Institute panelist Jon Barron. Several years ago, he teamed up with Ron Manwarren of Royal Botanicals in the development of a unique topical pain reliever that is safe and completely free of the side effects of dangerous pharmaceutical pain killers. While Barron was refining a revolutionary all-natural transport system that would send the power of herbal extracts deep into aching muscles and joints, Manwarren was working on a deep tissue oil based on a time-tested traditional formula. When Manwarren brought his formula to Barron, Barron suggested moving "tradition" into the 21st Century by combining their efforts in a revolutionary new formula, available in a product called Soothanol X2.

While over-the-counter topical products commonly contain one, two, or three pain-relieving substances, such as methyl salicylate, menthol, and camphor, Soothanol X2 is a proprietary blend of 12 ingredients that work together to fight pain on contact.

Because Soothanol X2 is an easy-spreading and potent liquid, only a few drops are needed. Soothing pain relief is delivered on contact. In fact, we tested it informally here at the Health Sciences Institute Baltimore office.

The scented ingredients in Soothanol X2 are mild—contrary to the overpowering smells of most over-the-counter products. Although cayenne can deliver a warming or hot sensation, much of that sensation depends on the type of injury you're treating and your sensitivity to cayenne. Of the five people who tested our sample bottle here in the office, only one commented that he felt an uncomfortable amount of heat.

Because a little goes a long way, the cost per application is extremely economical. See the Member Source Directory for ordering information. Unfortunately, this product is not available in Australia.

Please note: HSI doesn't accept fees from outside companies for editorial coverage. However, NorthStar Nutritionals is one of HSI's dietary supplement affiliate companies. Even though we would never recommend any product we don't believe in, you should know about that relationship when deciding whether to try their products.

CHAPTER SEVEN

Want relief from migraine headaches? A few drops under the tongue may be all you need

A new product called MigraSpray landed on my desk—and from the initial reports I'm getting, it sounds like it might be the answer to your prayers if you suffer from migraines.

A colleague of mine has been fighting migraines for nearly 30 years, and has tried everything from pills to injections to nasal sprays. She says her migraines are so intense, that she's willing to try almost anything. But unfortunately, nothing has given her much relief—until now.

Almost immediate relief—and no side effects

So I gave her the sample I was sent. She tucked it away, and probably forgot about it. But the next time she developed a migraine, she remembered and dug it out. A couple of quick spritzes under the tongue, and almost immediately she could feel the pain dulling. Before taking MigraSpray, she had been sitting in a pitch dark room, because she couldn't stand even the light of a single bulb. After taking MigraSpray, she was able to turn on the lights—a simple thing that non-migraine sufferers like me take for granted.

She didn't experience any negative side effects, either-no "rebound" headache, no nasty taste, no stomach upset. She said she'll definitely use MigraSpray again, only next time, she'll use it sooner, before her headache fully blooms into a migraine.

Unique blend of four traditional herbal medicines

So how does it work? It's a homeopathic blend of four traditional herbs: feverfew, goldenseal, dandelion, and polyporus officinalis. The lead ingredient, feverfew (tanacetum parthenium) is a traditional herbal remedy for migraines and clinical studies have supported its ability to prevent migraines and reduce their severity.[1,2] Research suggests that feverfew's active ingredients are phytochemicals called sesquiterpene lactones, particularly one component known as parthenolide. Scientists believe parthenolide may relieve migraines by inhibiting cerebral blood vessel dilation. Parthenolide exerts anti-inflammatory properties by inhibiting platelet aggregation and prostaglandin synthesis, as well as the release of serotonin from platelets.[3]

The other ingredients in MigraSpray are not traditional headache remedies, but each contributes factors that may complement feverfew's anti-inflammatory power. Goldenseal (hydrastis rhizoma), which contains the amebicide phytochemical berberine, has traditionally been used to treat cholera. But herbal authorities also report that goldenseal can work as a sedative and an anti-inflammatory, particularly relieving inflammation in the mucous membranes of the head and throat.[4] Dandelion (Taraxacum denleonis) is best known as a potent diuretic and laxative, and is a rich source of potassium. And P. officinalis, a fungus commonly known as white agaric or larch agaric, is known in herbal medicine to have effects on the sympathetic and spinal nervous systems, and is used as a remedy for spasmodic nerve pain and epilepsy.[5]

In a private study conducted by MigraSpray's manufacturer, 41 migraine sufferers were divided into two groups to test the effectiveness of MigraSpray against a placebo. Nearly 88 percent of the MigraSpray group saw some level of improvement from using the spray, while about 66 percent of them reported full to complete improvement. Even better, the average elapsed time between administration and relief in the MigraSpray group was just six and a half minutes.[6]

MigraSpray is safe for most people, but the product label does warn pregnant and lactating women not to use it. My research also indicates that feverfew can alter clotting time.[7] Therefore if you are taking warfarin or other blood thinners, consult your physician and get your clotting times checked. Your medical dose may need to be lowered or feverfew may be contraindicated. Also, one study indicates that non-steroidal anti-inflammatory drugs, or NSAIDS, can negate feverfew's efficacy in fighting migraines, so you may want to avoid taking NSAIDS together with MigraSpray (also probably a good idea in light of the blood-thinning consideration).[8]

MigraSpray is available at many drug retailers, via the Internet, or by phone (see the Member Source Directory on page 529 for complete ordering information). It's hard to say how long one bottle might last, as it depends on the frequency of use. The product label recommends administering 10 sprays under the tongue at the first signs of an impending headache. After administration, wait at least 30 seconds before swallowing. If you don't feel relief after five minutes, you can repeat the process one more time.

CHAPTER EIGHT

Tibetan medicine relieves chronic leg pain

There are few things worse than losing your freedom to walk—not being able to go where you want to go or do what you want to do. But it's what thousands face each day, due to the often excruciating pain of intermittent claudication, a condition in which a decrease in blood to the legs brings about a reduction in oxygen to your lower extremities (which triggers the pain). The more you walk, the more oxygen is needed by your legs, hence, the greater the discomfort. This disorder can lead, if left untreated, to gangrene, and is linked to other serious health problems, such as hardening of the arteries and heart disease.

Mainstream medicine has little to offer. You can try a medication like Pentoxifylline, with undesirable side effects (including extreme dizziness and vomiting) and questionable effectiveness.[1] Or, as is often the case with Western medicine, you can opt for the ordeal of surgery.

An effective solution without side effects

But thankfully, you don't have to settle for the limited choices of the West. Eastern medicine has a better option—one that's both effective and free of side effects. Padma Basic is an herbal mixture from Tibet that's quickly proving to be a powerful treatment for intermittent claudication. Formulated over 2,000 years ago, the preparation is a complex combination of 19 different herbs that combine to produce a powerful antioxidant.

While the mixture was originally intended to treat illnesses brought on by the overconsumption of meat, fat, and alcohol, its broader uses are now being discovered.

In a dramatic double-blind placebo study held in 1985, intermittent claudication patients on Padma were found to have a 100 percent increase in the distance they could walk pain free. In addition, the drug was well tolerated by the patients.[2] Since then, a series of studies have confirmed these original results.[3-6]

Not surprisingly, the phenomenon of Padma has spread from the mountains of Tibet through Israel, Switzerland, England, and the rest of Europe. Now, Padma Basic is available to HSI members through Econugenics. They've set up a U.S. order bank, to make it easier for our American members to obtain this fantastic product.

The recommended dosage for Padma Basic is two tablets taken three times a day for the first four weeks. After that, take two tablets daily. Please be aware that it could take a minimum of three months for you to receive the full benefit of this treatment. Refer to the back of this book for ordering information.

CHAPTER NINE

Raw bar favorite offers arthritis relief

Imagine if you didn't need pain relievers every day? Our research has uncovered something totally new—a completely safe and natural food extract that may be the most powerful anti-inflammatory compound ever discovered.

It's called Lyprinol, an active lipid fraction isolated from the New Zealand green-lipped mussel, or Perna canaliculus. According to centuries-old tradition, native Maoris believe that eating the green-lipped mussel leads to a long and healthy life. And, in fact, medical statistics show that arthritis and rheumatic disorders are unknown among the coastal-dwelling Maori.

Scientists have now determined that the anti-arthritic properties of the green-lipped mussel are due to the unique configuration of certain polyunsaturated fatty acids (or PUFAs) called Eicosatetraenoic Acids (ETAs). Related to the Omega-3 fatty acids found in fish, flaxseed, and perilla oil, ETAs display more intense and targeted anti-inflammatory and anti-arthritic activity than any other known PUFA or Omega-3 fatty acid.

Research in the 1970s and 1980s confirmed that something in the

New Zealand green-lipped mussel had the ability to erase arthritic pain and stiffness. A double-blind, placebo-controlled trial conducted in 1980 at the Victoria Hospital in Glasgow, England, tested a powdered mussel supplement on 66 arthritis patients.[1] At the start of the six-month trial, all of the subjects had failed to respond to conventional treatment and were scheduled for surgery to repair badly damaged joints.

At the close of the trial, the researchers reported improvements in 68 percent of the rheumatoid arthritis (RA) patients and in 39 percent of the osteoarthritis (OA) patients. The scientists also noted the low incidence of adverse side effects.

Nearly two decades later scientists perfect the solution

For the next 18 years, leading scientists from universities and research labs in Australia, Japan, and France worked together to understand the secret locked within the green-lipped mussel. Step by incremental step, the scientists managed to identify the active biological fraction of the green-lipped mussel, isolate it without destroying its essential properties, cleanse it of impurities, stabilize it, and standardize its potency for reliable results.

At every step of the way, clinical and laboratory studies confirmed that scientists were moving in the right direction. Their excitement mounted as each phase yielded a more potent and powerful compound. Even early versions of the green-lipped mussel extracts were found to be more effective than aspirin and ibuprofen in reducing inflammation.

But inflammation isn't the only thing it helped. In 1986, a trial of 53 RA patients, conducted by the Societé Française de Biologic et Dietique (SFBD) in Dijon, France, found that the greenlipped mussel extract reduced pain by 62 percent after six months, while those on a placebo had a 20 percent increase in pain.[2]

Lyprinol: 200 times more effective than high potency fish oil in controlling swelling

Ultimately, scientists zeroed in on the ETAs in the green-lipped mussel as the active ingredients responsible for its remarkable anti-arthritic effects. This specific grouping of ETAs is not found in any other known substance. The methods used to concentrate these active components in a pure and stable form have been granted patents in several countries. The final result is now available as Lyprinol.

Researchers at the University of Queensland in Brisbane, Australia, studied the efficacy of Lyprinol using laboratory animals with adjuvant-induced polyarthritis, which is the closest model for rheumatoid arthritis in humans.[3]

When administered as an oral supplement, Lyprinol reduced arthritis-related swelling in the animal's paws by more than 90 percent. It was also effective when rubbed directly into the affected area.

Comparisons of Lyprinol to other natural lipids, or fatty acids, known to be helpful in treating arthritis and inflammation, tested Lyprinol against flax oil, evening primrose oil, Norwegian salmon oil, and MaxEPA (a high potency fish oil product). Of these, Lyprinol was the most effective in preventing arthritis-related swelling, reducing swelling by 79 percent. MaxEPA was the next best at 50 percent. However, the real story is the dosages used to achieve these results.

Achieving a 50 percent effectiveness rate required a dosage of 2000 mg/kg body weight of MaxEPA. But the effective dosage of Lyprinol was only 20 mg/kg—or 1/100 the amount. Extrapolations from these results suggest that the anti-inflammatory compounds in Lyprinol are 200 times more potent than MaxEPA (and 350 times more potent than evening primrose oil).

Outperforms arthritis drugs without harmful side effects

Researchers also compared the effectiveness of Lyprinol to that of the prescription arthritis drug indomethacin, the mainstream drug of choice at the time of the study. A dosage of 5 mg/kg of Lyprinol was 97 percent effective in reducing swelling, while indomethacin was only 83 percent effective at the same dosage. Unlike indomethacin, Lyprinol is non-toxic and essentially free of side effects. In a 2000 study, researchers found that when compared to NSAIDs, three Lyprinol was "non-gastro toxic."[4]

Recommendations for use

Lyprinol is recommended for the alleviation of inflammatory conditions, including osteoarthritis, rheumatoid arthritis, and virally-induced arthritis.

While Lyprinol appears to be the most powerful anti-inflammatory and arthritis pain reliever yet discovered, it still won't rebuild or restore previously damaged cartilage. For the most complete healing of arthritis, we recommend you combine Lyprinol with a natural joint building supplement containing glucosamine and chondroitin.

Recommended amounts: The amount needed for optimal results can vary widely for each individual, but range between two and four capsules per day. A higher amount (up to six capsules per day) can be used for the first one to two weeks of use. It can take up to four weeks to evaluate the full benefit. In addition, the research suggests that rubbing Lyprinol onto swollen and tender joints can help relieve pain and swelling. To do this, simply open the capsule and squeeze the contents onto the affected area. See the Member Source Directory to learn how you can order Lyprinol.

Part II

Cancer

CHAPTER ONE

Cancer's kryptonite: HSI panelist tests breakthrough seaweed cancer treatment

It's a weed and a slimy weed at that. But unlike the ones that invade your lawn, this weed might actually do you some good. It has been credited as a primary cause for record-low cancer rates in Okinawa, Japan. It was used—with reported success—to treat and prevent radiation sickness following the Chernobyl meltdown in Russia. It has yet to be tested in a single human clinical trial. But according to panelist Kohhei Makise, M.D., the Japanese medical community is being inundated with reports of how this medicinal seaweed has helped thousands of patients fight cancer.

Dr. Makise recently wrote us a long, excited e-mail discussing several new natural remedies that are producing impressive results among Japanese patients. But in this report, we decided to focus on a natural immune builder and cancer fighter that's so new to North America that we'd never heard of it before.

It's called fucoidan, and it's a complex of polysaccharides (carbohydrates) found in brown seaweed, most commonly in an Asia-Pacific variety known as kombu or Laminaria japonica. The seaweed has been a dietary staple in Japan since the second century B.C. And in Okinawa—which posts Japan's highest per capita rates of kombu consumption—it has reportedly produced considerable health benefits. Okinawa residents who eat an average of 1 gram of kombu (containing roughly 5 mg of fucoidan) daily enjoy some of the longest lifespans in Japan and the single lowest cancer rate in the country.

Seaweed extract causes cancer cells to self-destruct

In the 1990s, scientists identified fucoidan as the primary immune-building substance in brown seaweed and began to test it.

In one case, researchers injected female lab rats with a carcinogen known to induce mammary tumors. They fed half of the rats a standard diet, fed the other half a standard diet plus daily helpings of brown seaweed containing fucoidan, and monitored the animals for 26 weeks. The fucoidan appeared to convey two substantial benefits. First, the fucoidan fed rats developed fewer tumors than the control rats: 63 percent developed breast cancer vs. 76 percent of control rats. Second, the fucoidan-fed rats resisted developing tumors for longer periods of time: control rats typically developed tumors within 11 weeks, whereas fucoidan-fed rats remained cancer-free for 19 weeks.

In other studies, oral and intravenous doses of brown seaweed proved anywhere from 61.9 to 95.2 percent effective in preventing the development of cancer in rats implanted with sarcoma cells. One group of researchers described fucoidan as a "very potent antitumor agent in cancer therapy" after it inhibited the growth and spread of lung cancer in rats. (That type of cancer is particularly resistant to chemotherapy.)

Various studies further demonstrated that fucoidan combats cancer in multiple ways:

- It causes certain types of rapidly growing cancer cells (including stomach cancer, colon cancer, and leukemia) to self-destruct (a process call apoptosis).

- It physically interferes with cancer cells' ability to adhere to tissue. That interference prevents the cancer from spreading (or metastasizing) to new areas.

- It enhances production of several immune mechanisms, including macrophages (white blood cells that destroy tumor cells), gamma interferon (proteins that activate macrophages and natural killer cells), and interleukin (compounds that help regulate the immune system).

Proof from the panelist's practice

But as Dr. Makise points out, fucoidan still needs to prove itself in large, double-blind, clinical trials involving creatures more evolved than guinea pigs.

Dr. Makise believes, however, that there is compelling evidence that fucoidan can help prevent cancer. Through his practice in Japan, Dr. Makise has seen that fucoidan can even help patients who already have cancer. He says that cancer patients benefit most by taking a combination of:

- fucoidan

- AHCC or other immune-enhancing mushrooms

- antioxidants, especially large doses of selenium

- Enterococcus faecalis—1 to 3 trillion dead bacterium (Enterococcus faecalis is a beneficial bacterial found in the intestine. In addition to promoting healthy digestion and controlling bile acids that can cause colon cancer, it delivers certain immune-enhancing vitamins—like biotin and certain B vitamins—to the blood stream)

- essential daily vitamins and minerals (Dr. Makise recommends his patients take triple the recommended daily dosage of essential vitamins and minerals. He says it's especially important that cancer patients take daily supplements of selenium and zinc)

- a healthy lifestyle and diet that avoids meat, milk, and other animal proteins and fats.

"It is very effective for cancers that already exist, even end-stage metastases," Dr. Makise told us. "Each substance of this combination has a different mechanism to fight against cancer, so we get synergistic effects."

Fucoidan can be found in a product called Modifilan, manufactured by Fucoidan Sales. The product contains fucoidan, along with organic iodine—shown to promote maturation of the nervous system and alginate—a natural absorbent of radioactive elements, heavy metal, and free radicals. See the Member Source Directory at the back of this book for ordering information.

CHAPTER TWO

News of astounding natural cancer killer nearly squashed forever

Recently, Health Sciences Institute uncovered a remarkable story about a natural cancer killer that had been kept under lock and key for over 20 years. With this information, the future of cancer treatment and the chances of survival look more promising than ever. There's a healing tree that grows deep within the Amazon rainforest in South America that could literally change how you, your doctor, and possibly the rest of the world think about curing cancer.

Since the 1970s, the bark, leaves, roots, fruit, and fruit seeds of the Amazonian Graviola tree have been studied in numerous laboratory tests and have shown remarkable results with this deadly disease.

Several years ago, a major pharmaceutical company began extensive independent research on it. They learned that certain extracts of the tree actually seek out, attack, and destroy cancer cells. Because the natural extracts themselves could not be patented, the company labored to create a synthetic copy that showed the same promise. After more than seven years of work behind closed doors, researchers at this company realized they couldn't duplicate the tree's natural properties with a patentable substance. So they shut down the entire project. It basically came down to this—if they couldn't make huge profits, they would keep the news of this possible cure a well-guarded secret. But one researcher couldn't bear that, and decided to risk his job with the hope of saving lives.

Seven years of silence broken

This conscience-driven researcher contacted Rainforest Pharmacy, a natural products company dedicated to harvesting plants from the Amazon. In the course of working with Raintree on another story, they shared the exciting Graviola breakthrough with us. Since then, we've been looking closely into the research to date on Graviola. One of the first scientific references to it in the United States was by the National Cancer Institute (NCI). In 1976, the NCI showed that the leaves and stems of this tree were effective in attacking and destroying malignant cells. But these results were part of an internal NCI report and were, for some reason, never made public.

Since 1976, there have been several promising cancer studies on Graviola. However, the tree's extracts have yet to be tested on cancer patients. No double-blind clinical trials exist, and clinical trials are typically the benchmark mainstream doctors and journals use to judge a treatment's value. Nevertheless, our research has uncovered that Graviola has been shown to kill cancer cells in at least 20 laboratory tests.

The most recent study, conducted at Catholic University of South Korea, revealed that two chemicals extracted from Graviola seeds showed comparable results to the chemotherapy drug Adriamycin when applied to malignant breast and colon cells in test tubes.

Another study, published in the *Journal of Natural Products*, showed that Graviola is not only comparable to Adriamycin—but dramatically outperforms it in laboratory tests. Results showed that it selectively killed colon cancer cells at "10,000 times the potency of Adriamycin."[3]

Perhaps the most significant result of the studies we've researched is that Graviola selectively seeks out and kills cancer cells—leaving all healthy, normal cells untouched. Chemotherapy indiscriminately seeks and destroys all actively reproducing cells, even normal hair and stomach cells, causing such devastating side effects as hair loss and severe nausea.

Grown and harvested by indigenous people in Brazil, Graviola is available in limited supply in the United States and is distributed through Rainforest Pharmacy. But now, you can be among the select few in the entire country to benefit from this powerful treatment. We encourage you to consult with your doctor before beginning any new therapy, especially when treating cancer.

Graviola has been combined with seven other immune-boosting herbs in a product called N-Tense. As a dietary supplement, you should take six to eight capsules of N-Tense per day. Graviola and N-Tense are completely natural substances with no side effects apart from possible mild stomach upset at high dosages (in excess of 5 grams) if taken on an empty stomach.

If you've been diagnosed with cancer, you and your doctor should look into all the available treatment options. Graviola could just make all the difference in beating cancer. See the Member Source Directory at the back of this book for ordering information.

CHAPTER THREE

Hybridized mushroom extract destroys cancer cells and provides powerful immune protection

Until now, the only way to get access to this remarkable immune booster was to live in Japan. For the last five years in Japan, people with cancer, AIDS, and other life-threatening illnesses—as well as healthy people who want to stay that way—have been revving up their immune systems, destroying tumor cells, and preventing cancer and other illnesses with a powerful extract called AHCC (activated hexose correlate compound). Now, AHCC is available to consumers in the United States.

AHCC is an extract of a unique hybridization of several kinds of medicinal mushrooms known for their immune-enhancing abilities. On their own, each mushroom has a long medical history in Japan, where their extracts are widely prescribed by physicians. But when combined into a single hybrid mushroom, the resulting active ingredient is so potent that dozens of rigorous scientific studies have now established AHCC to be one of the world's most powerful—and safe—immune stimulators.

In vitro animal and human studies confirm that AHCC effectively works against and, in some cases, even prevents the recurrence of liver cancer, prostate cancer, ovarian cancer, multiple myeloma, breast cancer, AIDS, and other life-threatening conditions, with no dangerous side effects. In smaller doses, AHCC can also boost the immune function of healthy people, helping to prevent infections and promote well-being.

Calling up your first line of defense

Our immune systems stand between us and the rest of the world. Without it, our bodies would be overrun by bacteria, viruses, parasites, fungi, and other invaders, infections would rapidly spread, and cancer cells would proliferate. Like a highly responsive and well-coordinated army, our immune systems are composed of a variety of specialized immune cells that identify, seek out, and destroy microbes, pathogens, and tumor cells.

First on the scene of possible trouble are the phagocytes and natural killer (NK) cells, which respond quickly to potential threats. Often referred to as the body's "front-line defense," these cells are constantly on the lookout for any suspicious substances. NK cells latch onto the surface of substances or the outer membranes of cancer cells and inject a chemical hand grenade (called a granule) into the interior. Once inside, the granules explode and destroy the bacteria or cancer cell within five minutes. Itself undamaged, the NK cell then moves onto its next victim. In its prime, a NK cell can take on two cancer cells at the same time, speeding up the process.

Recent research shows that as we age, our immune systems function less efficiently. In particular, the ability of our NK cells to respond quickly and effectively declines with age and illness. When NK cells lose their ability to recognize or destroy invaders, health can deteriorate rapidly. Moderately low to dangerously low NK cell activity levels have been found in people with AIDS, cancer, immune deficiency, liver disorders, various infections, and other diseases. Because measurements of NK cell activity are closely correlated with one's chances of survival, anything that helps increase NK cell activity may help people treat, recover from, and/or prevent these illnesses.

Research finds remarkable immune system boost in multiple ways

Scientific studies of the extract AHCC, published in respected peer-reviewed journals such as *International Journal of Immunology*, *Anti-Cancer Drugs*, and *Society of Natural Immunity*, have established the health benefits and safety of AHCC more conclusively than nearly any other natural supplement. What is especially remarkable about AHCC is that it consistently and effectively boosts immune system function. Specifically, AHCC:

- Stimulates cytokine (IL-2, IL-12, TNF, and INF) production, which stimulates immune function.
- Increases NK cell activity against diseased cells as much as 300 percent.
- Increases the formation of explosive granules within NK cells. The more ammunition each NK cell carries, the more invaders it can destroy.
- Increases the number and the activity of lymphocytes, specifically increasing T-cells up to 200 percent.
- Increases Interferon levels, which inhibits the replication of viruses and stimulates NK cell activity.
- Increases the formation of TNF, a group of proteins that help destroy cancer cells.

These dramatic immune effects translate into profound health benefits. A 1995 clinical trial reported in the *International Journal of Immunotherapy* showed that 3 grams of AHCC per day significantly lowered the level of tumor markers found in patients with prostate cancer, ovarian cancer, multiple myeloma, and breast cancer. This study documented complete remissions in six of 11 patients and significant increases in NK cell activity in nine of 11 patients. T- and B-cell activity levels also rose considerably.

AHCC now available in the United States

After years of successful use in Japan, AHCC is available in the United States as the active ingredient in a product called ImmPower. Distributed by The Harmony Company, ImmPower comes in gelatin capsules containing 500mg of AHCC (proprietary blend).

ImmPower can be taken in preventive or therapeutic doses and should be discussed with your personal physician. For prevention, the recommended dose is 1 gram per day taken as one 500mg capsule in the morning and again at night. This dose will help increase NK cell activity and support immune system functioning for good health and general well-being. For those with cancer, AIDS, or other life-threatening conditions, the research indicates a therapeutic dose of two capsules in the morning, two at mid-day and two at night for a total of 3 grams per day to jump start NK cell activity. After three weeks, the dose can be reduced to 1 gram per day (one capsule in the morning and one at night), to maintain the increased NK cell activity level. See the Member Source Directory for purchasing information.

CHAPTER FOUR

The lactoferrin miracle

We're on the verge of a major medical breakthrough with lactoferrin.

Because of this unique extract, much of what we now consider state-of-the-art medicine—such as radiation, antibiotics, and chemotherapy—may eventually seem as primitive as bloodletting.

If lactoferrin proves to be as powerful as it promises to be, many deadly diseases that haunt our thoughts today will no longer frighten us.

Where does lactoferrin come from and how does it work?

From the moment you were born, lactoferrin—an iron-binding protein found in breast milk (colostrum)—was your first shield against infection and disease and your primary source of immune-system chemicals. The primary task of your immune system is to survey your body—organ by organ, tissue by tissue, cell by cell—to make sure that only the cells that are supposed to be there... are. When a healthy immune system recognizes a foreign substance—a virus or cancerous cell—it immediately fights to eliminate it.

Researchers discovered the significance of lactoferrin to the immune system while researching another mysterious biological phenomenon: pregnancy.

What's so mysterious about pregnancy?

Until recently, scientists had been baffled by the fact that a woman's body doesn't normally reject a fetus, which naturally contains the foreign antigens of the father. But the puzzle is beginning to unravel: Science has discovered that shortly after conception, a woman's immune system is down-regulated.

This is why her body does not reject the fetus as "foreign" matter. (For this reason, pregnant women should not take lactoferrin.) Immediately after delivery, however, her body produces colostrum, or the first milk, which restores her immune system and provides powerful immune chemicals to the infant. Lactoferrin is the primary immune-system chemical in first milk.

Studies have shown that the mother's first milk is the only source from which an infant can get these significant immune substances. Synthetic formulas can't offer the same nutritional, immunological, or physiological value, despite efforts to produce formulas that mimic breast milk as closely as possible.

Unraveling the healing mystery of lactoferrin

Lactoferrin has at least two specific immune- boosting functions:

- It binds to iron in your blood, keeping it away from cancer cells, bacteria, viruses, and other pathogens that require iron to grow. The lactoferrin protein is able to sequester and release iron as needed, under controlled conditions. This property helps prevent harmful oxidative reactions, making lactoferrin a powerful antioxidant.

- It activates very specific strands of DNA that turn on the genes that launch your immune response. This is such a rare and surprising action that there is no other kind of protein like it. Lactoferrin is in a class by itself.

Lactoferrin also contains antibodies against a wide range of bacterial, fungal, viral, and protozoal pathogens. In effect, the lactoferrin protein backs budding cancer cells or bacteria into a corner . . . starves them and sends out a signal to your white blood cells that says, "It's over here! Come and get it!"

State-of-the-art techniques in cellular and molecular biology have recently allowed us to isolate lactoferrin from the "first food of life." The commercially available preparation is in a form in which the food hasn't been chemically altered.

Widely used to support recovery from malignancies in animals

Numerous studies on rats and patient case histories have documented the benefits of lactoferrin in helping to combat many types of malignancies.[1,2]

Many holistic practitioners use it and achieve great effects by combining it with other immune-enhancing natural tumor-fighting therapies. In one case, a leukemia patient (labeled the worst case the Mayo Clinic had seen in 20 years) had his condition reversed on lactoferrin. His white blood cell count rose, and his problems disappeared. This seemingly "hopeless" case was transformed into a remarkable recovery.

Other case histories indicate that the negative effects of conventional treatments like chemotherapy and radiation are drastically reduced or eliminated with supplemental lactoferrin. (The amounts of lactoferrin used in these reported cases range from 500 to 1500 mg a day.) Again, it should be noted that lactoferrin appears to be perfectly safe, even in high doses.

What else can you use it for?

Other clinical and case studies have shown that lactoferrin...

- contains an anti-inflammatory molecule—which means it can help if you suffer from the pain and debilitation of joint inflammation[3]
- plays a role in lessening ocular disturbance, which means it may help with vision problems[4]
- acts as a potent antimicrobial agent against Candida albicans[5]
- shows potent antiviral activity useful in reducing your susceptibility to viruses, including herpes and HIV[6]

If you're wondering how safe lactoferrin is, remember that it is nontoxic and is well tolerated by nursing infants.

Should you take it as a daily preventive?

There are many everyday threats that wear down the immune system—such as environmental toxins, emotional and physical stressors, and genetic problems. Taking 100 mg of lactoferrin each day at bedtime, however, can help upgrade your immune system, so you can take full advantage of your natural defenses in a world full of potential health threats. For use in cancer recovery, up to 1500 mg a day can be taken without fear of side effects. And unlike penicillin or other synthetic drugs, your body will not become immune to the effects of lactoferrin, because it's something your body is familiar with and knows how to handle.

Since lactoferrin is a natural substance, large pharmaceutical companies aren't able to patent it and make millions. But it's available from a limited number of suppliers in the United States, and it shouldn't be overlooked as a powerful tool in the fight against serious diseases. For information on purchasing lactoferrin, refer to the Member Source Directory at the back of this book.

CHAPTER FIVE

Discover the cancer-fighting potential of Brazil's "Mushroom of God"

Nearly 30 years ago researchers began investigating a medical curiosity among the people of Piedade, Brazil. Residents of the small community near Sao Paulo enjoyed extraordinarily good health. They developed few diseases and lived unusually long lives. Outsiders began to wonder what was enhancing the Brazilians' immunity and lifespan. In their quest for an answer, researchers stumbled upon the "Mushroom of God."

Depending on which account you believe, it was either two researchers from Penn State or Taktoshi Furumoto, a Japanese farmer living in Brazil, who solved the puzzle. He (or they) zeroed in on a small, wild mushroom that locals ate regularly, believing it fostered good health. It was commonly known as Cogumelo de Deus or Cogumelo do Sol—Mushroom of God or Mushroom of the Sun.

Regardless of who discovered it, it was Japanese researchers (doctors from Tokyo University and Japan's National Cancer Center, in particular) who eventually subjected the mushroom to pharmacological testing. They reported that the mushroom, which eventually acquired the botanical name *Agaricus Blazei Murill* (ABM), could be a potent immune-builder and cancer-fighter.

To date, ABM has not been used in any human clinical trials. All research has been performed in petri dishes or laboratory animals. However, news of this rare medicinal mushroom has already prompted between 300,000 and 500,000 Japanese people to supplement with ABM, hoping to prevent cancer or stop the disease from recurring. Numerous others consume it regularly reportedly to avoid infection, diabetes, hyperlipidemia, chronic hepatitis, and arteriosclerosis.

ABM enhances the immune response to protect you from cancer

In recent years, Japanese research has confirmed that ABM contains a host of health-promoting components: vitamins B1 and B2, niacin, phosphorous, iron, calcium, protein, amino acids, and ergosterol (which converts into vitamin D2 when the mushroom is dried). But most importantly, the researchers discovered that ABM contains large quantities of active polysaccharides—complex carbohydrates, most commonly found in foods like wheat, rice, and potatoes that stimulate the immune system to fight off bacterial and viral illnesses.[1]

ABM stimulates the immune system by triggering the production of:

- T-cells, which directly attack cells that have been taken over by viruses or cancers;[2]
- interleukin, which bolsters the immune system by stimulating the growth and activity of white blood cells;
- tumor necrosis factor (TNF), which activates white blood cells and fights tumors;
- and macrophages, which protect the body from infection by consuming foreign material.[3]

Obviously, a list of *in vitro* and animal studies (with no human trials in the mix) is not proof that ABM is an effective cancer treatment. Products, whether they are natural or pharmaceutical, need to pass more extensive and rigorous testing to support such a claim.

In several studies, however, ABM has stimulated animals' immune systems and arrested the growth of their tumors. And in the past, HSI has documented the ability of other medicinal mushrooms, such as AHCC, to build immunity and help people fight cancer (see the *HSI Members Alert* issues for January 2000 and January 2002 or search online at www.hsionline.com). We don't know yet if ABM will eventually rank with those health-promoting mushrooms. But the preliminary evidence was compelling enough that we decided to analyze it and report the findings to you.

Retard tumor growth by 90 percent in just three weeks

At Japan's Ehime University School of Medicine, researchers tested ABM's impact on tumors. Twenty days of treatment with certain ABM extracts (800 mg/kg per day taken orally) retarded tumor growth in cancerous mice between 80 and 90 percent. The researchers determined that the tumor-retarding agent was ergosterol, a steroid alcohol that occurs naturally in mold and yeast.

So they conducted a second experiment, giving oral doses of ergosterol (between 100 and 800 mg/kg) daily to tumor-bearing mice for 20 days. The treatment "significantly reduced tumor growth" in a dose-dependent manner. Mice given the largest doses experienced 85.5 percent less tumor growth than mice treated with placebos. The ergosterol, however, did not destroy cancer cells directly. Instead, it inhibited the development of new blood vessels within the tumor—a process that can stop and eventually reverse tumor growth. The treatment also produced another benefit: After 20 days of treatment none of the mice were suffering any of the side effects typically induced by chemotherapy drugs.[4]

Using guinea pigs as guinea pigs

Cancerous guinea pigs experienced even greater recovery rates—

over 99 percent—when they were treated with ABM. Researchers from Tokyo College of Pharmacy, Tokyo University, and Japan's National Cancer Center Laboratory injected cancer cells into the femur (thighbone) of each pig—a procedure that normally causes cancer to spread throughout the animal's body within four to five weeks.

Twenty-four hours later (once the cancer cells were embedded in the animals' tissue), the researchers gave the pigs ABM injections and continued to give them daily injections for 10 consecutive days. Five weeks later, 99.4 percent of the guinea pigs had fully recovered from the cancer.[5]

Could this Brazilian mushroom hold the secret to better chemo?

If ABM shows such promise on its own for fighting cancer, it seems logical to assume that it could enhance the effects of conventional cancer treatments. But when it comes to your health, assuming isn't nearly enough.

At Mie University in Japan, researchers conducted a series of tests with ABM and the cancer chemotherapy drug, 5-fluorouracil (5-FU). Administered alone (at a dosage of 10mg/kg for 30 days), the ABM extract moderately inhibited tumor growth in cancerous mice. Treatment with both ABM and 5-FU strongly inhibited tumor growth in the mice.

The more interesting results, however, centered around ABM's effects on 5-FU. First, it prolonged the action of 5-FU, which, like many chemotherapy drugs, is only effective on its own for a short period of time. Second, it offset the drastic immune-system weakening usually caused by chemotherapy. At the end of the experiment, mice treated with the ABM/5-FU combination showed "significantly increased" numbers of immune-modulating cells compared to the mice treated with saline only.[6]

Other scientists tested ABM's ability to fight cancer by first injecting tumor cells in both the right and left flanks of laboratory mice. The scientists then injected ABM fractions into the mice, but only into their right-flank tumors. The injections inhibited tumor growth in the right flank, and even caused regression in some cases. But the treatment also inhibited growth of left-flank tumors. The researchers, who were based at Japan's Miyagi Cancer Center Research Institute, speculated that the ABM had triggered the immune system to unleash more white blood cells to all cancerous areas, not just those specifically injected with the extract.

Granted, that's a lot of speculation. And all of these trials may make you want to give thanks you're not a rodent living anywhere near a Japanese laboratory. But the dramatic results shown by the mice and guinea pigs tested certainly seem reason enough to investigate ABM further to determine if it's anywhere near as promising for us humans with cancer.

Extreme growing conditions make mushroom a rare commodity

Unfortunately, accessing supplies of ABM mushrooms or ABM supplements has been difficult. For decades, growers were unable to successfully cultivate this wild mushroom. It typically thrives in extreme conditions—intense Brazilian sunlight, humidity averaging 80 percent, and temperatures that soar to 100 degrees during the day and drop to 68 degrees overnight. It was only in the early '90s that growers devised a method of producing biologically active ABM mushrooms in beds of pasteurized horse manure and sugar cane residue (hardly appetizing, but reportedly it creates a powerful growing medium).

Today, Japanese consumers purchase 90 percent of Brazil's yearly ABM crop. Consequently, you're not likely to find fresh ABM mushrooms in even the best produce markets in America.

A few supplement companies, however, have begun producing

ABM tablets (which are already hot sellers in Japan). No clinical trials have yet been published about these supplements. (All the published trials involve ABM extracts. The supplements typically contain whole mushrooms that have been freeze-dried and powdered.) So, the exact impact of ABM supplementation isn't known. But, again, our experience with other similar supplements makes us less skeptical.

If you try ABM, let us know about your experience with it. HSI will continue to search for information on this promising mushroom and for a source for the extract. Ordering information is in the Member Source Directory on page 529.

CHAPTER SIX

This overlooked "waste product" may be the cancer-fighting breakthrough of the century

I t was one of those moments that makes working for HSI so rewarding and exciting. I had received an email out of the blue, telling me about a new discovery with results that were nothing short of astounding…

Stage 4 cancer patients cancer free within two months.

Tumor metastasis reduced by 82 percent.[1]

A human study in which 31 percent of cancer cells were flat out killed. In thirty days.[2]

In another study, mice fed this substance ended up with half the tumors of the control group.[3]

Oh, and the incredible results weren't limited to cancer. People with Type 2 diabetes have stopped needing shots of insulin. Men with enlarged prostates have started sleeping through the night.

This intriguing email was from Wendy Selvig of the AIDS Research

Assistance Institute—a non-profit organization in Mansfield, TX. And as much as Wendy's email got my heart racing, it was tempered with a strong dose of skepticism. With HSI's worldwide reputation for uncovering the best health breakthroughs, we receive word of new products every single day. And we are extremely careful about choosing only the very best to introduce to you.

So I immediately picked up the phone and gave Wendy a call. And the story she told me—of an all-natural disease-killing dynamo backed up by some very impressive science—was astounding.

But it was the source of this miracle cure that just about made me drop the phone.

The latest breakthrough in cancer treatment is... flax?!

Wait, wake up; I can hear you snoring. Of course you've heard of flax seed. Nothing new there, right? But, this isn't the same flax seed you've been seeing on the health food store shelves. In fact, it's not flax *seed* at all.

The breakthrough that takes aim at cancer cells like a heat-seeking missile is Concentrated Flax Hull Lignans.

Concentrated Flax Hull Lignans are *not* flax seeds. Rather, they are concentrated directly—using a special process—from flax seed shells, or hulls, which typically don't make it into the bags of flax seed in the store.

Which is a shame, because it turns out the vast majority of the disease-fighting lignans in the flax seed are located in the hull that encases the seed.

The nutrients contained in flax seeds are highly concentrated in the shells—one teaspoon of Concentrated Flax Hull Lignans contains the nutritional equivalent of two gallons of flax seed. Yes, gallons. And flax seed oil? Forget it. There are practically no lignans contained in the oil.

You might be wondering what these lignans are, exactly. Lignans are a group of chemical compounds found in plants. They're one of the major classes of phytoestrogens (you might have seen that word before in discussions about soy), which are chemicals that act as antioxidants. Flax seed is the richest source of lignans in the plant kingdom, containing up to 800 times more than any other plant source. There are 27 different lignans in the flax seed and scientists believe they all work together to provide their amazing health benefits.

The major lignan in flax seed is called secoisolariciresinol diglucoside (SDG). It's actually a lignan precursor, which means its power isn't unlocked until it is metabolized by your body. In the intestines, SDG becomes two lignans. These lignans have the power to wipe out cancer, as well as do battle against diabetes, shrink enlarged prostates, boost the immune system... in fact, as my research went on, I found there's not much these lignans can't do.

A new process unlocks this superfood's disease-fighting prowess

Though scientists have known for some time that the flax seed hulls have an amazing nutritional profile, they've been at a loss as to how to unlock those nutrients. Finally, a farmer by the name of Curtis Rangeloff invented a chemical-free method of mechanically separating the lignan-rich hulls from the rest of the flax.

The Concentrated Flax Hull Lignans sold through Flax Lignan Health boast a pure lignan content of up to 65 percent. Each scoop of the product contains 150-300 mg of SDG per serving. That's 70 times the amount of SDG typically contained in the same amount of traditional ground flax seed.

In addition to their lignan content, flax seed hulls contain high levels of omega-3s, as well as off-the-charts antioxidants. To put it in perspective—kale has one of the highest ORAC values (this is the measurement of a food's antioxidant content) at 1,770 per 100 g. Concentrated Flax Hull Lignans? They come in at a whopping 19,600 per 100 g. The hulls also contain 4.3 g of fiber and 2.8 g of protein in each tablespoon.

And while the nutritional value of Concentrated Flax Hull Lignans is certainly a bonus, the true value of the product is in its promise as a potent cancer-killer.

The evidence I found for SDG's effects on cancer is nothing short of incredible. The most exciting study was carried out in Canada on a group of postmenopausal women with newly diagnosed breast cancer.

Each day for a month, the women in the test group ate a flaxseed muffin containing a predetermined concentration of SDG. After only one month, the growth of the cancer cells was reduced by 34.2 percent. Even better, 31 percent of cancer cells were completely killed, and the expression of the cancer growth receptor Her2 (c-erB2) decreased by 71 percent.[2]

Her2 is part of a family of genes that help to regulate cell growth. Some breast cancers, for reasons no one really understands, undergo a gene amplification. So, instead of having two gene copies of the Her2 gene as in a normal cell, there are multiple copies.

This results in cell growth regulation going haywire. Tumors grow more quickly, are more aggressive, and are less sensitive to chemotherapy. This can also occur in other cancers such as ovarian cancer and stomach cancer. It seems that SDG is able to hinder this process considerably.

Driving cancer cells to mass suicide

In two studies on breast cancer cells implanted into immune deficient mice, flax lignans again proved deadly to cancer. Both tumor growth and metastasis were significantly reduced. In one of the studies, metastasis to the lungs was reduced by 82 percent. The average number of tumors was also considerably lower in the test group than in the control group.[3]

The promising studies don't stop at breast cancer. A study in California demonstrated that SDG reduced risk of endometrial cancer in some women by 32 percent. This reduced risk was most evident among postmenopausal women who consumed high levels of both isoflavones and lignans.[4] Other studies have shown similar reduced risk for uterine and ovarian cancers.

A clinical trial in Canada found that higher dietary lignan intake was linked to considerable reduction in colorectal cancer risk.[5] And, according to studies with human colon cancer cells, lignans stunt the growth of tumor cells and actually drive them to what can only be described as mass suicide.[6]

Supplementation with SDG reduced tumors significantly in mice with melanoma. The average number of tumors in the control group was 62, while the average number in the groups of mice receiving SDG was around half that. Tumor size was also decreased.[3]

Even the Mayo Clinic, the American Cancer Society, and the FDA acknowledge the cancer-fighting power of flax lignans. The Mayo Clinic says flax seed lignans may inhibit the growth of some breast cancers, and the American Cancer Society cites a study in which the growth rate of cancer cells was slowed in men suffering from prostate cancer.

Perhaps most surprising of all is the support flax lignans have gotten from, get this, the FDA. Apparently even the FDA can't miss a sure thing. They have stated that flax seed lignans have anti-tumor activity and are potentially the richest source of phytoestrogens, and that their significant ability to prevent cancer is recognized by the National Cancer Institute.[7]

A survivor's tale: Concentrated Flax Hull Lignans beat back cancer for 'hopeless' cases

Personally, I find that one thing speaks even more loudly than the many exciting studies I've talked about so far. And that is the words straight from the mouths of people who have seen their lives changed as a result of including flax lignans in their diets.

A 52-year-old woman started taking Concentrated Flax Hull Lignans two years after she was diagnosed with bone cancer. At that point, she was only able to walk with crutches, and painfully at that. After just one month with the lignans, she stopped taking her pain medication, ditched the crutches, and found her energy level returning to normal.

And then there's the story of 84-year-old Tony. Last September, he was told his lung cancer was so advanced that he wouldn't make it to Christmas. His daughter-in-law was distraught, knowing her daughter's December wedding would be a sad event without him. She learned about the Concentrated Flax Hull Lignans from a friend and had some sent to Tony.

Come December, he was a happy guest at his granddaughter's wedding. When one of his doctors found out that he had been treating his cancer with Concentrate Flax Hull Lignans, she became angry with him. She was convinced that the cancer had spread throughout both lungs and his esophagus. She thought more "aggressive steps" should have been taken.

However, the doctor had to eat her words when a scan showed the cancer had not spread and actually was reduced to one tiny nodule in his lung. This was after Tony had been taking the Concentrated Flax Hull Lignans for only six months.

These are just two of the many stories that demonstrate the incredible healing power of flax lignans.

If its power against cancer isn't enough, that's just the start

Amazingly, the scientific evidence for Concentrated Flax Hull Lignans doesn't stop at its cancer-fighting abilities. Diets rich in foods containing plant lignans have long been associated with reduced risk of cardiovascular disease. In a 12-year study of Finnish men, it was found that those with the highest intake of plant lignans were significantly less likely to die from cardiovascular disease than their counterparts who ate the least amount of foods containing plant lignans.[8]

Flax lignans have also been shown to suppress the development of atherosclerosis (chronic inflammation of the arteries due to an accumulation of plaque) in a study on rabbits. The development of atherosclerosis in rabbits treated with the lignans was reduced by 34.4 percent. The lignans also lowered LDL cholesterol and raised levels of HDL cholesterol.[9] In a study concerning Native American postmenopausal women, it was found that flax seed lowered LDL cholesterol by 10 percent.[10] Mind you, that was just with flax seed, not the nutritionally rich hulls.

There is discussion in the scientific community that flax lignans may help to lower sugar levels in people with diabetes. While there are no specific studies to this effect, people who are living with diabetes have been vocal about the results they've seen taking Concentrated Flax Hull Lignans.

One woman noticed that her blood sugar has been regular, and that she's been feeling healthier in general.

A 26-year-old man who was diagnosed with type 2 diabetes a few years ago has been struggling to manage his illness ever since. Unable to keep his blood sugar down, he watched helplessly as it regularly spiked to 600, despite taking 40 units of insulin with every shot. Two weeks after he began including Concentrated Flax Hull Lignans in his diet, he noticed a change in how he felt. Now, his blood sugar stays under 200, and he hasn't had to give himself a shot in two months.

Finally, no more late-night bathroom trips

If you're living with an enlarged prostate, you know what agony it can be. A recent study demonstrated that flax lignans could reduce prostate size. Rats given the human equivalent of 50 mg per day of SDG (remember, Concentrated Flax Hull Lignans contains up to 300 mg per serving) had significantly smaller prostates than those without the SDG supplementation. The SDG didn't just stop prostate growth— it actually helped reduce the size of the prostate.[11]

Lee, who describes himself as having a "bad prostate," has been using Concentrated Flax Hull Lignans for a couple of months. He has been making less and less trips to the bathroom in the middle of the night, and says he generally feels better. His wife is happy, too-with Lee getting so little sleep, he'd been "a real grouch," and she jokes that she may keep him if the Concentrated Flax Hull Lignans keep working!

G.E. wrote about her husband, Hugh, who suffers from both an enlarged prostate and irregular heartbeat. She was amazed when, after only two weeks, there was a complete reversal in Hugh's nightly routine. She said he doesn't get up more than once a night, and his heart has been beating steadily.

Previously a candidate for a pacemaker, Hugh reports his doctor has not mentioned the surgery since he started taking the Concentrated Flax Hull Lignans. Rather, his doctor was flat-out astonished at his progress, stating he'd never seen such a dramatic improvement. At 71, Hugh is now "bouncing along and mowing and putting up hay and working with his horses and cattle."

Though there are no conclusive studies concerning flax lignans and prostate cancer, there are a few that are promising. In a trial using mice, flax inhibited the growth and development of prostate cancer. In a study of 25 men who were scheduled for prostatectomy, supplementation with flax brought significant changes in serum cholesterol, total testosterone, and the free androgen index. Researchers concluded that flax lignans may be a very beneficial food for men battling prostate cancer.[12]

Fight the flu with a super-charged immune system

All of what I've just reported was enough to convince me to buy my own supply of Concentrated Flax Hull Lignans. But, as I delved even deeper, I began to uncover more amazing benefits to a diet that includes flax lignans.

In a 90-day anecdotal test on 100 people with HIV (75 percent exhibiting full AIDS symptoms), 97 percent reported positive health changes, with energy and appetites increasing. Most amazing is the fact that, after 6 weeks, 28 percent had viral loads drop to non-detectible levels. Their super-charged immune systems were fighting the virus like they never had before.[13] And it works against another virus, too...

As you may know, flu shots don't actually do much for preventing the flu, and at their worst are actually harmful. And flu drugs? Forget it! The virus builds resistance almost as soon as the drugs are put on the market. In 2005, 14.5 percent of flu viruses were resistant to major flu drugs. That might not sound like a lot, but compare it to the fact that only 1.9 percent of flu viruses were resistant just one year earlier.

Luckily, it seems flax lignans can do the same thing for influenza that they are doing for the HIV virus in Africa.

When a virus enters the cells of the body, it stimulates hormones that activate the gene for p53. When this gene is activated, it actually induces virally infected cells to shut down, thereby preventing the virus from spreading. If this is activated shortly after infection, further viral replication is completely stopped.

Based upon recent studies, influenza virus infections can be stopped in this way. Flax lignans, through a series of interactions with the inner workings of the body's cells, can increase the level of p53 in cells. Long story short, flax lignans can actually help to both prevent flu infections and fight those that already exist.

And the amazing abilities of flax lignans don't end there, Canadian study also suggests that SDG may have a therapeutic role in treating lupus. A Dutch human study showed that flax lignans could be the answer for men and women with hair loss and thinning hair. Yet another, this one on rats, showed potential for liver protection.

If you're ready to try this wonder food, ordering information is in the Member Source Directory.

CHAPTER SEVEN

The metal that shrinks tumors within weeks—your blood will actually repel cancer

Imagine a cancer treatment so powerful it could bring a comatose patient back to consciousness in a matter of days—and needing only $70 per month to get it.

This very miracle does exist, and it's been around since the 1930s, when Dr. Hans Nieper began using cesium chloride to treat his patients in Germany. It was Dr. Keith Brewer, though, who took this therapy to the next level by combining it with a chemical called dimethyl sulfoxide, or DMSO.

Cesium is nature's most alkaline metal and when it's combined with DMSO, it directly targets cancer cells, stopping the metastasis of the cancer, shrinking tumor masses within weeks, and stopping the pain of cancer within 24 to 48 hours.

This amazing protocol is touted by many alternative practitioners as one of the most effective treatments for bone and brain cancers and other fast-growing cancers too. Read on to learn more about this incredible cancer treatment combo.

The secret's in the water

Conventional medicine has a lot to learn from the populations of the world that haven't yet been touched by Western civilization about how to maintain vibrant wellness and health.

Many of these populations boast very low incidences of cancer, and it so happens that in the environments where they live, there are high levels of strong alkaline minerals in the water supplies. For example, the Hopi Indians' water contains rubidium and potassium and the Hunzas of northern Pakistan have water high in cesium and potassium.

It's this high mineral content that keeps their blood alkaline—an internal environment that cancer steers clear of.

Around 1900, this concept of an alkali (low-acid) therapy for treating cancer was developed in the West, and though it worked quite well for cancer, it was forgotten about when only a few practitioners were willing to face the opposition that the medical establishment directed toward them.

But one brave German practitioner, Dr. Hans Nieper, believed strongly in the use of strong alkali like cesium chloride. In fact, in his Hannover, Germany practice, Dr. Nieper used this therapy to treat hundreds of cancer patients, including many celebrities, executives, and even a U.S. President.[1]

Dr. Nieper found that when cesium is taken up by cancer cells, it raises the pH of the cells and kills them. Then, they are eliminated by the body.

Cesium chloride selectively targets cancer by taking advantage of the fact that most types of tumor cells need much more glucose than do normal cells. In order to get more glucose into the cancer cells, the sodium-potassium (Na-K) pumps on the cell walls must run 20 times faster than normal, pumping more sodium out and more potassium in.

Since cesium acts like potassium, the Na-K pump brings lots of it into the cells. But once cesium is in a cell, it can't get out because it blocks the channels through which potassium leaves. This buildup of cesium then kills the cancerous cell.[2]

The addition of DMSO allows the cesium chloride to target the cancer cells even more effectively since it's what is known as a super-solvent. DMSO also has the ability to penetrate every single cell of the body, and whatever is administered with DMSO tends to bind with it and get carried to the inside of cells along with it—which makes the treatment even more powerful.[3]

How the American Cancer Society dropped the ball on this cancer breakthrough

One of the more important studies on cesium chloride was conducted by Dr. H.E. Sartori, who began his research in April 1981 at Life Sciences Universal Medical Clinics in Rockville, MD. His subjects were 50 patients with widespread metastatic tumor deposits that represented a variety of cancers—including breast, colon, prostate, pancreatic, lung, and liver.

Forty-seven of these 50 patients had already completed surgery, radiation, and multiple courses of chemotherapy before trying the cesium. But after treatment with cesium chloride, approximately 50 percent of the patients survived—including the three patients who were comatose when the therapy was initiated. Pain also disappeared in all patients within one to three days of beginning the cesium therapy.

Thirteen patients did die within the first two weeks of therapy; however, autopsy results in each of these 13 showed a reduction in tumor mass size.[4]

Even the American Cancer Society (ACS) concluded that "studies conducted in several experimental tumor models in the 1980s found that the use of cesium chloride led to less tumor growth and fewer deaths of certain tumor-bearing mice such as those with sarcoma or breast cancer."[5] Furthermore, they noted that "recent research in rats has shown that DMSO may deserve further study as a drug carrier used to enhance the effectiveness of some chemotherapy agents for the treatment of bladder cancer."

Studies done in animals since 1988 have found that adding DMSO to some chemotherapy drugs helped the bladder absorb them better. Research has also shown that "DMSO does appear to have some effect in reducing pain, swelling, and inflammation, as well as some other properties that may make it useful in treating certain condition."[3]

What this revelation from the ACS says to me is that (at the VERY least) someone there has most seriously "dropped the ball," as they say. That such a therapy—admittedly effective in animal studies and lacking in serious side effects—would be known to conventional medicine for so many decades, and subsequently ignored, seems to me to smack of some serious negligence (or worse) on someone's part. But, I digress…

The cesium chloride and DMSO protocol

If you decide to try it, the cesium chloride and DMSO combo can be used topically or orally. The protocol can be self-administered, but I strongly suggest that you opt to do it under the guidance of an experienced professional.

If you use the duo topically, it can be applied to the skin in a localized area (such as the abdomen) via a spray bottle. You should know, though, that DMSO is sulfur-based and has a pungent sulfuric smell that is definitely noticeable—and not very pleasant.[3]

Cesium chloride supplements are also available in pill form in a wide range of doses. Keep in mind, though, that cesium chloride in combination with a high pH diet causes potassium depletion, so it's essential to get plenty of potassium (from food and supplements) while you're on the protocol.

The recommended dosage of cesium chloride is 1 to 6 grams per day. Most patients take 3 g per day, always with food. Below is one version of a cesium chloride protocol, but as always, DO consult with an experienced practitioner before starting!

Breakfast: cesium chloride (1 gram), vitamin C (1,000 mg), zinc (25-30 mg), one potassium capsule as prescribed by a physician

Lunch: vitamin C (1,000 mg)

Dinner: cesium chloride (1 gram), vitamin C (1,000 mg)

Before bed, after eating two slices of bread: cesium chloride (1 gram), vitamin C (1,000 mg)

Side effects and important notes

As mentioned above, you'll need to add potassium to your diet to increase your blood potassium levels. If, however, your serum potassium gets too high, then hyperkalemia (excess potassium) can result, so be sure to have this delicate balance of serum potassium checked every couple of weeks to avoid damage to your kidneys if you choose to try this treatment.

Cesium chloride does stay in the body for a couple of months even after you stop taking it, so be sure to continue potassium supplementation for a couple of months after you discontinue cesium therapy.

Since cesium chloride and DMSO cause the death of many cancer cells at once, your body's ability to process and eliminate the byproducts of this massive cellular death may cause a "detoxification reaction" that can involve flu-type symptoms like headache, nausea, and skin rash. For some people, the herb milk thistle can be very helpful to the liver in the elimination of toxins.[4]

In rare cases, cesium capsules can cause perforation of the stomach or small intestine if the capsules become positioned against the wall of either organ. This is the reason cesium must always be taken with food. Personally, I would use the liquid form of cesium to avoid this problem altogether.

Another condition observed after cesium therapy is a striking rise in blood uric acid levels caused by the release of DNA from all of the dead cancer cells (DNA is metabolized into uric acid). This has the potential to cause decreased kidney function because large amounts of uric acid appearing in kidney tubules can form crystals that block those tubules. This can be prevented by using the pharmaceutical drug Xyloprim (allopurinol) before and with cesium treatment, so that excessively high values of uric acid do not build up.[4]

I must also mention that in a small number of people, cesium chloride has also been linked with ventricular tachycardia, a rapid and irregular heartbeat that can lead to sudden cardiac death.[2]

Also, some physicians believe that the administration of just 0.5 g per day of cesium can actually enhance the rate of tumor growth, since this low amount raises a cell's pH into the "high mitosis," or cell division, range. But the data so far reveal that any quantity of 3.0 g or above will be effective in treating cancer.[2]

And one more important note for brain-cancer patients: Brain cancer presents a difficult problem for any cancer treatment, whether orthodox or alternative. When a cancer cell is dying, from whatever cause, it can create inflammation in the brain, which can cause a seizure, so it is even more important for you to solicit the care of a knowledgeable practitioner to support you during this treatment.

This seems like a long list of caveats, but if you're interested in trying cesium chloride, getting the help you need may only be a phone call or mouse-click away. Check out the professional support from www.shopthewolfeclinic.com or (877)359-6950. Information on where to get cesium chloride is in the Member Source Directory on page 529.

CHAPTER EIGHT

"Choking" weed starves tumors by cutting off blood supply

Diagnosed with ovarian cancer, a woman walked out of her doctor's office in search of an alternative treatment. Her mother had died of the same disease seven years earlier, and this woman's doctor felt her chances were equally bleak.

So she traveled to Oklahoma from her home in Kansas, where she met a shaman who gave her a tincture made from a common (and—among gardeners—universally hated) plant. She faithfully used the tincture every day. She started to feel her symptoms melting away, and after a year had passed her shocked doctor pronounced her cancer-free.

This woman, though she's never shared her name, couldn't wait to share her story. One day, she showed up at The Center for the Improvement of Human Functioning International, a Kansas clinic dedicated to cancer research and treatment. She eagerly told her story, and the team at the clinic found her tale so compelling that they immediately began research.

But they were puzzled at first. The plant didn't seem to kill tumor cells or boost the immune system. It took almost four years for them to find the answer—and, in a twist out of the movies, it turned out that what made the plant so hated was just about the same thing that made it a breakthrough in cancer treatment.

Miracle extract inhibits all tumors—not just certain kinds

Gardeners and farmers absolutely hate it. Bindweed (Convolvulus arvensis) may feature lovely flowers, but it will methodically invade, entwine, and choke surrounding plants, costing over $350 million in crop losses in the United States alone each year.

But, as these things usually happen, there's an ironic twist.

That same choking action, loathed by farmers, is loved in the cancer lab. Because an extract of bindweed, comprised of proteoglycan molecules (PGMs), has demonstrated an ability to do the very same thing to tumors.

You see, in order to survive, tumor cells have to have a blood supply. The body isn't interested in providing them with one, so they have to trick it by releasing chemicals that shift the body's production of blood vessels into overdrive.

The new blood vessels help tumors to grow unnaturally fast. As they feed off these new nutrient supplies, they grow stronger and harder to fight. But PGMs bring this growth to a screeching half.

After finding their answer, the team at the clinic tested the extract in animal models of various tumors. In each case, it was able to inhibit growth by 70-99.5 percent. Triumphantly, they classified it as an all-tumor inhibitor, equally effective in inhibiting the progression of all tumors. Used with an immune stimulant, it was even more impressive.

100 times more effective than the leading natural "tumor starver"

It all comes down to angiogenesis, the process in which new blood vessels are created from existing networks in the body. In a healthy body, it's a stop and go process—blood vessels grow, and the brakes are put on before the new growth gets out of hand.

In women, this process occurs monthly during the menstrual cycle, as the lining of the uterus is rebuilt. And in both men and women, angiogenesis is essential to tissue repair after an injury.

But in the case of a tumor, blood vessel growth gets completely out of hand—cells divide more rapidly and spread more quickly than they normally should. This is because tumors secrete substances that block the normal "braking" that should be part of the angiogenesis process.

PGMs work on a particular chemical involved in angiogenesis. Called vascular endothelial growth factor (VEGF), it helps tumors' blood vessels thrive.

Research has shown that cancer, particularly breast cancer, is linked to too much VEGF showing up in the blood. It's thought that this overexpression is an early step in metastasis, as tumors feed off the new blood vessels and grow larger. Basically, the more VEGF in the blood, the more likely angiogenesis is going haywire.

Inhibiting VEGF cuts off angiogenesis, leaving the tumor to starve.

For a while, shark cartilage seemed to be the gold standard when it came to natural inhibition of angiogenesis. But the supporting data was conflicting, and resources are limited, making it expensive. However, PGMs have been found 100 times more effective than shark cartilage when it comes to regulating angiogenesis.[1]

Researchers working on PGMs knew they were onto something when they conducted a chicken egg chorioallantoic membrane assay. This is a way to test human tumor cells in conditions similar to those in the human body. In this test, PGMs inhibited new blood vessel growth up to 73 percent, and cut abnormal cell growth by up to 98.6 percent.

In a test on mice, the extract inhibited tumor growth by an impressive 70 percent when taken orally.[2] In another, the inhibition was at 96.8 percent, regardless of how the dose was administered. Researchers declared PGMs "a potent angiogenesis inhibitor" and also noted its support of the immune system.[3]

Tumor growth in various studies was stunted at non-toxic doses (you can't say that about chemo, can you?). In fact, no toxicity was found in test animals in doses up to a human equivalent of a whopping 1,400 g.

It is important to note, though, that bindweed does contain toxins before the extraction process. So you can't use the whole plant—the good stuff is in the extract.

Keep new tumors from developing after conventional treatment

It's a frightening and disheartening pattern: A tumor is surgically removed, the patient is declared cancer-free, and then it returns. Nearly 50 percent of cancer patients experience growth of metastases—and it can be years after the original tumor is removed.

A group of doctors at Harvard struggled for years with the question of why new tumors develop after treatment—and, more importantly, how to keep it from happening. They found that cells in the body normally produce, in balance, proteins that both inhibit and stimulate blood vessel growth. Cancerous tumors put those proteins out of balance, turning down the inhibitors.

Directly around the primary tumor, stimulators prompt blood vessel growth. Both stimulators and inhibitors leak into the bloodstream, where stimulators break down, but inhibitors reach microscopic secondary tumors. Those tumors can't grow new blood vessels, and so they lie dormant.

But—remove the first tumor, and those microscopic tumors suddenly don't have anything keeping them from growing their own networks of new blood vessels. In one experiment on mice, researchers removed the primary tumor from mice with lung cancer, and saw an "explosion" of metastatic growth within just five days. Within two weeks, there were so many tumors that lung function was completely taken over.

So, finding a substance that prevents tumors from building this network of blood vessels is essential to people undergoing conventional treatment. Researchers started developing angiogenic inhibitors in an effort to block metastatic growth.

This led to a few mainstream solutions, most notably Avastin, which puts the brakes on angiogenesis, but can lead to a whole slew of potentially devastating problems (see sidebar on the following page).

Why use the mainstream's flawed and dangerous drugs when a safe and natural option is available? An extract of bindweed, rich in PGMs, is available in a product called C-Statin.

Choke out cancer with the most effective angiogenesis suppressor out there

Doctors and patients alike are impressed by C-Statin's ability to choke out cancer. Dr. Freidrich R. Douwes, of the St. George Clinic in Germany (a clinic devoted to alternative cancer treatments), is a big supporter of C-Statin. He praises it for being the most effective suppressor of angiogenesis he's come across, and uses it with most of his patients at the clinic.

Jeff Marrongelle, who has been in practice in Schuylkill, PA for 15 years, has found bindweed extract an invaluable tool in his clinic. If it doesn't shrink the tumor, he notes, it stops the progression and growth long enough to add other therapies. Every one of his patients who has used it has had positive results.

Another naturopath, Mary Shackelton of Boulder, CO, reports that her patients feel better and find their symptoms reduced on PGM.

Nancy Taylor, a 52-year-old woman from Arizona, has stage 4 metastatic breast cancer. Her white blood cell counts have only been

Mainstream might buy you a few months, but at what cost?

Of course, the mainstream has their own answer to angiogenesis—but it invites a whole slew of other serious problems.

Once research showing that cutting off the blood supply could starve tumors started rolling in, the race began. At one point several years ago, more than 60 angiogenesis inhibitors were in clinical trials for the treatment of cancer.

And out of those trials came Avastin. Touted as a landmark in the battle against cancer, Avastin couldn't cure cancer, but it did increase survival by a few months. Now it's used to treat brain tumors as well as cancers of the colon, rectum, lung, or breast.

Given by injection every couple of weeks, Avastin might buy you a few more months of life (20 months vs. 16 months with just standard treatment in one study). But the possible side effects are disturbing.

You may have problems with wound healing, which could result in infection. Avastin can affect fertility, and can also cause a serious neurological disorder that may not show up for a whole year after treatment starts.

And the list of serious side effects is shockingly long, ranging from "vomit that looks like blood or coffee grounds" to completely ceasing to urinate to chest pains. And at the end of the list, this shows up: "This is not a complete list of side effects and others may occur." There are so many serious side effects, they can't even tell you what they all are! Not exactly comforting, when I'm supposed to "tell my doctor immediately" if any of these unnamed side effects are observed.

No matter how many things like this I come across, I never get used to it—here you have a promising angle in the fight against cancer. And the mainstream is content to turn a blind eye to a *safe* and *natural* treatment that does the job without side effects.

considered low once in the past six months, and she fully believes it is due to taking C-Statin.

Ordering information for C-Statin is in the Member Source Directory on page 529.

CHAPTER NINE

The magic mushroom formula that can conquer breast cancer

Most traditional Asian medicine is thousands of years ahead of Western medicine... and that's glaringly obvious in the fight against cancer.

And now, one ancient remedy has been married with today's technology, creating a cancer-fighting agent so powerful that it can take on breast cancer cells before they grow and multiply—literally stopping the disease in its tracks.

In fact, if you lived in Korea instead of the United States, this potent natural cure could very well be the treatment your doctor prescribed for cancer rather than chemotherapy.

Japanese doctors have also seen remarkable results: In one breast cancer patient, doctors saw a pingpong ball-sized tumor disappear after just two months of treatment with Meshima... a medicinal mushroom brought to a new level by a few extremely insightful scientists.

And thanks to a man with a strong belief in natural medicine, you finally have access to the most powerful cancer-fighting medicinal mushroom... along with other supportive natural compounds that could help you win the fight against breast cancer, maybe even stop the disease in its earliest stages before it can fully develop.

MWI brings medicinal mushrooms to the U.S.

Other than as an occasional pizza topping or in a traditional green bean casserole, Americans don't really eat a lot of mushrooms—and when we do, it's the standard white button variety.

And while we can find more exotic mushrooms (like portabella and shiitake) in the grocery stores, medicinal mushrooms are virtually nowhere to be found—and they still might be off our radar if it weren't for the work of Mushroom Wisdom, Inc (formerly known as "Maitake Products, Inc.").

Back in 1991, Mike Shirota founded MWI to bring the one of the most powerful medicinal mushrooms on earth—the maitake—to the United States. Since then, the company has branched out with even more healing products… and they're now introducing one that might just wipe out breast cancer.

Breast-Mate™ was specifically formulated to support healthy breast cells—but it appears to do much more than that.

Man on a mushroom mission
uncovers potential breast cancer cure

Dr. Daniel Sliva has a mission: To let the world know about the simplest, safest way to prevent and treat cancer. Through years of research, Dr. Sliva has come up with the answer, and he's got stacks of proof to back it up. The answer is mushrooms, and it seems that certain mushrooms may be able to stop cancer before it gets a chance to start taking over.

After completing his post-doctoral work in Sweden, Dr. Sliva set off on a research path that surprised and amused his colleagues. "They thought I was crazy to study mushrooms," he said. "But I went ahead, and looked to 4,000 years of medicinal mushroom use in traditional Chinese medicine. I wanted to prove that they worked on a molecular level."

And that he did.

For ten years, Dr. Sliva studied the molecular biology of medicinal mushrooms like maitake and reishi—and found they could have stunning results when pitted against breast cancer cells. Then he came across what may be the most powerful cancer suppressor yet: phellinus linteus (PL).

In one of the most stunning studies to date, Dr. Sliva and his team found undeniable evidence in the lab that an extract of PL has a four-fold anti-breast-cancer effect:[1]

1. It inhibits cell adhesion, meaning it keeps breast cancer cells from joining together to form tumors.

2. It restricts cell migration, so breast cancer cells can't move to other areas of the body (known as metastases).

3. It curbs cell invasion, meaning the PL extract doesn't let breast cancer cells take over healthy cells.

4. It suppresses angiogenesis, which is the formation of new blood vessels—something tumors can't live without

---

By any other name...

In Japan, the mushroom got its name—Maitake, which translates to 'dance mushroom'—because it's shaped like a dancing nymph. Legend has it, though, that it got the name because when people stumbled across this rare and precious mushroom deep in the forest, they began to dance with joy.

Then there's its scientific name, *Grifola frondosa*—referring to the mythical half-lion, half-eagle griffin, considered to be an especially powerful creature that's well-known for guarding treasure.

On top of that, the PL extract decreased cancer cell multiplication by up to 78 percent! PL extract appears to halt the invasive behavior of abnormal breast cells—it can literally stop breast cancer cells dead in their tracks.

While PL mushrooms are edible, and simply eating them might help prevent or treat cancer, the extract contains more concentrated biologically active compounds—making it that much more powerful as an anti-cancer agent. And, so far, PL extract appears to be completely safe.

Once PL has been confirmed as safe and effective in animal trials, toxicology studies will begin. After that comes human clinical trials—and hopefully a new way to treat cancer without harming patients will emerge.

And while successfully—and safely—treating cancer is critically important, Dr. Sliva is even more focused on prevention. "Help needs to start sooner. Signal pathways are activated before cancer even starts. And if we can close them down, the cancer will never get a chance to start. That is much better than treating cancer."

PL Mushroom extract shows off its anticancer powers

It turns out that Dr. Sliva wasn't the only one who'd seen phenomenal anticancer effects with PL extract:

- Back in 1970, a group of Japanese researchers induced sarcoma 180 (cancerous tumors) in mice. PL mushroom extracts caused complete tumor regression in more than half of the mice... and demonstrated inhibition ratios (meaning that tumor growth stopped) over 95 percent... with absolutely no toxicity.[2]

- In 2009, researchers uncovered yet another key component of PL, called hispolon, that causes apoptosis (cell death) in breast and bladder cancer cells.[3]

- A cultured version of PL was approved as a medicine in 1997 in Korea, and has been used there as medication ever since— sometimes in conjunction with standard chemotherapy, and sometimes as a stand-alone treatment for cancer patients.

Building on Dr. Sliva's Success

The MWI research and development team already knew about the powers of medicinal mushrooms, but when they learned of Dr. Sliva's work with the meshima mushroom (the Japanese name for PL), they knew it would become the centerpiece of their new formula—Breast-Mate.™

With PL-fraction (the same extract used in Dr. Sliva's research) as their key ingredient, the team sought out other supportive natural ingredients—all proven to have anti-cancer benefits, particularly when it comes to breast cancer. Because these natural compounds attack breast cancer at the cellular level, they make superior preventives... and potent treatments.

Five proven cancer-fighters join the PL fraction

While PL is the centerpiece of the Breast-Mate™ formula, it's not the only ingredient proven to have a powerful impact on breast cancer. In fact, all of the ingredients in this formula have been shown to combat breast cancer—in the lab, in animal studies, and in people. *Maitake Standardized Extract PSX Fraction*™ Maitake mushrooms, the cornerstone of MWI, have a long and rich history when it comes to fighting cancer... and that includes breast cancer. But it turns out that a special extract, the PSX Fraction, can take on breast cancer from another angle entirely.

For decades, scientists have been studying the maitake's anti-cancer properties, and learning about the many different ways these mushrooms can protect you against cancer—from boosting your immune system function to taking on the tumors themselves.

Then in 2003, researchers discovered another important benefit these mushrooms could offer, this time using a distinct extract, different than the one they'd been pitting against cancer cells. This extract could lower blood sugar—even better than a prescription drug.

In fact, one study found that maitake extract (in a form called WS-fraction, which would later be concentrated and renamed SX fraction) lowered blood sugar in mice by a full 70 points in just one week… compared to a 43-point drop with popular diabetes drug glipizide.[4]

Another study found that maitake SX-fraction improved insulin sensitivity, reducing both insulin resistance and blood glucose levels, in rats. In fact, the SX-fraction performed as well as pioglitazone (a common diabetes drug)… with no adverse side effects.[5]

You may be wondering what lower blood sugar and increased insulin sensitivity have to do with breast cancer—I did, too, and that's why I asked the Dr. Cun Zhuang of MWI about the choice to use the PSX fraction (an extract standardized to contain 18 percent SX-fraction) instead of the proven cancer-fighting D fraction.

"It is said that cancer feeds on sugar, and the relationship between high blood sugar and cancer (especially breast cancer) has been discussed more and more these days. Maitake SX-fraction is out proprietary extract that improves insulin resistance, making it effective for people with Metabolic Syndrome and Type 2 Diabetes."

So I looked at the research, and it turns out there's quite a lot of evidence linking Type 2 diabetes and Metabolic Syndrome to breast

---

Metabolic Syndrome, a.k.a. Syndrome X

Metabolic Syndrome (which is also known as Insulin Resistance Syndrome or Syndrome X) comes with a variety of symptoms—all of which can put your good health at risk. It involves such dangerous symptoms as high blood pressure, high blood sugar, high triglycerides, and insulin resistance.

cancer. In fact, according to an Israeli study, women with Type 2 diabetes appear to face up to a 20 percent higher risk of developing breast cancer... especially postmenopausal women.[6]

A review of the Women's Health Initiative found that women with Metabolic Syndrome faced nearly double the risk of developing breast cancer.[7] And an Italian study found that women with Metabolic Syndrome were more likely to suffer breast cancer recurrence than women without the condition.[8]

Since the maitake extract included in the Breast-Mate™ formula is proven to lower blood sugar and improve insulin resistance, it may nullify the cancer-promoting effects of Type 2 diabetes and Metabolic Syndrome—giving you a unique way to conquer breast cancer.

Note: If you're taking any medication to lower your blood sugar, please consult with your health care provider before taking any supplement containing Maitake SX-fraction.

Broccoli extract

For your whole life, people have probably been nagging you to eat your broccoli. Turns out they were offering some very good advice—because in the fight against cancer, you definitely want broccoli on your side.

Broccoli, like its other cruciferous cousins, contains a compound known as indole 3 carbinol (I3C)—a compound that's been found highly beneficial in the fight against breast cancer. In fact, back in 1995, scientists found that I3C could actually prevent breast tumors in rodents.[9]

Then in 1999, researchers found that using I3C in combination with tamoxifen (a common chemotherapy used on breast cancer patients) better halted the growth of estrogen-dependent breast cancer cells (known as MCF-7 cells) than the drug on its own.[10]

Finally in 2004, scientists figured out just how it works. It turns out that I3C activates a pathway that stops the cycle of human breast cancer cells (specifically, MCF-7 cells).[11] It also produces a substance called DIM (3,3'-Diindolylmethane) during digestion, and DIM performs a critical job… it converts a potentially dangerous hormone into a super-safe version instead.

That's right—DIM prevents estrone from turning into its cancer-causing form, 16-hydroxyestrone. Instead, it helps the hormone turn into 2-hydroxyestrone, a completely non-cancer-causing form… stopping cancer cells before they can get started.

Green tea extract

Green tea is well-known around the world for its cancer-fighting properties, along with plenty of other health benefits. And over the past ten years or so, researchers have focused on the green tea-breast cancer connection.

In a nutshell, several population studies have found that people who drink green tea enjoy a decreased risk for breast cancer and cancer recurrence. One study in particular found that women with breast cancer who drank green tea had the least cancer spread… and that women who drank at least 5 cups a day before their diagnoses were less likely to have their cancer recur.[12]

Green tea seems to get its cancer-fighting powers from a component called EGCG (epigallocatechin gallate)… which has been studied vigorously in the lab, with a lot of success. Back in 1998, researchers discovered that EGCG inhibited the growth of cancer cells without doing any damage to healthy cells.[13] And even further back, in 1995, scientists discovered that EGCG could inhibit breast cancer cells transplanted into mice by up to 99 percent.[14]

Fast forward to 2007, when researchers learned that EGCG along with other polyphenols found in green tea could slow down breast cancer tumor growth, shrink tumors, and set off breast cancer cell death in mice (who'd been injected with human breast cancer cells).

And while it may seem that green tea on its own—and especially in combination with mushroom and broccoli extracts—can fight off breast cancer, the researchers at MWI took their formula two steps further.

The formula rounds out with two vitamins that have gotten a lot of press over the past few years: *vitamin D3* and *folic acid*. Both of these nutrients have been studied and found to have connections with breast cancer.

Vitamin D's role comes in prevention—women who get more dietary vitamin D and more exposure to sunlight seem to have a substantially reduced risk of developing breast cancer. But it also comes with a treatment component, where using vitamin D to treat breast cancer may keep tumors from growing.

Folic acid also helps lower the risk, especially for postmenopausal women and women who drink alcohol. Studies have shown that higher intake of folic acid is linked with a decreased risk of breast cancer—a decrease of up to 29 percent.[15] And the benefit is even stronger when women get plenty of 'folate cofactors' (other nutrients that work together with folic acid), like vitamins B6 and B12.

Using Breast-Mate™ to take on breast cancer

Breast-Mate™ can be used for both breast cancer prevention and treatment. (For treatment, better results may be seen when Breast-Mate™ is used together with Maitake D-fraction.) The recommended dose of Breast-Mate™ for treatment is two tablets, twice per day. For breast cancer prevention, the manufacturer recommends one to two tablets, twice a day.

You can find ordering information for Breast-Mate™ in the Member Source Directory on page 529.

CHAPTER TEN

Defeat even advanced prostate cancer with "killer" herbs

If you know someone who's suffering from prostate cancer, you'll want to read this article *right now*.

Because no matter what else they've tried, no matter whether their cancer is androgen-dependent or (much more difficult to treat) androgen-independent, this combination of time-tested and cutting-edge formulas can turn things around... even if the cancer has gotten to the advanced stage.

Making a natural cancer killer even more effective

When we first introduced you to PectaSol® back in 2004, we knew it had potential beyond what science had so far shown. And we were right...

Developed by HSI panelist Dr. Isaac Eliaz, PectaSol (a special form of modified citrus pectin, or MCP) showed great promise against a variety of cancers. In fact, one early study found that seven out of ten patients with recurrent prostate cancer significantly slowed their PSA doubling time (a measurement that shows how fast prostate cancer is growing) by using Pecta-Sol.[1]

But Dr. Eliaz knew he could make it even more effective. And he did.

After years of research, Dr. Eliaz realized that people would be able to absorb pectin more effectively if its molecules weren't so big. So he developed a special process that could make those pectin molecules smaller—and PectaSol-C® was born.

And with those miniscule molecules, more of that pectin can travel through your bloodstream and latch on to their targets: cancer cells.

It worked. In fact, it worked so well that the newly shrunk MCP molecules were able to take on advanced cancers, even cancers that had spread rampantly to cause even more damage.

Killer citrus stops even treatment-resistant cancer in its tracks

In August 2008, we told you about another astonishing MCP breakthrough: In a groundbreaking trial[2], PectaSol-C was shown to work miracles for people with even advanced and treatment-resistant cancers. The patients in the trial all had terminal cancer (of various kinds), and almost 90 percent of that cancer had metastasized—and they'd all suffered through the ineffective 'solutions' offered by mainstream medicine (like chemotherapy and surgery) with no success.

Then they tried the PectaSol-C, and it literally turned their lives around. After just 16 weeks, 35.7 percent of the patients had shown a positive response (measured in pain status, functional impairment, and weight loss). On top of that, 28.6 percent of the patients remained stable after 16 weeks of treatment.

"I believe PectaSol-C has prolonged my life."

One of those patients had advanced prostate cancer, and his results were nothing short of miraculous.

"I believe PectaSol-C has prolonged my life," said R.F. of California, a man stricken with advanced prostate cancer.

Over that 16-week trial period, R.F. saw his PSA drop 50 percent. He also experienced significant increases in clinical benefit, quality of life, and decline of pain.

These impressive results show that MCP rivals the power of many prescription cancer drugs. But what makes PectaSol-C even better is that it doesn't appear to have any dangerous side effects or interactions. In fact, very few people who take MCP experience flatulence or loose stools, due to its soluble fiber content. But this can be easily managed by lowering the dose and slowly working back up to the therapeutic level. But when you compare that to the toxic side effects of most conventional cancer treatments, these problems are very minor.

Now PectaSol-C brings more compelling new cancer-fighting science to the table

It's clear that PectaSol-C can wreak havoc on prostate cancer, and now we know exactly how that happens.

In a just-published *in vitro* study[3], scientists discovered that PectaSol-C actually stops the production of new prostate cancer cells, and even brings on their apoptosis (cell death). So at the same time it's killing off old cancer cells, it's also preventing the creation of new ones.

But it gets better...

PectaSol-C has the same impact on both androgen-dependent *and* androgen-independent (AI) prostate cancer cells (see sidebar). That's very good news for men suffering from AI prostate cancer, which is much harder for mainstream medicine to treat.

So you can see just how PectaSol-C can work miracles for prostate cancer patients. And when it's teamed up with a second prostate cancer-fighting formula, the results are even better.

Thirty-three prostate supporting ingredients join forces to wipe out cancer

Dr. Eliaz could have been satisfied with the overwhelming success of PectaSol-C, but he didn't rest on his laurels. Instead, he was instrumental in creating a prostate-specific supplement, one that would complement the cancer-killing powers of MCP and join in its fight to wipe out prostate cancer.

ProstaCaid® contains an impressive, comprehensive collection of ingredients, thirty-three of the most potent prostate supporters in existence. This complex blend of healing herbs and nutrients provides a wholly integrative approach to conquering prostate cancer.

The formula helps promote and maintain long-term prostate health—and that can go a long way toward preventing prostate cancer from striking. ProstaCaid contains several ingredients that help control hormone levels, especially to positively balance the estrogen/testosterone ratio, which is critical to prostate health.

And its comprehensive antioxidant profile helps prevent DNA damage and protect your prostate cells.

According to Dr. Eliaz, "The ability of this specific combination of ingredients to kill both hormone-sensitive prostate cancer as well as hormone-resistant prostate cancer (the type that metastasizes) is truly unusual. The research shows this specific combination of ingredients can save lives, prevent prostate cancer and prolong the lives of those suffering from prostate cancer."

ProstaCaid kills off cancer cells in just 72 hours

ProstaCaid, like its partner PectaSol-C, can stop prostate cancer in its tracks—but it does it in a different way, as a brand new trial demonstrated.[4]

This formula actually interrupts the life cycle of prostate cancer cells (a process called G2/M cell cycle arrest). ProstaCaid cancels the cycle before the *mitosis* (or M) stage, the point where a cell would normally divide and replicate. Without mitosis, prostate cancer cells can not multiply.

Like PectaSol-C, ProstaCaid also causes prostate cancer cells to die by setting off apoptosis. And ProstaCaid has the same killer effect on both androgen-dependent and androgen-independent prostate cancer cells.

That's especially important, as lead study author Dr. Jun Yan tells us. "The results we saw with this formula are very important for cancer therapy because currently there is no effective treatment for hormone resistant prostate cancer."

And in this trial, the formula was able to stop prostate cancer cell multiplication *and* induce cancer cell death after only 72 hours of treatment—just three days!

Even better, it only took minute doses to knock out the cancer cells. The synergistic effect of the ProstaCaid formula brings on a response at much lower concentrations than you'd see with any single ingredient.

The amazing killing powers of this formula come thanks to its comprehensive range of ingredients. But since delving into each ingredient's prowess would take an entire double issue (remember, there are 33!), we'll focus on just some of the key players.

DIM slows tumor growth with no toxic side effects

Diindolylmethane (commonly called DIM) is a proven cancer-fighting nutrient—especially when it comes to hormone-related cancers.

There are numerous studies proving DIM's effectiveness against prostate cancer specifically. One *in vitro* study found that DIM, on its own, could cause prostate cancer cell death.[5] A second *in vitro* study[6] found that the nutrient prevented prostate cancer cell proliferation, leading the researchers to conclude that DIM may "reduce disease recurrence." Another study[7], this one involving mice, showed that DIM inhibited prostate tumor growth with no toxic side effects.

How does DIM get the job done? It inhibits the creation of a particularly dangerous type of estrogen known as 16-Hydroxyestrone, instead producing a safer version of the hormone.

Stinging nettle root prevents benign cells from turning malignant

Stinging nettle may not sound like something you want involved with your prostate, but it is a highly effective cancer treatment and preventive.

In fact, nettle appears to keep the benign cells of an enlarged prostate from heading down the path of malignancy and turning into prostate cancer.[8]

On top of that, an *in vitro* study[9] showed that stinging nettle can keep prostate cancer cells from multiplying, which may help keep cancer in check.

Chinese skullcap: Treating prostate cancer for ages

Long used in traditional herbal medicine, Chinese skullcap (scientifically known as *Scutellaria baicalensis*) has a long history of being used to treat the prostate. And modern science has finally caught up, with numerous studies supporting that traditional use.

A key compound in Chinese skullcap known as baicalin is the main powerhouse here. This flavonoid appears to inhibit prostate cancer cell growth, whether those cells are androgen-dependent or independent, and stimulates apoptosis at the same time.[10]

A study[11] involving mice injected with human cancer cells demonstrates just how well this staple of Chinese herbal medicine works. The researchers saw a 66 percent decrease in tumor mass after just seven weeks of treatment with Chinese skullcap.

Berberine knocks out tumors
and inflammation all at once

Berberine is a compound found in many medicinal herbs. And this alkaloid substance sets off apoptosis in prostate cancer cells, whether or not they're androgen-dependent. And, like other powerful cancer killers in the ProstaCaid formula, berberine also keeps those cancer cells from multiplying and taking over.[12]

This compound works by interrupting the prostate cancer cell life cycle, which keeps those malignant cells from running rampant in the prostate. At the same time, though, it had no negative impact on healthy prostate cells—meaning it targets only the bad guys.

Pomegranate: A proven prostate protecting fruit

Pomegranate has it all: brilliant color, sweet-tart taste, and pros-tate-saving powers. And there are numerous studies showing just how effectively this fruit fights against prostate cancer. Here are some of the highlights…

- A 2005 study[13] found that prostate cancer patients who simply drank eight ounces of pomegranate juice per day saw increased PSA doubling time

- In the lab,[14] several forms of pomegranate (like fermented juice, and seed oil) prevented prostate cancer cell growth

- A 2005 lab study[15] found that pomegranate fruit extract stopped prostate cancer cell growth and set off apoptosis in those cells

- Pomegranate fruit extract was shown to decrease PSA levels and inhibit tumor growth in mice implanted with prostate cancer cells[16]

Ganoderma lucidum interrupts the
cancer supply line so tumors can't survive

Medicinal mushrooms have been fighting disease for centuries, and the *Ganoderma lucidum* (more familiarly known as the reishi mushroom) is among the most powerful. The reishi has been shown to prevent proliferation and bring on apoptosis in prostate cancer cells.[17]

One way this magic mushroom defeats this disease is by cutting off the blood supply to prostate cancer cells[18]—and without supplies, they simply can not thrive and survive. It turns out that reishi can stop a process called *angiogenesis*, which is the creation of new blood vessels, so that tumors never get a chance to grow and spread.[19]

In addition, the reishi mushroom prevents highly aggressive prostate cancer cells from spreading by interrupting special cellular signals[20]—a key factor in getting the cancer under control.

Pygeum boosts prostate health while stopping cancer cells in their tracks

Pygeum bark has long been a superstar in the prostate protection arena, easing symptoms (like frequent night-time urination) and promoting prostate health.

In fact, even in the early days, more than twenty-five years ago, researchers believed this pine-like tree held the answer to healthy prostate. Back then, scientists conducted a placebo-controlled study[21] which included 120 patients, and found that pygeum extract significantly improved prostate-related urinary problems.

But pygeum doesn't stop with prostate support—it also actively takes on prostate cancer cells, and keeps them from multiplying beyond control. An *in vitro* study[22] showed that pygeum can interrupt the prostate cancer cell cycle and prevent cell division and reproduction.

ProstaCaid doubles the cancer-killing powers of PectaSol-C

You've seen just how effective both ProstaCaid and PectaSol-C are at destroying prostate cancer. But even Dr. Eliaz was amazed by how much stronger they are when they work as a team.

Ongoing work[23] (which will be submitted in a paper for publication in the future) shows that when both products are used together, the anti-cancer effects of PectaSol-C are doubled.

Researchers are now studying the impact of PectaSol-C alone, and then the MCP combined with ProstaCaid against highly invasive prostate cancer cells. The MCP alone, as expected, had a powerful effect, stopping the migration of those invasive cells.

And when the research team added ProstaCaid to the MCP, they saw an enormous decrease in that invasive behavior.

That remarkable discovery took place in the lab. But Dr. Eliaz saw the incredible impact of the combination on advanced prostate cancer in one very sick patient.

The case study presented by Dr. Eliaz clearly shows just how well these two supplements work together. The patient in this case had hormonal-resistant, metastatic prostate cancer. He suffered through multiple mainstream therapies with no success. But the mix of ProstaCaid and PectaSol-C lowered his PSA significantly *and* substantially slowed his PSA doubling time—a remarkable result considering the aggressiveness of his disease.

Protect your prostate with ProstaCaid and PectaSol-C

Your prostate can reap the benefits of these two powerful cancer-fighting weapons, especially when using both together. According to Dr. Eliaz, though, if you plan to try only one, choose ProstaCaid.

With ProstaCaid, Dr. Eliaz recommends taking 6 capsules, twice a day with food for active support. For long-term support, the suggested dosage is 3 capsules, twice a day with food. And for prevention, Dr. Eliaz suggests taking 3 capsules once or twice daily with food, depending on the risk level, with a recommended loading dose of six capsules per day (with food) for the first two weeks.

As for PectaSol-C, this needs to be taken on an empty stomach, whether you choose the powder or the capsules. For active support, Dr. Eliaz recommends using 5 grams of powder or 6 capsules, three times per day. For long-term support, he suggests taking 5 grams of powder once daily or 6 capsules.

You can find ordering information for ProstaCaid and PectaSol-C in the Member Source Directory on page 529.

The Complete Cancer-Fighting Roster of ProstaCaid

Nutrients	Prostate Support Proprietary Blend		Immune & Hormonal Supprt Proprietary Blend		Liver Support Proprietary Blend	MycoCaid® Proprietary Herbal Enhanced Mushroom Blend
Vitamin C	Saw palmetto berry	Pygeum bark extract	Job's tears seed extract	Stinging nettle root extract	Broccoli extract	*Phellinus linteus*
Vitamin D-3	Grape skin extract	Lycopene	Chinese golden thread rhizome extract	Alpha lipoic acid	Skullcap root extract	*Ganoderma lucidum*
OptiZinc®	Pomegranate	Berberine	Citrus bioflavanoid complex	Eleuthero root extract	Chinese skullcap root extract	*Coriolus versicolor*
Selenium	Pumpkin seed oil extract	Tumeric root extract	*Astralagus membranaceus* root extract	Green tea leaf	Dandelion root extract	
Beta sitosterol	Chinese Similax rhizome extract	Quercetin				
DIM	Knotweed					
Boron						

CHAPTER ELEVEN

Vietnamese medicinal herb shows promise in healing prostate and ovarian disease

We talk a lot about traditional Chinese medicine and the inroads it's made as a modern approach to healing. But we never focused much on traditional Vietnamese medicine until we learned about one of its most valuable herbs called crinum latifolium. Apparently, it's so revered in Vietnam that it used to be reserved only for royalty and was known both as the "Medicine for the King's Palace" and the "Royal Female Herb."

Those traditional references actually highlight one of crinum's most unique aspects—its ability to target both prostate and ovarian health concerns. But crinum seems to be an equal opportunity herb. And its benefits seem to go beyond just sex-specific diseases too.

First, let's talk about what it can do to protect you from prostate or ovarian diseases.

Picking up where PC Spes left off—without the risk

Although most of the research on crinum focuses on men, it all started when the Hoang family studied its effect on ovarian health.

Dr. Kha Hoang was the Chief Teacher and medical doctor for the Vietnamese royal family. In 1984 his daughter had so many cysts on her ovary that surgery was planned to remove it. Dr. Hoang had her start drinking a tea made with crinum leaves, and about six weeks later the cysts were gone.

Today, three generations of the Hoang family are integrated medicine practitioners. The family has used crinum together with other supportive herbs in treating a variety of prostate and ovarian conditions. Biopsies confirmed 16 cases of advanced prostate cancer were completely cured regardless of prostate specific antigen (PSA) levels. In fact, sometimes PSA levels go up in men taking crinum, even though testing shows that their prostate cells are normal and healthy. That is exactly what happened to Ken Malik, the co-founder and Executive Director of the Prostate Awareness Foundation, a non-profit organization based in San Francisco, California.

In his own battle with prostate cancer, Malik chose to take the natural approach—opting for a therapeutic regimen of nutrition and exercise. He also used the herbal supplement PC Spes for eight years and found doing so stabilized his condition. PC Spes was marketed as an herbal formula that had shown remarkable results in treating prostate problems. Recently though, it was pulled from the market after researchers discovered that some PC Spes products claiming to be all-natural actually contained synthetic, potentially harmful substances. Malik was one of millions of men worldwide affected when PC Spes was taken off the market. When he stopped taking it, his PSA level started to creep upward. So he began his search for a replacement. That led him to crinum.

He started taking it in January 2002, and, over the course of the next 10 months, his PSA actually continued to go up. Most of the time, this would be cause for concern. But Malik's most recent biopsy showed only healthy tissue. His experience might add some support to recent reports that claim the PSA test might not be the best indicator of prostate cancer risk.

Malik was excited enough about his own experience to organize an informal trial with 10 members of the Prostate Awareness Foundation. Participants were told to take nine crinum tablets each day for three months. All 10 noted some kind of functional improvement.

Not everyone using crinum experiences elevated PSA levels. Sometimes its benefits follow a more predictable path, like the testimonial the manufacturer shared with me from a 58-year-old man who had a PSA of 93 when he went to his urologist for treatment. He'd waited so long that his cancer had spread to his bones, intestines, and lymph nodes. He was placed on an aggressive herbal program that included crinum. After just four months, his PSA was down to 0.9 and the symptoms he'd been experiencing—difficulty urinating, swelling in his legs, and extreme fatigue—had all disappeared.

92.6 percent success for BPH symptoms

Crinum isn't just for prostate cancer or extremely advanced cases of prostate disease. It also appears to alleviate the symptoms of one of the most common male problems—enlarged prostate, or benign prostatic hyperplasia (BPH). The main symptom of BPH is frequent and sometimes painful urination. There are over 500 individual case histories of successful crinum treatment for BPH. And after seven years of research, the International Hospital in Vietnam reported that 92.6 percent of patients had good results using crinum for BPH (confirmed by measurements of prostate size and clinical evaluation by urologists).[1] However, these results have not been confirmed in Western studies.

Helping your cells communicate

As effective as crinum appears to be, there's still no official consensus as to why or how it works. Researchers think it may have something to do with how it affects you at the simplest level—the cellular level. The human body contains about 70 trillion cells. With a few exceptions, each of these individual cells is a living entity with its own complete set of genes. Each of these cells maintains its own existence and also makes a vital contribution to your life and health. But in order for your body to function properly, all of those cells must communicate. For instance, your muscles must contract only when your brain sends a message to contract and not any other time.

Cells also communicate with one another to determine the correct balance of cell proliferation and apoptosis, or death. Basically, they're constantly working together to regulate how many cells you have—and how healthy they are—at any given moment. But if your cells aren't communicating properly, apoptosis may not happen the way it should, which means that unhealthy, even cancerous, cells can continue to thrive and mutate. Recent experiments show that crinum extract helps cells produce a substance called neopterin, which they send out to communicate with immune cells, calling them into action against cancer and other foreign invaders.

Five more ways to knock out disease

I found a crinum supplement called Healthy Prostate & Ovary that also contains five other herbal ingredients—alisima plantago-quatica, astragalus, momordica charantia, carica papaya leaf, and annona muricata leaf—all known for their immune- and energy-boosting effects as well as their abilities to regulate abnormal body functions.

Crinum is so established and widely used as a treatment for prostate and ovary diseases in Vietnam that their crops of the herb are generally prohibited from being exported. So Healthy Prostate & Ovary is one of the first crinum products we know of to be made available in the U.S. See the Member Source Directory on page 529 for complete ordering information.

If you decide to try the Healthy Prostate & Ovary formula, the recommended dose is three 600-mg tablets three times daily. And, as always, if you're battling cancer or any other serious illness, please consult with your physician before using this or any other product.

CHAPTER TWELVE

How you can take advantage of the AMAS Cancer Test

The AMAS Cancer Test stands for Anti-Malignan Antibody in Serum test. Malignin is a peptide found in people with a wide range of cancers. If the anti-malignan antibody is detected in the blood, it means that the body detected the presence of this peptide, and launched an immune response against it. Clinical studies have shown that the AMAS test is up to 95 percent accurate on the first reading, and up to 99 percent accurate after two readings.

In one study at Beth Israel Hospital in New York, the AMAS test demonstrated amazing accuracy. Within the study group of 125 people, the test was positive for 21 people who were later confirmed to have cancer, while it was negative for 97 people who showed no signs of cancer. The remaining seven people produced positive readings on the AMAS test but showed no signs of cancer; yet the study notes that all were symptomatic, had a family history of cancer, or both—indicating that the AMAS test may have detected a problem that conventional screening methods could not find.

This simple blood test can detect precancerous and cancerous cells with up to 99 percent sensitivity. Many of our members wrote in to say they were having difficulty finding a doctor willing to do the test—because they had never heard of it.

At HSI, we're committed to bringing you breakthrough information on the latest health discoveries. Our research often brings information directly to you before it even reaches your doctor. We realize there's no benefit to providing you with cutting-edge information if you can't use it. So our team did some research to learn more about the availability of the AMAS test and how you can take advantage of it.

Luckily, we were able to speak directly with Dr. Samuel Bogoch, one of the two doctors who first discovered the anti-malignin antibody and developed the AMAS test. He said that the test has been available for some time, but so far, doctors have only learned of it through word of mouth. Recent efforts have started getting the word out—but there is a still a long way to go.

You don't need a doctor's permission to order the AMAS test

But the good news is that ANYONE can order an AMAS test. Just call 1-800-922-8378 and leave your name and address to receive a free kit in the mail. The kit includes the materials and instructions you need to complete the test, and a packet of scientific literature supporting its benefits. Then, take the kit to your doctor, and ask him to order a blood sample and sign the analysis form. All AMAS tests are analyzed by Dr. Bogoch's staff in Boston (overnight shipping instructions are included in the kit). As some members have found, some labs refuse to draw specimens for tests that will be performed at another lab. According to Dr. Bogoch, that's more often the case with smaller labs; larger labs usually send specimens to other labs on a daily basis. If your doctor's lab is not willing to process the AMAS test, and your doctor is not willing to find one that will, do some research on your own. Check the Yellow Pages and call around to larger labs in your area.

Some readers also asked about the availability of the AMAS test outside the U.S. Anyone from anywhere in the world can order the test. The only unique challenge is the shipping. Samples sent from outside the U.S. may need to ship in dry ice to ensure a valid sample. The analysis costs $165 (not including extra lab fees or shipping costs), but the test is Medicare approved; and remember, ordering the kit is completely free.

The AMAS test can detect the presence of cancerous cells, but can't pinpoint their location. So a positive reading must be followed up by additional testing to locate the cancer and determine its stage. But the test does come much closer to offering true early detection than many other screening methods, and does so in a non-invasive way. To learn even more about AMAS, you can visit this website: www.oncolabinc.com.

If you're interested in the AMAS test, you don't have to wait for your doctor to hear about it. Call and order the free kit, and review the research. If you're still interested, take the kit and the literature to your doctor.

CHAPTER THIRTEEN

Is it really from heaven above? The cancer miracle that leaves healthy cells healthy

Cancer treatment has come a long way since the use of mustard gas derivatives in the early 1900s—or has it? When doctors discovered during World War I that mustard gas destroyed bone marrow, they began to experiment with it as a way to kill cancer cells. Although they had little success with the mustard gas, it did pave the way for modern chemotherapy—which involves the most toxic and poisonous substances anyone deliberately puts in his body. These treatments kill much more than cancer cells—they have a devastating effect even on healthy ones.

Sometimes it seems as if only a miracle could provide a cure that's both safe and effective. And a miracle is just what Dr. Mate Hidvegi believed he found when he patented Avemar, a fermented wheat germ extract. Studies have shown that Avemar reduces cancer recurrence, cuts off the cancer cells' energy supply, speeds cancer cell death, and helps the immune system identify cancer cells for attack.

A miracle in the making

Back in World War I, Dr. Albert Szent-Györgyi (a Nobel Prize recipient in 1937 for his discovery of vitamin C) had seen the effects of mustard gas up close and personal and was determined to find a safer alternative for cancer treatment. His goal was to prevent the rapid reproduction that is characteristic of cancer cells. He theorized that supplemental quantities of naturally occurring compounds in wheat germ called DMBQ would help to chaperone cellular metabolism, allowing healthy cells to follow a normal course but prohibiting potentially cancerous ones from growing and spreading. His early experiments, published in the *Proceedings of the National Academy of Sciences USA* in the 1960s, showed effects of naturally occurring and synthetic DMBQ against cancer cell lines, confirming his theory.

But it was then that the science community shifted its focus to killing cancer outright—at any cost. His approach, seen as negotiating with the enemy as opposed to destroying it outright, was cast to the side.

It wasn't until the fall of communism in Hungary in 1989—when scientists were allowed for the first time to pursue independent, personal interests—that Dr. Hidvegi picked up where Szent-Györgyi left off.

But when Hidvegi's funding ran out, it seemed as if the research would once again be set aside. He had no money, he had no prospects, and his wife insisted he give up his research and find a paying job.

They were desperate. Yet he did still have one thing at that time—faith. Being a devout man, Dr. Hidvegi prayed to the Virgin Mary for guidance—and an investor.

Miraculously, the very next day a stranger wrote Hidvegi a check somewhere in the $100,000 range. With that money, he was finally able to patent a technique of fermenting wheat germ with baker's yeast. He named this fermented product Avemar in tribute to the Virgin Mary (*Ave* meaning hail and *Mar* meaning Mary). It became the standard compound for research and later commercialization because it assured a longer shelf life while maintaining its live food status.

Avemar is supported by more than 100 reports (written for presentation or publication) conducted in the U.S., Hungary, Russia, Australia, Israel, and Italy and is validated by the publication of more than 20 peer-reviewed publications describing *in vitro*, in vivo, and human clinical trials.

Reduce cancer recurrence

Since 1996, over 100 studies done on Avemar have impressed oncologists and cancer researchers. Studies have shown that when Avemar is used as an adjunct treatment, it enhances the effects of the standard treatment agents. It's particularly effective in reducing the chances of cancer recurrence.

In a controlled study, 170 subjects with primary colorectal cancer either had surgery and standard care with chemotherapy or the same plus 9 g of Avemar taken once a day. Only 3 percent of the people in the the Avemar group experienced a recurrence, vs. more than 17 percent of those in the chemo-only group. The Avemar group also showed a 67 percent reduction in metastasis and a 62 percent reduction in deaths.[1]

In a randomized study, 46 stage III melanoma patients with a high risk of recurrence either had surgery and standard care with chemotherapy or surgery plus standard care and 9 g of Avemar taken once a day. Those taking Avemar showed approximately a 50 percent reduction in risk of progression.[2]

In a one-year, non-randomized trial of 43 patients with oral cancer, 21 patients received surgery and standard care while 22 others received the same plus Avemar. The Avemar group showed an 85 percent reduced risk of overall progression. Plus, only 4.5 percent of the patients in the Avemar group experienced local recurrences as opposed to more than 57 percent of the people in the standard care group.

Avemar also reduced the frequency and severity of many common side effects, including nausea, fatigue, weight loss, and immune suppression.

Rejuvenate your immune system

Although Avemar was born out of cancer research, it can also help if you don't have cancer. In fact, since one of its main actions is to keep your immune system operating at peak performance, there really isn't anyone who can't benefit from it. The biological state of aging counteracts your immune function, particularly after the age of 40. Many of the symptoms generally associated with simply "aging" are due to the declining ability of the immune system to differentiate between "foreign" proteins and natural ones. When this happens, the immune system not only becomes less capable of resisting infection and cancer but also begins to attack the body's own healthy tissues.

Avemar has been shown to normalize the imbalance in the immune system that results from age and stress. It has also been shown to improve the ability of T-cells to respond to antigens and the ability of B-cells to produce antibodies. And it enhances the functioning of macrophages—the key players in the immune response to foreign invaders like infectious microorganisms. So Avemar supports and enhances overall immune strength, coordination, and function.[7] In a sense, it rejuvenates your aging immune system.

Cut off cancer cells' energy supply

One of Avemar's most unique benefits is that it cuts off cancer cells' energy supply by selectively inhibiting glucose metabolism. Cancer cells love glucose: It fuels the voracious growth and spread of tumors. In fact, cancer cells utilize glucose at a 10-to 50-times higher rate than normal cells do.

Cancer cells that have a higher rate of glucose utilization have a greater chance of spreading. It's on these cells that we see Avemar's most dramatic effects. In fact, the greater the metastatic potential of the cancer cell line tested, the higher the glucose utilization rate and the more dramatic Avemar's effect.

Typical cancer treatments like chemotherapy kill off all cells—cancerous and healthy ones alike. But because of how Avemar interacts with glucose, it can selectively attack cancer cells while leaving healthy cells alone. Studies have shown that it would take a 50 times higher concentration of Avemar than is in a normal therapeutic dose to inhibit glucose utilization in normal healthy cells.

Avemar speeds cancer cell death

The second way Avemar works against cancer is to keep cancer cells from repairing themselves. Cancer cells reproduce quickly and chaotically, producing many breaks and other mistakes in the cellular structure. Because of this, cancer cells need a lot of the enzyme known as PARP (poly-ADP-ribose) to repair breaks in DNA before the cells divide. Without adequate PARP, cancer cells cannot complete DNA replication. When there's no PARP to repair the damage, an enzyme called Caspase-3 initiates programmed cell death.

Avemar has been shown to speed up the death of cancer cells by inhibiting the production of PARP and enhancing the production of Caspase-3.[3]

Researchers at UCLA also showed that Avemar reduces the production of RNA and DNA associated with the rapid reproduction of cancer cells. It also restores normal pathways of cell metabolism and increases the production of RNA and DNA associated with healthy cells.[4]

Undercover cancer cells exposed

Avemar also acts as a biological bounty hunter for disguised cancer cells. Healthy cells have a surface molecule called MHC-1 that tells natural killer (NK) cells not to attack. Virally infected cells don't display this molecule, which makes them targets.

But cancer cells have also been shown to display the surface molecule MHC-1, which means that cancer cells can actually hide from NK cells. Avemar helps the immune system identify cancer cells for attack by suppressing their ability to generate this MHC-1 mask, which allows the NK cells to recognize it as a target for attack.[5]

Children with cancer get a fighting chance

Possibly one of the most powerful studies on Avemar shows its effectiveness on children with cancer. Most forms of pediatric cancer have high cure rates from chemo-therapy as compared with adult cancers, but one of the limiting factors in using chemotherapy to treat children is the infection that can often occur during treatment.

Infection often sets in because chemotherapy kills large numbers of the child's infection-fighting white blood cells and destroys many of the bone marrow cells that produce them.

Doctors aware of the immune-enhancing properties of Avemar wanted to learn if it could possibly prevent the life-threatening infections that often occur in pediatric cancer patients.

A recent study published in the prestigious medical journal *Pediatric Hematology Oncology*, showed that such infections and the fever that accompanies them (called febrile neutropenia) were reduced by 42 percent in the children given Avemar after chemotherapy, compared to those not getting Avemar.[6]

Avemar has this effect because it helps rebuild the immune system, increasing the number and activity of functioning immune system cells. It's clear that, unlike conventional cancer therapy, Avemar does not produce side effects—it reduces them. It also allowed the children in the study to take more cycles of chemotherapy, increasing the chance of a cure.

As toxic as a slice of bread

As dangerous as Avemar is for cancer cells, it won't harm the rest of your body. In fact, according to an independent panel of medical, food safety, and toxicology experts: "Avemar is as safe as whole wheat bread."[8]

In Hungary, where it was developed and is manufactured, it is classified as a "dietary food for special medical purposes, for cancer patients" and is a standard therapy for patients with cancer. It is available as a food or dietary supplement in several other countries as well, including Austria, Australia, Switzerland, Italy, Slovakia, Czech Republic, Russia, Israel, and South Korea.

Avemar is made using a patented process that yields a uniform, consistent, all-natural dietary supplement. Although it is not certified organic, it is free of chemicals and synthetics. According to our contacts at The Harmony Company, the exclusive North American distributor of Avemar, there is simply no comparison between their product and other wheat germ products on the market because it is the only one supported by research demonstrating its effectiveness in maintaining normal, healthy cellular metabolism and immune regulation.[9]

But since this is a wheat product, there is the potential for allergic response. Although the process of making the product removes all gluten, the principal allergen in wheat, the product can still come in contact with gluten-containing wheat. The Harmony Company says that Avemar should not be consumed by people who have had an organ or tissue transplant, those who have malabsorption syndrome, or those with allergies to foods containing gluten, such as wheat, rye, oats, and barley.

It's also not recommended for people with fructose intolerance or hypersensitivity to gluten, wheat germ, or any of the components or ingredients of this product.

If you suffer from bleeding ulcers, you should stop using Avemar two days before undergoing a barium X-ray contrast examination and resume taking it two days after the completion of the examination. This precaution is necessary because wheat germ contains lectin, which can potentially cause red bloods cells to clump.

If you are currently taking medications or have any adverse health conditions, you should consult with your pharmacist or physician before taking Avemar.

Unique delivery system makes fighting cancer easier—and even tasty

The Avemar product our contacts at The Harmony Company offer is an instant drink mix called AvéULTRA, which combines Avemar with natural orange flavoring and fructose in pre-measured packets.

As a dietary supplement, the recommended usage is one packet per day mixed with 8 oz. of cold water (or any other beverage containing less than 10 mg of vitamin C). I found that the best way to mix it is to shake it in a closed container. When I tried it, it reminded me of Tang, though it wasn't quite as sweet.

You should consume it within 30 minutes of mixing a batch. Also note that it's a good idea to take AvéULTRA one hour before or after a meal and two hours before or after any drugs or other dietary supplements.

If you weigh over 200 pounds, use two packets per day. If you weigh under 100 pounds, only use half of a packet per day. Consult with a healthcare professional for recommended usage levels for children, for guidance on alternative usage levels, and for use in combination with other dietary supplements.

Most people who use AvéULTRA daily notice an effect within three weeks, reporting improvements in appetite, energy, and general quality of life.

If you work with your health care professional to use AvéULTRA as an adjunct cancer treatment, you should know that it will take a good three months before you will see a change in objective measurements—such as blood markers, CAT scans, MRIs, etc. Although some people reported uneasiness in their stomachs during the first few days of using Avemar, the effect only lasted a few days. No vomiting, diarrhea, or any other symptoms were reported.

Part III

Heart

CHAPTER ONE

Prevent heart attack and stroke with potent enzyme that dissolves deadly blood clots in hours

The ability of blood to coagulate can be a crucial part of survival in cases of severe injury. But when blood clots occur at the wrong times, in the wrong places within the body, they can have serious—even deadly—consequences. Unfortunately, your treatment options in these circumstances are limited, and treatment must be administered quickly. Which is why prevention and knowing all of your options now—before problems occur—is crucial.

Blood clots (or thrombi) form when strands of protein called fibrin accumulate in a blood vessel. In the heart, blood clots cause blockage of blood flow to muscle tissue. If blood flow is blocked, the oxygen supply to that tissue is cut off and it eventually dies. This can result in angina and heart attacks. Clots in chambers of the heart can mobilize to the brain. In the brain, blood clots also block blood and oxygen from reaching necessary areas, which results in senility and/or stroke.

In Japan, the levels of disease and fatalities caused by blood clots are alarming. Researchers estimate that blood clots that diminish blood flow to the brain are responsible for 60 percent of all senility cases in that country.[1] Consequently, Dr. Hiroyuki Sumi—a Japanese researcher doing work at the University of Chicago's medical school— began searching for a substance that could dissolve and even prevent blood clots.

His team of researchers tested roughly 173 foods, including several types of liquor, before examining a traditional Japanese food called natto, made from boiled and fermented soybeans. The Japanese have consumed natto for centuries under the belief that it fosters cardiovascular health.

In Dr. Sumi's lab that folk remedy turned into a clinically scrutinized piece of modern medicine. He isolated an enzyme inside natto, called nattokinase, and showed that it can prevent and dissolve blood clots and may be able to safeguard people from hardened arteries, heart attack, stroke, angina, and senility.

Natto may help where modern medicine— and the human body—fall short

While the human body contains several enzymes that promote the creation of blood clots, it produces only one enzyme, plasmin, that dissolves clots, and production of that enzyme diminishes as we age.

Modern medicine includes several thrombolytic or clot-busting drugs. The leading variety is t-PA (tissue plasminogen activators), such as activase, urokinase, and streptokinase. Each year, hospitals give these drugs to more than a million stroke and heart attack patients. The treatment saves between 300,000 and 500,000 lives annually. But it's not a perfect cure. TPAs are expensive (a dose of urokinase costs approximately US$1,500) so many patients don't receive the treatment. And the drugs' impact can be short-lived. Urokinase, for example, begins to lose effectiveness within four to 20 minutes after administration.

But when Dr. Sumi's researchers dropped natto onto an artificial thrombus (a blood clot) in a petri dish and allowed it to stand at body temperature, the blood clot gradually dissolved and disappeared completely within 18 hours. Dr. Sumi commented that nattokinase—the active enzyme in natto—showed "a potency matched by no other enzyme."[2]

The HSI network has played a key role in making this information available in North America. Through their relationship as panelists, Dr. Martin Milner of the Center for Natural Medicine in Portland, Oregon, and Dr. Kouhei Makise of the Imadeqawa Makise Clinic in Kyoto, Japan, were able to launch a joint research project on nattokinase and write an extensive paper on their findings. "In all my years of research as a professor of cardiovascular and pulmonary medicine, natto and nattokinase represents the most exciting new development in the prevention and treatment of cardiovascular related diseases," Dr. Milner said. "We have finally found a potent natural agent that can thin and dissolve clots effectively, with relative safety and without side effects."

Blood clots dissolve almost 50 percent faster with nattokinase—in as little as two hours

Nattokinase has been the subject of 17 studies, including two small human trials.

Dr. Sumi and his colleagues induced blood clots in male dogs, then orally administered either four capsules of nattokinase (250 mg/capsule) or four placebo capsules to each dog. Angiograms (X-rays of blood vessels) revealed that the dogs who received nattokinase regained normal blood circulation (free of the clot) within five hours of treatment. Blood clots in the dogs who received only placebos showed no sign of dissolving in the 18 hours following treatment.

Researchers from Biotechnology Research Laboratories and JCR Pharmaceuticals Co. of Kobe, Japan, tested nattokinase's ability to dissolve a thrombus in the carotid arteries of rats. Animals treated with nattokinase regained 62 percent of blood flow, whereas those treated with plasmin regained just 15.8 percent of blood flow.[3]

Researchers from three organizations—JCR Pharmaceuticals, Oklahoma State University, and Miyazaki Medical College—tested nattoki-nase on 12 healthy Japanese volunteers (six men and six women, be-tween the ages of 21 and 55). They gave the volunteers 200 g of natto daily (before breakfast), then tracked fibrinolytic activity in the volun-teers through a series of blood plasma tests. The tests indicated that the natto generated a heightened ability to dissolve blood clots: On average, the volunteers' ELT (a measure of how long it takes to dissolve a blood clot) dropped by 48 percent within two hours of treatment, and volun-teers retained an enhanced ability to dissolve blood clots for two to eight hours. As a control, researchers later fed the same amount of boiled soy-beans to the same volunteers and tracked their fibrinolytic activity. The tests showed no significant change.[4]

Enhance your body's ability to fight clots without IV treatment

According to Dr. Milner, what makes nattokinase a particularly potent treatment is that it bolsters the body's natural abilities to fight

Studies suggest natto may prevent osteoporosis

Some researchers suggest that natto might help prevent the on-set of osteoporosis.

Chemical analyses of natto have revealed the fermentation pro-cess generates substantial quantities of vitamin K2. Natto actually ranks as one of the richest sources of the vitamin. Animal studies have concluded that a diet rich in vitamin K2 can prevent bone loss.[5] Japanese research has shown that people with osteoporosis have lower K2 levels than people who don't have the disease.

To get the benefit of vitamin K, however, you have to eat the food version of natto. Nattokinase supplements do not contain the vita-min. If you decide to try adding natto to your diet, talk to your doctor first. Vitamin K can interfere with the normal functioning of certain medications, especially blood thinners such as Coumadin.

blood clots in several different ways. It closely resembles plasmin and dissolves fibrin directly. In addition, it also enhances the body's production of both plasmin and other natural clot-dissolving agents, including urokinase.

In some ways, he says, nattokinase is actually superior to conventional clot-dissolving drugs. T-PAs like urokinase are only effective when taken intravenously and often fail simply because a stroke or heart attack victim's arteries have hardened beyond the point where they can be treated by any clot-dissolving agent. Nattokinase, however, can help prevent that hardening with an oral dose of as little as 100 mg a day.

Reduce blood pressure by 10 percent

Many Japanese have long believed that regular consumption of natto tends to lower blood pressure. Over the past several years, this belief has been substantiated by several clinical trials: In 1995, researchers reported that they had confirmed the presence of angiotensin converting enzyme (ACE) inhibitors in natto.[6] ACE causes blood vessels to narrow and blood pressure to rise. Consequently, substances that inhibit the production of ACE help lower blood pressure.

Researchers from two Japanese institutions—the Miyazaki Medical College and the Kurashiki University of Science and Arts—launched studies to test natto's impact on blood pressure in both rats and humans. They administered a single dose of natto extract (the equivalent of 25 mg of natto) into the peritoneal cavity of six male rats. On average, the rats' systolic blood pressure fell by 12.7 percent within two hours.[7]

The researchers then tested natto extract on humans. Five volunteers with high blood pressure each received the extract daily (an oral dose equivalent to 200 g of natto) for four consecutive days. In four of the five volunteers, both systolic and diastolic blood pressure dropped. On average, systolic blood pressure fell by 10.9 percent and diastolic fell 9.7 percent.

Supplement brings Japanese discover to America

Since natto is traditionally a Japanese food, and one that is referred to even there as "an acquired taste," it isn't readily available in the United States. However, Nutricology, one of the first American companies to investigate natto, arranged to bring a nattokinase supplement, called NattoZyme, to the U.S. market. The supplement is available through Nutricology and its Allergy Research Group, and through Dr. Martin Milner's Center for Natural Medicine. Contact information is listed in the Member Source Directory on page 529.

CHAPTER TWO

Reverse Metabolic Syndrome—high blood sugar, high cholesterol, high triglycerides—with this rare Italian fruit

Imagine throwing out your potentially dangerous (but also effective) medications—your statin, your blood sugar medicine—and replacing them with a single, effective, side-effect-free remedy. One that helps keep your numbers in normal range, and causes no negative side effects.

That dream is a reality—as finally there's a single comprehensive solution for many symptoms of Metabolic Syndrome.

This bitter fruit can make your life much sweeter—without increasing your blood sugar

In a tiny region on the southern coast of Calabria, Italy, a unique super citrus fruit grows. This small area boasts 80 percent of the world's bergamot production—and its polyphenolic extract is exclusively used to make a remarkable antidote to Metabolic Syndrome.

Bergamot is different than any citrus fruit you've ever seen. It's yellow like a lemon, but the size of an orange. It's less sour than a lemon, but much more bitter than grapefruit. And while you wouldn't really want to snack on bergamot, you will want to make it part of your daily diet.

What makes this bitter fruit so remarkable? In just thirty days, you could see results of up to

- a 37 percent plunge in your LDL cholesterol
- a 49 percent decrease in your triglycerides, and
- a 22 percent drop in your blood sugar levels

All that from a single, safe solution… instead of a handful of potentially dangerous drugs.

Hard-to-control symptoms need a nudge from nature

Sometimes, your body needs a little help to get things right. Unfortunately, the mainstream approach often uses a battering ram where a gentle nudge would do the trick—and bergamot fruit can provide just the right nudge.

For one thing, this citrus fruit helps your body by naturally blocking one of the enzymes (HMG-CoA reductase) needed for cholesterol production. Now, your body needs cholesterol—that's why your liver makes it—but sometimes production can get a little out of control. The powerful flavonoid compounds in bergamot help keep that in check by inhibiting that enzyme (which, by the way gets more active when blood sugar levels are high).

Those flavonoids also impact high blood sugar levels in a very positive way. By acting directly on glucose transporter proteins and glucose-regulating enzymes, these compounds can help rein in high blood sugar—as well as improving insulin sensitivity, a key factor in healthy glucose levels.

In addition, these plentiful flavonoids have well-documented antioxidant properties that contribute to your overall good health.

Bergamot is chock full of powerful, natural healing compounds

Like virtually everything produced by Mother Nature, bergamot fruit contains a wide range of healthy compounds, the most potent of which include:

- Naringin
- Rutin
- Narirutin
- Hesperidin
- Neoeriocitrin
- Eriocitrin
- Neoesperidin

Some of these have been the subject of extensive study (naringin, in particular), while others quietly do their jobs without attracting a lot of research attention. And when you put them all together—as nature did in bergamot fruit—they combine to substantially affect your cholesterol, triglycerides and blood sugar.

The bitter pill turns out to be a better pill

Bergamot gets its distinct bitterness from a super powerful bioflavonoid called naringin. This natural compound has been put to the test against high cholesterol, diabetes, and high triglycerides… and come out victorious in multiple studies.

First, let's look at cholesterol. One study[1] found that naringin on its own was able to lower LDL cholesterol by 17 percent and total cholesterol by 14 percent in patients struggling with high cholesterol.

Next, high blood sugar, another defining symptom of Metabolic Syndrome—one that can lead to full-blown diabetes, and its many dangerous complications. And researchers discovered that naringin (along with hesperidin) can have a significant impact on blood sugar levels. One animal study[2] showed that supplementing with this flavonoid substantially lowered blood glucose in mice modeled with type 2 diabetes.

And then there's the way naringin knocks down high triglyceride levels, which is critical to optimal cardiovascular health. Two animal studies[3,4] found that adding naringin into the diets of rats effectively lowered their serum cholesterol levels.

Bergamot extract knocks down cholesterol, triglycerides, and blood sugar in staggering numbers

When it comes to fighting Metabolic Syndrome, bergamot extract may be your best bet. Because while a single one of its main compounds (naringin), its combination of powerful flavonoids really takes the symptoms to task.

In one stunning clinical trial[5], researchers uncovered the true power of bergamot polyphenolic extract (BPF). This 30-day placebo-

---

Metabolic Syndrome Can Kill You

While there's no one established definition of Metabolic Syndrome (aka Syndrome X), the basic core symptoms include some of the worst risk factors for premature death:

- Elevated blood pressure (130/85 or higher)

- Low HDL cholesterol level (Less than 50 in women, less than 40 in men)

- Elevated Triglyceride level

- Elevated C-reactive protein level

- Fasting glucose level that indicates insulin resistance/ glucose intolerance

- Excessive abdominal fat

This constellation of symptoms can lead to full-fledged diabetes, and a whole host of serious cardiovascular problems—significantly increasing the risk of death.

controlled interventional study included 238 patients, all of whom had high cholesterol, and some of whom also had high blood sugar.

At the end of 30 days, most of the patients in the BPF group had substantially lower total cholesterol—up to 38 percent lower! And their LDL cholesterol plunge was just as impressive, with an average 37 percent drop.

And, according to the researchers, the most impressive changes were seen in a subgroup of patients identified as having Metabolic Syndrome. Those patients saw a huge dip in their triglyceride levels— up to a 49 percent drop—and an average 22 percent drop in blood sugar levels. In just one month!

Citrus Bergamot

While you might not want to suffer through eating the extremely acrid bergamot fruit—even to get results like that—you can get its benefits without taking a single bitter bite. Bergamot polyphenolic extract comes in one unique supplement called Citrus Bergamot (formerly Bergamonte).

The manufacturer recommends a therapeutic dose of two to four Citrus Bergamot capsules daily, before dinner, on an empty stomach for the first thirty days. After that, they recommend a maintenance dose of one capsule daily (still before dinner, on an empty stomach).

You can find ordering information for Citrus Bergamot in the Member Source Directory on page 529.

CHAPTER THREE

Sugar cane extract rivals popular cholesterol-lowering drugs, without the dangerous side effects

Amid reports of health problems and deaths caused by statin drugs, we've learned that an extract of a commercial crop—sugar cane—can lower cholesterol just as effectively.

As we've told our readers over the past couple of years, cholesterol isn't the primary cause of heart disease… homocysteine levels are. Nevertheless, cholesterol *does* play an important role in coronary health, and any good program for reversing heart disease must address that as well. So you can imagine how excited we were when our researchers discovered that a sugar cane extract could *dramatically* reduce cholesterol levels.

While it's drawn from the same plant that produces table sugar, policosanol doesn't affect blood sugar levels when ingested. Cuban scientists, however, have discovered that it can have a cholesterol-reducing effect[1] without creating the uncomfortable and even dangerous side effects associated with statin drugs.[2,3] Statin drugs lower elevated cholesterol by limiting cholesterol production in the liver, but they also have side effects ranging from heartburn to potentially fatal cases of muscle breakdown. This widely prescribed class of drugs—statin sales topped $14 billion last year—includes the brand names Lipitor, Lescol, Zocor, Mevacor, Pravachol, Prevastatin, and Baycol (which was recalled after being linked to over 40 deaths).

In several studies that compared both cholesterol-lowering methods, policosanol surpassed the performance of statin-drug therapy. One Cuban study compared the effects of policosanol to Pravastatin on patients who had elevated cholesterol levels and were considered to be at high risk for coronary disease. Patients took 10 mg of either policosanol or Pravastatin with their dinners for eight weeks. The group taking statins saw their LDL levels fall by 15.6 percent and their total cholesterol by 11.8 percent. But those in the policosanol group exceeded those numbers, and dropped their LDL levels by 19.3 percent and their total cholesterol by 13.9 percent. **The HDL levels of the statin test subjects remained the same, while the policosonal group increased their HDL by 15.7 percent.** Because HDL cholesterol aids in the removal of fat from arterial walls, an increase in these levels is beneficial.

Thousands of people struggle with cholesterol problems, and the chance of developing high cholesterol increases as we age. As we grow older, our hormone levels drop, making it easier for cholesterol levels to rise in our bodies. Researchers believe policosanol may be a safe method of reducing and regulating LDL. In a clinical trial involving 244 post-menopausal women with high cholesterol, researchers first attempted to bring down elevated lipid levels through six weeks of a standard lipid-lowering diet. When this proved unsuccessful, they gave the women 5 mg of policosanol daily for 12 weeks, then 10 mg daily for another 12 weeks. Researchers found that the supplement was effective in significantly lowering LDL levels (25.2 percent) and total cholesterol (16.7 percent). In addition, the women experienced a 29.3 percent increase in HDL levels.[4]

Extract relieves painful leg cramps

One of the common—and debilitating—side effects of high cholesterol is a syndrome known as intermittent claudication—a cramping pain in the calves. This is often linked to poor circulation and the presence of arterial fat deposits (atherosclerosis). Intermittent claudication occurs only during certain times, such as after walking. Removal of arterial fat deposits has been found to decrease claudication.

Researchers at the Medical Surgical Research Center in Havana, Cuba tested policosanol patients who suffered from moderately severe intermittent claudication. In this two-year long study, 56 patients were randomly assigned to receive either policosanol or a placebo.

Researchers determined if the policosanol was relieving the claudication by conducting treadmill walking tests on each subject before the study and again on 6, 12, 18, and 24 months after beginning treatment. Although both test groups showed some progress during the interim tests, the final results indicated that policosanol had a significant benefit for sufferers of intermittent claudication. After two years of treatment, patients in the placebo group were able to walk a maximum of 0.15 miles while the group taking policosanol could walk 0.40 miles before having to stop. **The 21 people taking policosanol increased their walking distance by at least 50 percent.** Only five members of the placebo group showed a similar improvement.[5]

And it's possible that policosanol could do more than alleviate the risk of heart disease, circulatory problems, and other ailments commonly associated with high cholesterol…

A possible defense against Alzheimer's

Dora M. Kovacs, Ph.D., a researcher at Massachusetts General Hospital, recently received a $200,000 research grant to study the side effects of cholesterol on the development of Alzheimer's Disease (AD). She found that even normal levels of cholesterol may increase the risk of senility-causing plaques and neurofibrillary tangles in the brain, which are associated with the development and progress of AD.[6]

Dr. Kovacs' research is focusing on the development of drugs that inhibit the production of ACAT, an enzyme that enables cholesterol and other lipids (fats) to enter cells and form solid lipid droplets there. Those droplets can hinder the normal functioning of the cell. They can also increase amyloid beta production, which is associated with the progress of mind-robbing plaques and tangles. When lipid droplet levels increase, amyloid beta production increases... and so does the risk of Alzheimer's. Dr. Kovacs and her research team believe that ACAT-inhibiting drugs are the keys to halting the process of cholesterol and lipid buildup that results in AD. But the related research is in its early stages. Dr. Kovacs plans, but has not yet started, to test ACAT inhibitors on mice specially bred to have AD. Other researchers have developed a potentially safe class of ACAT inhibitors to treat atherosclerosis. But it may be another five to 10 years before this family of drugs is thoroughly developed, tested, and made available to the public.

There may be an alternative therapy available right now, however. In an interview with Emma Hitt, Ph.D. for the Reuters news service, Dr. Kovacs indicated that several studies have shown that patients who take statin drugs have lower rates of AD and other types of dementia. Cholesterol-lowering statins do not appear to hinder the ACAT enzyme, but the act of maintaining low cholesterol levels lowers the risk of dementia. Since statin drugs can induce serious side effects, policosanol may prove to be a better alternative. In double-blind trials, policosanol produced mild, short-term side effects—such as insomnia, headache, diarrhea, nervousness, and weight loss—in less than 1 percent of test subjects. So policosanol may prove to be an efficacious mind-saver as well as a life-saver.

Caution: Researchers warn that policosanol can interact with blood-thinning drugs. So if you try policosanol (after consulting your doctor), your dose of blood-thinning medication may have to be adjusted with careful medical monitoring. If you would like to purchase policosanol, see your Member Source Directory on page 529. If you're already taking cholesterol-lowering drugs or being treated for any other health condition, you should consult with your doctor before trying policosanol or discontinuing any prescription drug.

CHAPTER FOUR

The amazingly simple way to slash your stroke risk in half

W e've just uncovered a way to slash your risk of getting a stroke by 55 percent. And you can do it without dangerous drugs. This might even be the secret to getting off those blood pressure meds—or not having to start on them in the first place.

Because what researchers have discovered about this common food component and its unique powers is nothing short of miraculous. Especially what it can do for your heart and blood vessels.

And best of all, it's probably in your refrigerator right now—hiding in one of your favorite condiments! Remember all those jokes anti-Reagan liberals made back in the '80s about ketchup being called a vegetable?

Well, it looks like the joke is on them. Because ketchup, it turns out, contains an amazing compound. One so potent you could even call it a "super vegetable!" It's called lycopene. You've probably heard of lycopene for prostate health.

But that's just the beginning. Researchers from the University of Cambridge recently found that the lycopene in tomatoes is so potent that it can significantly improve functioning of the vascular system in people who already have heart disease.

These were people on regular doses of drugs, including statins, but whose blood vessels still weren't working normally. And that's very dangerous. Because blood vessel constriction is a major factor in strokes…and heart attacks.

The English researchers discovered that just 7 mg of lycopene could widen the blood vessels of those in the study with heart disease. And not by an insignificant amount either, but by a whopping 53 percent!

And here's the amazing part. It's what separates the real foods and compounds Mother Nature gave us from risky drugs created in a laboratory. The lycopene didn't widen the blood vessels of the healthy people in the study. So it seems to work only when the body needs it!

And that brings me back to ketchup. The lycopene in tomatoes becomes even more potent, and easier for your body to use, when it's pureed, like tomatoes are to make ketchup! In fact, just a tablespoon of this super condiment will give you almost 3 mg of lycopene. That's close to half the dose the researchers used in their study.

Just incorporating some tomato products into your daily diet might be all it takes not to have your doctor constantly nag you about taking Lipitor or other dangerous meds. As for high blood pressure medications—well, you can throw a tomato at them as well.

In Israel, researchers found that those who took a daily tomato extract dose were able to drop their top blood pressure number—the systolic one—by 10 points, and lower the bottom diastolic number by 4 points.

But for the icing on the lycopene cake, another published study has shown that men who had the highest levels of lycopene in their blood had a 55 percent lower risk of getting a stroke compared to those who had low levels. And these were men in their mid to late 60s, not twenty-somethings!

So the next time ketchup is on your shopping list, here's a good reason to try an organic brand. Organic ketchup has been found to have 57 percent more lycopene than non-organic varieties. And that's a heart-saving "vegetable" everyone can agree on.

CHAPTER FIVE

The link between homocysteine and heart disease

The truth is that cholesterol is NOT the deadly threat you may think it is. Aside from the fact that it's necessary for everything from the production of sex hormones to bile synthesis... it does *not* clog your arteries unless it has something to attach to: a tear, a rough surface, a ridge, a sharp turn.

When the homocysteine levels in your blood become too high, the perfect conditions are created for plaque buildup. An amino acid, homocysteine, promotes the growing of smooth muscle cells just below the inner wall of the artery. Multiplying rapidly, these cells create a deadly bulge that protrudes into the artery itself. On this bulge, cholesterol, blood products, and calcium begin to accumulate. These are the blood traps that lead to problems like impotence, poor memory, heart attacks, strokes, and even death. And research indicates that you should be just as concerned—if not more so—over your homocysteine level as you are over your cholesterol level.

Destroys arterial walls

A team of Seattle researchers showed that injections of homocysteine rapidly caused early signs of arteriosclerosis in baboons. The researchers reported that in their test, the cells just beneath the animals' artery walls were mutating and reproducing at a wild rate, and this growth was destroying the arterial walls.

After just one week of high levels of homocysteine in the baboons' blood, 23 percent of their artery walls were lost. The researchers found that the higher the level of homocysteine and the more severely injured the inner artery wall, the more severe the signs of arteriosclerosis.[1]

Homocysteine can kill—if you don't know how to control it

Your body forms homocysteine when you eat food containing an amino acid called methionine, which is present in all animal and vegetable protein. As part of the digestive process, methionine is broken down into homocysteine. As long as certain helper nutrients are present, homocysteine subsequently converts back into one of two harmless amino acids. However, when these helper nutrients aren't present, homocysteine levels become dangerously high.

Research shows that vitamin B6 is one of the key helper nutrients necessary for normalizing homocysteine levels. In a study at the University of Wisconsin, participants given daily supplements of B6 (2mg/day) experienced dramatic drops in their homocysteine levels. And at the Titus County Memorial Hospital in Mount Pleasant, Texas, patients given vitamin B6 were able to reduce their risk of chest pain and heart attack by 73 percent.[2] More importantly, they lived an average of eight years longer than those who didn't take the supplements!

Unfortunately, the typical American diet is low in vitamin B6 and high in methionine. And because of food processing, it's almost impossible to get enough B6 in the North American diet.

Recent research has uncovered similar links among homocysteine, folic acid, and B12 and has found that you need all three nutrients to keep homocysteine levels down.[3]

Here's what you need to do TODAY!

You can't ensure healthy, effective levels of B6, B12, and folic acid through diet alone. Americans are so deficient in these nutrients that even the Food and Drug Administration (FDA) and the Centers for Disease Control in Atlanta (CDC) have launched campaigns to increase your intake through supplementation.

Unfortunately, we've discovered that most multivitamin formulas fall short. They simply don't have enough B6, B12, or folic acid to be effective in reducing homocysteine levels.

There are a number of specialized formulas now available that specifically address the homocysteine threat. Check your local health-food store, or, you can try a high-quality supplement called Homocysteine Formula that is based on the latest homocysteine research. Each tablet provides 800 mcg of folic acid, 2,000 mcg of B12, and 100 mg of B6. In addition, the formula includes beneficial components that aid in the metabolism of these crucial heart protective nutrients. For information on ordering Homocysteine Formula, refer to the Member Source Directory at the end of this book.

CHAPTER SIX

The single-ingredient formula rivaling a major class of blood pressure drugs

In many cases, you can control your blood pressure with some simple diet and lifestyle changes. But unfortunately sometimes drugs are necessary. Necessary because some cases of dangerously high blood pressure stay that way no matter what you do to try to lower them. And unfortunately because the only drugs that seem to work come with a nasty list of side effects. So we always keep an eye out for natural hypertension alternatives for those of you who need that helping hand. The latest one to cross our desks is called Vasotensin, a product formulated from a single ingredient that appears to rival one of the leading classes of hypertension drugs—but without the potential risks.

Japanese fish alleviates hypertension

Vasotensin is made from a substance called bonito peptides. That's it—one ingredient. But the manufacturer, Metagenics, claims that bonito peptides have been shown to have such significant effectiveness as a single ingredient that there's no need to add any others. So what exactly are bonito peptides? Well, in general, peptides are short chains of amino acids. Specifically, bonito peptides are amino acid chains isolated and extracted from the bonito fish, which is a member of the tuna and mackerel family.

Bonito peptides have been shown to inhibit Angiotensin Converting Enzyme (ACE) activity. ACE spurs the formation of angiotensin II—a potent compound responsible for blood vessel constriction. ACE also has a negative effect on a substance called Kinin, which lowers blood pressure by relaxing blood vessels. So, in other words, bonito peptides seem to slow down the process responsible for high blood pressure.[1]

Now, it must be some powerful stuff—but I wondered just how it was discovered. It turns out that it was a case of one man's (well, in this case, one industry's) trash being another's treasure.

Fish food finds its way to the research lab

The type of bonito peptides used in Vasotensin is actually a by-product of the Katsuobushi manufacturing process.

Katsuobushi is a traditional Japanese seasoning that has been used in soups and other dishes for over 1,500 years, and it's made from the flesh of the bonito fish. To get a better understanding of how the Katsuobushi industry is connected to Vasotensin, it helps to know a bit about how Katsuobushi is processed. The *Reader's Digest* version goes something like this: the fish meat is heat-treated in water and stirred. The result is the seasoning and the remaining residue. Yet it is from this residue that (typically discarded or used as organic fertilizer) we get this promising compound because one creative (and curious) researcher, Dr. Masaaki Yoshikawa of Kyoto University, decided to take another look at its potential. He discovered that this part of the bonito fish's muscle has strong ACE-inhibiting properties. Apparently, through careful purification and separation, nine active bonito peptides have been identified and sequenced.

But you can't get the anti-hypertensive response by simply eating the bonito fish itself or by eating Katsuobushi.

As Dr. Yoshikawa's research uncovered, there are actually nine specific active peptides that contribute to bonitos' ACE-inhibiting effects. The research I read focused on two of them, one called LKPNM and one called LKP. On its own, LKPNM only slightly inhibits ACE. But when ACE interacts with LKPNM, it gets converted into the peptide LKP, ACE-inhibitory activity of LKP is eight times higher than LKPNM. This unique property gives it a longer sustainable effect; accidentally skipping a dose would not produce a quick spike of blood pressure.

But in order to be "activated," these peptides are dependent on specific enzymatic reactions. The problem is, our bodies don't produce the right enzymes to separate the active parts from the rest of the fish, so the only way to get those blood pressure lowering benefits from the bonito peptides is to have them separated from the fish for you. In other words, you need to take a supplement like Vasotensin to get the ACE-inhibiting effect.

Limited—but promising—results

In a human study out of Japan, researchers tested the anti-hypertensive effects of bonito peptides against a placebo in 61 borderline and mildly hypertensive subjects for 10 weeks. For the first half of the trial, 31 subjects (group 1) took 1.5 grams per day of a bonito peptide mixture. The other 30 subjects (group 2) received a placebo. In the second five-week period, the order was reversed: group 1 subjects took the placebo and group 2 subjects received the bonito peptide mixture. During both phases, the placebo group failed to show any significant decrease in blood pressure. And researchers reported that the anti-hypertensive activity was demonstrated without any side effects.[2]

I also managed to get my hands on a study that showed how bonito peptides stack up to mainstream hypertension drugs. In this study, researchers examined the anti-hypertensive activity of LKP, LKPNM, and Captopril (a common prescription ACE-inhibitor) in rats. The group fed LKP showed an immediate response, but the blood pressure started to go back up after two hours. But in the group fed LKPNM, the anti-hypertensive effect was almost the same as Captopril. And the effects lasted over six hours.[3]

The bottom line on Vasotensin is it has potential. Even though the majority of testing seems to have been done by the manufacturing lab in small, short-term studies, all results were positive and showed no bad reactions. Of course, you should keep in mind that it is an ACE-inhibitor, and with these types of products there is always a possibility of potassium buildup and kidney problems. So you still need to work closely with your doctor to regularly monitor your potassium and blood pressure levels, as well as your kidney function.

The dosage recommendation is two tablets twice daily with meals. See the Member Source Directory at the end of this book for ordering information.

CHAPTER SEVEN

The silkworm's secret: Ease inflammation and respiratory illness with this enzyme

At some point or another, you've probably seen a nature film showing a caterpillar turn into a butterfly: It weaves a cocoon around itself, and eventually it breaks through the hardened chrysalis, having sprouted wings and changed form almost completely. In the case of the silkworm, there is a specific enzyme called serrapeptase that helps break down the cocoon, letting the newly-transformed moth emerge.

Serrapeptase works by dissolving non-living tissue. This ability captivated researchers around the world, who have subsequently studied its effects in the human body. Some of the claims made about serrapeptase (also known as serratia peptidase) may be stretching it just a tad—we've heard reports that it helps with rheumatoid arthritis, ulcerative colitis, psoriasis, uveitis (eye inflammation), allergies, and may even help fight some forms of cancer. While some of those claims make sense logically, we haven't found enough clinical evidence just yet to tell if they're valid.

But many studies do verify serrapeptase's ability to perform two key functions: it dissolves dead tissue and reduces inflammation. And those functions can ease numerous medical conditions. In human trials overseas, people using serrapeptase have found relief from inflammation, carpal tunnel syndrome, bronchitis, sinusitis, and other ear, nose, and throat ailments. According to one alternative medicine practitioner in Germany, it may even dissolve arterial plaque.

Surgical patients treated with serrapeptase experience rapid reduction of swelling

In Europe and Japan, clinical studies have shown that serrapeptase induces anti-inflammatory activity, anti-edemic activity (the lessening of fluid retention), and fibrinolytic activity (the dissolution of protein buildups).[1] Consequently, physicians and patients in Japan, Germany, and elsewhere around Europe have begun taking serrapeptase to ease inflammation.

In a multi-center study involving 174 patients, Japanese researchers tested serrapeptase's ability to ease post-operative swelling. One day prior to surgery, 88 of the patients received three oral doses of 10 mg of serrapeptase. The evening following surgery, they received one dose. Then for the next five days, they received three doses per day. The other 86 patients received placebos. The researchers reported that "the degree of swelling in the serrapeptase-treated patients was significantly less than the placebo-treated patients at every point of observation after the operation up to the fifth day." None of the patients reported any adverse side effects.[2]

Ease respiratory disease in three to four days

Researchers in Italy tested the impact of oral serrapeptase on 193 people aged 12 to 77 who were suffering from acute or chronic disorders of the ear, nose, or throat. In a multi-center, double-blind, placebo-controlled study, subjects took 30 mg of serrapeptase a day for seven to eight days. "After three to four days' treatment, significant symptom regression was observed in peptidase-treated patients," the researchers reported. In particular, the treatment eased pain, fever, nasal obstruction, difficulty in swallowing, and anosmia (reduced sense of smell).[3]

Serrapeptase knocks out carpal tunnel and varicose veins 65 percent of the time

Not surprisingly, researchers have also tested serrapeptase's ability to ease other disorders involving inflammation, fluid-retention, and buildup of fibrous tissue. Carpal tunnel syndrome and varicose veins may seem as unrelated as two conditions could get. But as different as they are, symptoms of both have been dramatically reduced using serrapeptase.

The painful symptoms of carpal tunnel syndrome are caused primarily by inflammation. At the SMS Medical College in Jaipur, India, researchers tested serrapeptase on 20 patients with carpal tunnel. After assessing the subjects' conditions, they instructed the patients to take 10 mg of serrapeptase twice a day for six weeks, then return for reassessment. Sixty-five percent of the patients showed significant improvements. No one reported any adverse side effects.[4]

Fluid retention in and around the veins of the legs causes varicose veins. Researchers in Federico, Italy tested serrapeptase on another 20 people with this condition. The patients took two serrapeptase tablets three times a day (for a total daily dosage of 30 mg) for 14 days. The supplement generated good to excellent improvement also in 65 percent of the subjects. It reduced pain in 63.3 percent of cases, fluid buildup in 56.2 percent, abnormal skin redness in 58.3 percent, and nighttime cramps in 52.9 percent.[5]

Few participants in clinical trials have reported suffering from any side effects from serrapeptase. In the varicose vein study, one patient experienced diarrhea, which was alleviated by temporarily decreasing the daily dosage. In other trials, there have been at least two reported cases of serrapeptase-induced pneumonia. However, patients in both cases fully recovered. Serrapeptase is a blood-thinning agent. Consequently, it may impact anticoagulant therapy and other medications. To avoid any potential complications, consult your doctor before taking serrapeptase. Serrapeptase is available from a number of Internet sources, including the Green Willow Tree. Ordering information is listed in the Member Source Directory on page 529.

CHAPTER EIGHT

Ayurvedic herb fights angina, heart disease, atherosclerosis, and more

Once in a blue moon, HSI uncovers a supplement that does so many things, it's hard even for us to believe it's real. Such is the case with arjuna. The Terminalia arjuna tree is found throughout India, and its bark has been pulverized and used for heart conditions for over 2,700 years. Researchers are now investigating other diseases that may benefit from this Indian herb, but it's already a well-proven cardiovascular "cure."

If you're under a doctor's care or taking prescription drugs for any cardiovascular condition, you should consult with a practitioner before supplementing with arjuna. Because the herb is so potent and effective, the combination of arjuna and drugs may cause too sudden or too severe an effect.

Lower LDL cholesterol by at least 25 percent

Although vitamin E has been shown time and again to be an effective supplement for controlling cholesterol levels, the antioxidant capacity of arjuna outperformed the vitamin in a recent randomized placebo-controlled trial in India. After only 30 days of supplementation with arjuna, the test group decreased its average LDL ("bad") cholesterol levels by 25.6 percent with a corresponding 12.7 percent drop in total cholesterol. The groups receiving either the placebo or 400 IU of vitamin E had no significant change in either measurement.[1]

At SMS Medical College in India, scientists gave 500 mg of arjuna per day to a group of rabbits suffering from high blood-fat levels. After 60 days of therapy with the herb, the rabbits' average total cholesterol dropped from 574 to 217 and their LDL levels dropped from 493 to 162.[2] A group of rabbits receiving only 100 mg of arjuna also experienced lower cholesterol levels, although the drop in cholesterol levels was not as significant.[3]

Reduce angina attacks without the side effects of drugs

More than 6.2 million Americans suffer from angina (chest pain) due to an insufficient supply of blood to the heart. While nitroglycerin is a drug often prescribed for this condition, its effectiveness is reduced with each use. Arjuna, however, can continue to relieve angina regardless of how long it's used.

Researchers at Kasturba Medical College in Mangalore, India, tested arjuna against ISMN (Isosorbide Mononitrate), a nitroglycerin-based drug commonly prescribed for stable angina. While ISMN was effective over a 12-week period, it didn't perform as well as arjuna. The arjuna group had a 30 percent reduction of angina attacks, while the group taking ISMN had a 27 percent reduction. While this is not a significant difference, the performance of arjuna is considerable when you take into account the possible side effects of ISMN—lightheadedness, dizziness, a rapid pulse rate, and blurred vision. Scientists found none of these side effects with the group taking the herb.[4] And, of course, arjuna can be used without fear that it'll stop working when you need it most.

Another study found that 15 stable angina sufferers taking arjuna

for three months experienced a 50 percent reduction in angina episodes. A treadmill test administered before and after the subjects took
the herb showed that angina symptoms were significantly delayed after
supplementation. Subjects also reduced their systolic blood-pressure
levels, had a marked decrease in their body-mass indexes —which
indicates weight loss—and experienced an increase in HDL ("good")
cholesterol levels. The researchers concluded that treating stable angina patients with arjuna was an effective way to relieve symptoms.[5]

Patients with congestive heart failure improve in just two weeks

The New York Heart Association has developed a classification system that helps doctors determine the appropriate treatment depending on the severity of a patient's condition. Classes I and II are mild,
class III is moderate, and class IV is severe and sufferers are completely
incapacitated. In a recent double-blind, crossover, placebo-controlled
study, 12 class IV patients with refractory chronic congestive heart
failure received arjuna for two weeks in addition to traditional medication. The placebo term of the trial included only traditional medication. During the short treatment with the herb, the patients were
reclassified as class III patients due to improvements in a number of
cardiac factors. The results were so impressive that during a later third
phase of the study, the same patients continued supplementing with
arjuna for 20 to 28 months in addition to conventional medications.
Their conditions continued to improve, and they were able to tolerate
additional physical effort.[6]

Protect yourself from ischemic heart disease

If heart disease runs in your family and you'd like to take preventive measures, arjuna may do the trick. Scientists gave laboratory rats
a supplement containing the herb for 60 days, and after that time gave
them isoproterenol, a synthetic chemical that causes an irreversible
destruction of heart tissue. Researchers found that pretreating the
subjects with arjuna offered "significant cardioprotection." They also

found that there was a remarkable reduction in the loss of high-energy phosphate (HEP) stores, a protective factor against ischemia.[7] (Ischemia is a reduction in the supply of oxygen to an organ.)

Keep your arteries flowing free and clear

If the cholesterol circulating in your bloodstream isn't removed on a regular basis, it can deposit on the walls of your arteries. While this happens to everyone to a certain extent, thicker cholesterol deposits reduce the volume of blood flowing through your vascular system and decrease the oxygen reaching your organs. Blood vessels with significant deposits become inflexible and hard, which is why atherosclerosis is also called "hardening of the arteries." This can cause a deterioration of tissues and organs. Your arteries also deteriorate from the accumulation of cholesterol. If left untreated, atherosclerosis can kill you. But arjuna has been shown to turn around this life-threatening condition.

In one study, rabbits were fed a cholesterol-rich diet to create atherosclerosis and then divided into three groups to compare the effects of cholesterol-lowering supplements. One group of rabbits was treated with arjuna while the other two groups were supplemented with pharmaceuticals proven to lower cholesterol levels. In a comparison of all three groups, arjuna was pronounced as "the most potent hypolipidemic agent" and proved to induce "partial inhibition of rabbit atheroma."[8] These findings indicate that arjuna may help prevent the buildup of fat deposits in your arteries and possibly correct the deadly effects of atherosclerosis.

The same herb may fight cancer as readily as bacterial infections

One of the unique benefits of herbal therapies is their adaptogenic property. Many times, a single herb can conquer diseases and medical disorders with seemingly different origins and mechanisms. (Drug therapy is much more targeted and thus limited.) Doctors prescribe antibiotics for bacterial infections and must use completely different types of drugs to fight cancer. Although bacteria and cancer seem to start and spread by different means, arjuna has been shown to successfully fight both.

According to the Entomology Research Institute of Loyola College in India, E. coli, which is a dangerous food-borne pathogen, is no match for arjuna. Researchers tested 34 traditional tribal plants of India and found that arjuna had "significant antibacterial activity" against E. coli as well as the bacteria responsible for pneumonia, cystitis (a bladder infection), and pyelonephritis (a kidney infection).[9]

Salmonella typhimurium is the culprit behind paratyphoid fever, which is a milder form of typhoid fever, as well as salmonella gastroenteritis, a type of food poisoning. But researchers found that ellagic acid, one of the constituents of arjuna, is quite effective against it and stops it from mutating, thus preventing the spread of disease.[10]

While antibacterial drugs have not been proven to work against cancer, it appears arjuna can live up to this double duty—and without the damaging effects of chemotherapeutic drugs. Many of the side effects of prescription drugs, especially those used to treat cancer, may damage organs or have a serious negative impact on general health. But according to studies at the University College of Medical Sciences and SMS Medical College, both in India, researchers have not found liver or renal damage in either human or animal test subjects receiving arjuna.[11,12]

While no one drug or therapy works against all types of cancers, arjuna may help fill in the gap for some forms of the disease. According to scientists at the Department of Botanical Sciences at Guru Nanak Dev University in India, arjuna has cancer-fighting properties and may be a promising agent for stopping cell mutation[13]—believed to be one of the first steps in cancer development. By preventing this initial process, arjuna may cut off one of the most common routes used to convert normal cells into cancerous ones.

In research conducted by the National Institute of Bioscience and Human Technology in Japan, even osteosarcoma, a type of malignant bone tumor, was found to be no match for arjuna. By inhibiting the growth of osteosarcoma cells, arjuna may be able to prevent the growth and spread of this type of cancer.[14]

T. arjuna is not only effective—it's inexpensive!

Scientists still don't fully understand the many disease-fighting mechanisms of arjuna, so research on this herb continues. We've only scratched the surface of this incredible tree and will continue to keep you updated as new uses for it are discovered. T. arjuna is available from Himalaya Herbal Healthcare under the name of "Arjuna." Refer to the Member Source Directory on page 529 for ordering information.

CHAPTER NINE

One miracle molecule can stop heart attack, stroke... even pull you back from the brink of death

D r. Scott Chirault's grandmother was literally at death's door.

At 99 years and 11 months old, she became feverish and unresponsive, and was brought to the emergency room. With a declining heart rate, barely registering blood pressure (70/30), and a case of pneumonia, all hope was lost.

Mawmaw, as she was called, did not want IV medications to keep her alive. But just a few days earlier, Dr. Chirault had received a sample of a unique new supplement, and he believed it could help turn things around.

He placed a dissolving tablet in her mouth, then went out to the nurses' station. Just 40 minutes later, the nurse came to get him—Mawmaw's blood pressure was increasing, along with her heart rate.

A few hours later, Mawmaw woke up...sat up... talked to her grandson. And since they didn't know how long this would last, he called the family in to see her. They came, and she got to see and talk with everyone she loved.

After a couple of weeks, she asked to stop taking the supplement. And just five days later, she slipped into a coma, and then she died.

And while this supplement did not save her life—it couldn't cure the pneumonia—it gave her two more weeks to spend with her family, and a chance to say goodbye to everyone she loved.

One amazing molecule can turn everything around

That supplement did one simple thing: increase Mawmaw's nitric oxide levels.

It's just one little molecule, but it has the power over life and death. If your body is flooded with too much of it, there can be toxic effects. If you don't have enough, your body starts to break down, becoming ever more vulnerable to coronary heart disease, heart attack, stroke, diabetes, Alzheimer's disease, and so much more.

And this amazing molecule can literally pull someone back from the brink of death.

But that's not all it can do.

Prevent horrible health problems & reverse existing damage with NO

Nitric oxide didn't win "Molecule of the Year" for nothing. Here are just a few of the very important ways it keeps you alive.

- Stops artery-clogging blood clots from forming
- Reverses arterial plaque build-up
- Prevents high blood pressure
- Lowers C-reactive protein
- Slashes triglyceride levels

And with that protection, NO reduces your risk of heart attack and stroke… two of the top three killers of Americans. On top of that, the miracle molecule can reduce your risk of devastating diabetes complications, including kidney disease, blindness, and amputations.

How does one molecule do so much to keep you alive and well?

Nitric oxide sends signals between the cells in your body, and extremely pretty important signals at that. In fact, there's not a single cell in your body that isn't sending or receiving messages via NO. But its most important work is in your circulatory system… and should those messages go haywire, the consequences can be deadly.

It all centers around your endothelium (the cells that line every blood vessel in your body) which have the critical job of producing NO. The NO enters the smooth muscles of your arteries, and signals those muscles to relax (the technical term is vasodilation). That lets your blood flow increase to healthy levels, giving your body its full supply of oxygen and nutrients.

When you don't have enough NO to go around, your arteries can't relax, they remain small and tight. And when your blood has a smaller, cramped space to flow through, it forces your blood pressure higher. That high pressure can cause some serious damage to your artery walls, allowing dangerous plaques to move in.

And once this cycle kicks off, your risk of heart attack and strokes increases dramatically.

Lack of NO has other consequences, too. In addition to setting off a plaque attack, it also leads to very damaging chronic inflammation in your arteries. Then, oxidative stress sneaks in. On their own, inflammation and oxidation are bad. Together, they help plaque burst open to release its toxins which can trigger blood clots in your arteries.

But restoring your NO levels can stop this from happening at all.

NEO40 Daily™ brings back the NO

Dr. Nathan Bryan knows a little something about nitric oxide—he's been studying it for more than ten years. And when he realized its role in disease prevention, he knew he had to come with a way to help people (especially those of us over 40) improve their NO status.

So he, along with Dr. Janet Zand, started screening hundreds of herbs and foods for their NO content. They took the best of those, and formulated a lozenge called NEO40 Daily. Then Dr. Bryan and his research team set out to learn just how well their new NO-boosting supplement really worked.

First, they tested the NEO40 lozenges to make sure they could really generate NO. To do that, they had some people test the lozenges. The researchers drew blood to get a baseline level, then the subjects each let one lozenge dissolve in their mouths. After five minutes, the post-lozenge blood testing began. And when all the data was in, nitrite levels (a key indicator of NO levels) had doubled.[1]

And when they took their research to the next level, they found even more good news than they'd expected.

Reduce triglycerides by up to 55 percent while increasing your NO

The next phase of their study[2] lasted 30 days, and this time included subjects with at least known cardiovascular risk factors (like high triglycerides, high blood pressure, and diabetes, for example). Every day, these subjects took either a NEO40 lozenge or placebo twice a day for 30 days.

As expected, in the NEO40 group that led to a substantial increase in their blood levels of nitrite and nitrate, meaning more NO. The people in the placebo group actually saw a slight decrease in their levels.

But that's not all that happened. The NEO40 supplements also had made quite a direct difference in some very important cardiovascular risk factors.

- 72 percent of subjects with high triglyceride levels saw that drop dramatically

- Triglyceride levels (fasting) plummeted by up to 55 percent (with an average drop of 27 percent)

- Up to 37 percent reduction in C-reactive protein (CRP) levels in subjects with elevated CRP

- An average 7 point drop in systolic blood pressure (in subjects with hypertension), and a 2.7 point drop in diastolic pressure

- Plus, more than half the subjects reported feeling more energetic and less anxious

What's more, nearly 80 percent of those participants said that they wanted to keep taking NEO40 lozenges.

NEO40 can help you cut back on pharmaceutical drugs...and their side effects

While the studies offer up a lot of impressive numbers, you really need to know how taking NEO40 Daily can help change your life. And the most dramatic impact may be that you'll be able to cut back on— and maybe get off of—pharmaceutical drugs. Especially when it comes to blood pressure medication.

In fact, one of the first people to enjoy that was Dr. Bryan's father, who had very poor circulation due to a car accident that left him paraplegic. He'd been taking three different drugs to manage his blood pressure, along with metformin for his diabetes. So Dr. Bryan (working with his dad's cardiologist) started his father on the lozenges. Over a period of months, his blood sugar normalized, and he began to wean off the blood pressure drugs—now he only needs one.

And then there's Dr. Zand's father (remember Dr. Zand, one of the researchers working with Dr. Bryan). Her 90-year-old father was also taking three medications to control his blood pressure. But within six weeks of starting the NEO40 lozenges, he didn't need any of them anymore.

Impressive—but they're far from the only two who've experienced this miracle. Elizabeth Shirley, compounding pharmacist for the People's Pharmacy, has seen it happen time and again. In fact, that's one reason people go to her, to get off pharmaceutical drugs and avoid their negative side effects. And with NEO40 lozenges, she's been able to help many customers reduce their dependency on blood pressure medication.

In fact, she advises anyone taking blood pressure medication who starts using the lozenges to monitor their blood pressure regularly and to work closely with their doctors. Chances are, the doses will need to be lowered to make sure pressure doesn't drop down too far.

She does advise us of one pretty common side effect, though. Increasing your NO with NEO40 Daily will probably increase your sex drive, too.

NO side effect: a much better sex life

You've heard of Viagra, no doubt. Well it works by increasing circulation to the penis…by increasing NO, albeit in an unnatural way.

When you take NEO40 Daily, you increase NO, and improve circulation everywhere. That's right, when you let a lozenge dissolve in your mouth, it will kick off a chain reaction down below. And even if it's been a while since you've been able to achieve an erection on your own, those days will be over.

But NO isn't just for the men, ladies. It also plays an important part in female sexual desire and performance. So if you haven't been interested lately, NO can help turn that around.

Because satisfying sex really comes down to blood flow, and you'll get plenty of that from increased NO, thanks to the carefully selected formula that makes up NEO40 Daily.

Hawthorn and beet root boost NO and total heart health

The formula starts with a proprietary herbal blend which includes hawthorn and beetroot, both of which increase NO activity. When Dr. Bryan and his team were testing all those herbs and foods, these two scored the highest when it came to nitrate content (which your body uses to generate NO). But that's not where these two stop helping your heart.

Hawthorn does so much for your cardiovascular system, it's no surprise they included it in the NEO40 formula. And unlike many traditional remedies, this one has tons of science to back it up. In fact, this herb

- cuts down on angina attacks[3]
- treats atherosclerosis by shrinking plaque and lowering cholesterol[4]
- improves circulation to the heart by dilating coronary blood vessels[5]
- lower blood pressure[6]
- prevents heart attack[7]

And then there's the beet root, which in addition to its nitrate content has been shown to lower high cholesterol[8] and lower blood pressure.[9]

But the NO-producing formula doesn't stop there.

Four NO-boosting ingredients round out the NEO40 formula

NEO40 Daily also includes magnesium, vitamin C, vitamin B12, and L-citrulline. Together, along with the herbal blend, these ingredients work to provide your body with a source of nitric oxide when your endothelium just can't product enough.

Magnesium is an essential mineral with a huge impact on your cardiovascular system. Among other things, magnesium helps directly counteract atherosclerosis[10] and provides serious protection against heart attack and stroke.

Vitamin C promotes the availability of NO in your body, so you can use it most effectively. It also strengthen your arteries, and protects their structural integrity[11]. And like magnesium, it can help prevent heart attack and stroke. On top of all that, let's not forget that it's a potent antioxidant, with very powerful free radical scavenging capabilities.

Vitamin B12 plays a very important role in your cardiovascular system: you can't make red blood cells without it (in fact, vitamin B12 deficiency can cause anemia).

L-citrulline is directly involved in NO production. It does that by naturally converting to L-arginine, a form that's much easier for your body to use than if the L-arginine comes from supplements. Plus, L-citrulline has been shown (in an animal study) to reverse the progression of atherosclerosis.[12]

With this unique blend of NO-increasing ingredients, all of which

---

Is low NO killing dialysis patients?

Dialysis patients have an especially high death rate from cardiovascular events, and Dr. Bryan thinks he might know why. His theory: Dialysis decreases NO. And this soon-to-be-published study backs it up.

You see, low concentrations of nitrite and nitrate in the blood and saliva translates to lower NO in the body. So Dr. Bryan and his fellow researchers measured nitrite and nitrate levels in dialysis patients before, during, and after the procedure. And they learned that dialysis could remove up to 90 percent of the patients' nitrite and nitrate, which in turn could have a profound negative on their NO levels.[13]

do double duty to directly protect your cardiovascular system, NEO40 lozenges may just save your life.

Take NEO40 Daily to prevent—maybe even reverse—cardiovascular disease

NEO40 Daily can improve your NO status and help prevent cardiovascular problems...even if you're riddled with risk factors. And according to both careful research and customer response, it's very likely that you will feel better instantly when you use it.

The manufacturer recommends taking one NEO40 lozenge once or twice a day. Put the lozenge on your tongue (move it around) and just let it dissolve—don't chew or swallow it!

And for those of you who like to see exactly how well something is working, you can. There's a very simple NO measurement strip that can help you find out your NO status, and literally watch those lozenges work to improve it.

One little thing: the lozenges can make you burp (usually right after it's dissolved). That's totally normal, and actually makes a lot of sense. After all, nitric oxide is a gas, so that's one way to see it's really working.

You can find ordering information for NEO40 Daily lozenges and the nitric oxide test strips in the Member Source Directory on page 529.

Part IV

Asthma and COPD

CHAPTER ONE

Stamp out even the worst asthma: A breakthrough approach to easy breathing without devastating side effects

I doubt I need to say too much to sum up the terrors of asthma—the pressure of that invisible elephant that's permanently parked on your chest, the persistent but unproductive cough, the wheezing that keeps you awake like some never-ending nightmare. Then, as if all that weren't enough, there's the panic that tags along with all of these symptoms.

But I'll bet I also don't have to tell you that this is one case in which the "cure" is a whole lot scarier than the culprit. Steroids are not the kind of thing that anyone would consider safe for daily use—and yet that's just what many doctors might prescribe for you following an asthma diagnosis. And the real kicker is that they don't even fix your condition—they simply cover it up, while packing on the pounds, interfering with your adrenal function, and manhandling your immune system in the process.

With the FDA attack on ephedra, natural medicine doctors scrambled to find another effective herbal supplement that would control asthma. One doctor didn't stop until he discovered Phytocort.

Brand new to the market (and free of the super-dosing side effects that got its notorious predecessor into trouble) this blend of four Chinese herbs is poised to break through the all-too-common prednisone prison-not only safely, but just as successfully.

Works as well as prednisone— and benefits the immune system, too

Dr. Ba X. Hoang, working with the Allergy Research Group in Alameda, California, has made the research of natural asthma alternatives a lifelong mission, always staying on the lookout for the latest studies and continually scouring sources for potential breakthroughs in product development. It was a year ago now when he and his associates came across an all-too-rare published study of the effects of herbal treatment on asthma symptoms.[1]

The randomized, double-blind, placebo-controlled study was performed at Weifang Asthma Hospital in China between 2003 and 2004. Ninety-two nonsmoking patients (43 men and 49 women) between the ages of 18 and 64 with symptoms of moderate to severe asthma were recruited to participate in the study. A combination of three herbal extracts—all of which are the main components of another formula that has been used to treat asthma in China for decades—was pitted against prednisone in a four-week measure of asthmatic symptom relief.

The final results of the study showed that the herbal extract significantly reduced the participants' symptom scores, increased lung function as measured by forced expiratory volume/second (FEV1) and peak expiratory flow (PEF), and reduced the patients' use of an emergency inhaler. There was also a marked reduction of peripheral blood eosinophils (the white blood cells that often accompany allergic responses) and in levels of serum IgE antibodies (the immunoglobulin released in the reactions of hypersensitive individuals).

While lung function in the extract-treated group was not as high as lung function in the prednisone group, the herbal treatment's performance was comparable to the corticosteroid (the use of which is meant to mimic a class of hormones produced in the adrenal cortex) in every other category. But what's even more striking is that the herbal formula actually had an immune-boosting effect on the patients taking it.

Cases of asthma often involve an imbalance in the types of immune responses your body has. Typically, the T-helper 2 (Th2) response, which is associated with hyper-reactive allergic conditions, dominates. The other type of immune response, called T-helper 1 (Th1), doesn't produce these sorts of drastic reactions, but if your body's Th1 response isn't as strong as it should be, you'll wind up with any number of allergic reactions, or, in this case, an asthma attack. Prednisone works by suppressing overall immune function, which, in turn, lowers the Th2 response. But it also lowers the Th1 response even further—digging the hole deeper and not really solving the problem. But the herbal formula used in the study actually boosted Th1 response, balancing out the immune system.

The formula also increased the participants' cortisol levels—the suppression of which is yet another pitfall of prednisone. Regular use of corticosteroids can do irreversible damage to your adrenal glands over time, ultimately leaving your body unable to produce enough cortisol on its own. And this side effect is seriously bad news: Low cortisol levels can lead to a spike in pain and fatigue, often accompanied by a hefty dose of depression and difficulty in dealing with emotions in the face of stress.

The missing link between epilepsy and asthma

With years of clinical experience behind him, Dr. Ba knew that he and the team at the Allergy Research Group could replicate this formula—improve upon it, even. Which is exactly how they ended up with Phytocort. It wasn't sheer luck—in fact, Dr. Ba had begun his studies of the key herb, Sophora flavensis, nearly 10 years ago.

It's this component, he tells me, that holds the lion's share of responsibility in Phytocort's formula—though the reason behind its use might come as a bit of a surprise. As it turns out, Sophora flavensis is commonly used to treat another frightening and potentially dangerous condition: epilepsy.

Dr. Ba believes that the similarities between these two diseases, asthma and epilepsy, are strong—even if they appear to have nothing in common. We have all grown accustomed to hearing about asthma as being strongly related to the allergic responses mentioned earlier—a nasty byproduct of some inherent or acquired immune imbalance. But while those allergies are indeed triggering factors, Dr. Ba explained, it isn't an immune modulator that we need the most—it's something called an excitatory modulator.[2]

Excitatory modulators calm overexcited neurons—the unruly electrical activity of which is responsible for many of the symptoms of epilepsy. Cell signals run amok, and synapses fire in an abnormally synchronized manner, resulting in the volatile jerking motions common to even the mildest seizure. According to Dr. Ba, the non-neuronal cells in our airways react in much the same way in the throes of an asthma attack—be it mild or severe. And the culprits behind these uncontrolled motions are your cells' ion channels gone haywire.

As it turns out, these ion channels don't just exist in your brain cells—they also exist in cells from other places throughout your body, including the lungs. And relatively recently, scientists also found that a specific type of receptor normally thought of as strictly part of the central nervous system, called the N-methyl-D-aspartate (NMDA) glutamate receptor, is also present in the lungs and airways. According to the research paper I read, the NMDA glutamate receptor "might be an important, previously unrecognized mechanism of the airway inflammation and hyper-reactivity found in asthma."[3]

Exactly how all this works is extremely complicated. We're talking molecular physics and biology here—not topics you're likely to encounter at your next dinner party. And after trying to wade through and make sense of the science enough to explain it to you, I can see why. So, fair warning: The following paragraphs might be tough to wrap your head around. But let's give it a try.

Soothe aggravated airways by resting your stressed cells

Much like a battery, all neuron membranes must maintain a certain charge composition in order to keep up the electrical charge that's necessary for energy and motion-and even for life itself. Voltage-gated ion channels in the cell's membrane are essential to this process—acting as a "velvet rope" of sorts, allowing the entrance of only certain ions based on their charge. At rest, our nerve cells have more potassium (negatively charged) inside of them, and more sodium (positively charged) outside of them, a condition maintained by your ion channels, when such opposite charges would normally seek to diffuse each other.

The balance begins to shift away from this charged state when some stimulus (in the case of epilepsy, it could be something as simple as flashing lights) causes the two amino acids glutamate and aspartate to be set into action. They activate the NMDA glutamate receptor, which opens the ion channels back up again—but this time to let sodium in and to usher potassium out. This exchange continues until there's an explosion of electrical energy—the official starting point for any of your body's thoughts or movements.

Needless to say, if those ion channels aren't functioning properly, a whole lot of trouble breaks loose.

Too much sodium in a nerve cell too often will provoke hyperexcitability—meaning that even the smallest stimulus will create unwanted synaptic movements. Much as you would feel when you're burning the candle at both ends, these stressed cells suffer from a lack of energy accompanied by a desperate need to keep moving. But there's no end in sight—not enough potassium is being allowed in and not enough sodium is being expelled to return the neuron to its optimally charged resting state. It's a vicious cycle.

Such is the case with asthma, claims Dr. Ba, when the NMDA glutamate receptors in the airways are activated (and in this case, the finger might be pointed at prolonged exposure to certain toxins—the polluted air we breathe or the preservatives we eat every day). This excitability leads to an increase of fluid in the lungs and a constriction of the airways.

That's why severe asthmatics are so unresponsive to conventional treatment, such as prednisone or some other allergy-oriented medications—they merely address inflammation without digging to the root of the problem. And that's exactly why Sophora flavensis is such an effective treatment. Research has shown that two alkaloids found in the herb—matrine and oxymatrine—act as excitatory modulators, treating hyperreactive asthmatic airways.

These alkaloids have a relaxing and analgesic effect on the central nervous system. They have tranquilizing properties, promoting the influx of relaxing neurotransmitters (gamma-aminobutyric acid and glycine) and inhibiting the overactive NMDA receptors that result in such unwanted responses as seizures, tremors, hypertension, and asthma attacks. With the action potential diffused, aggravated cells—both neurons and non-neurons alike—are finally able to rest.

A balanced formula to help you breathe easier for good

With Sophora flavensis as the lead herb in Phytocort, Dr. Ba and his associates included the two supporting herbs in the original clinically tested formula for additional allergy and immune support, as well as a fourth, balancing, herb:

- *Ganoderma lucidum* is a medicinal mushroom with a wide range of uses, noted for its strong anti-inflammatory, immune strengthening, and general healing properties.

- *Glycyrrhiza uralensis*, or licorice root, offers support as an expectorant, an anti-spasmodic, an anti-inflammatory, and a soothing agent, also enhancing the effects of naturally occurring cortisone in the body.

- *Morinda citrifolia*, also known as noni, was added for its kidney support and diuretic qualities, to eliminate any possibility of bloating that could accompany licorice root.

The recommended initial dosage of Phytocort is three capsules three times a day, with a maintenance dosage of two capsules twice a day. And Dr. Ba tells me that, unlike ephedra, which can pose risks to cardiovascular and nervous function when taken in very large doses, this formula is considered safe for long-term use in any asthma patient.

While Dr. Ba has found that many asthmatics will experience a calming of their symptoms within two weeks, he advises that three to six months be allowed for the best restorative results. He recommends that you start with the maximum dosage, work with your doctor, and consider a gradual tapering off of prednisone use by 2.5 to 5 mg every two to three days until you have eliminated it altogether. Given enough time, even the most difficult-to-treat patients may eventually be able to toss away their steroids for good.

CHAPTER TWO

Fighting asthma or COPD? Increased lung capacity means no more wheezing and struggling for air

It's a disease that still has the mainstream scratching their heads. They don't have a cure, or even an effective treatment, for COPD. But that doesn't keep them from trying to make a buck off it—so they throw inhaled steroids at the problem. Never mind the fact that those drugs don't really work for COPD... or the fact they can raise your risk of heart attack or stroke by 58 percent.

And of course, those are the same drugs they throw at asthma, putting your health at severe risk.

Of course, I wouldn't be writing this if I didn't have an answer for you. And, as we often find here at HSI, the natural, steroid-free answer to COPD, asthma, and other lung conditions (including allergies, colds, and sinus headaches) lies in a formula that was stumbled upon purely by chance.

23 recently rediscovered herbs proven by centuries of use

As the CEO of a telecommunications company, Tom Long never thought he'd find himself marketing the latest breakthrough in respiratory health. But that was before the owner of his company got sick. Unable to breathe and fearing a heart attack, he checked himself into the hospital.

The doctors ran the usual tests and said there was nothing wrong. But he knew they were missing something—he felt awful and couldn't believe the pain in his chest was "nothing."

A friend suggested he see an acupuncturist and herbalist in Chicago. The herbalist knew what the problem was right away—he couldn't breathe properly. Stress and a lack of exercise contributed to the problem, leaving his lungs "locked up." And then he gave him something that started working almost immediately.

The herbalist let him in on the secret—Resprin. It's a formula made of a blend of 23 herbs, specially formulated to support clear breathing. The herbs falls into three categories:

- Vaporizing herbs like peppermint and schizonpeta herba.
- Expectorant herbs that flush out mucus and dust—these herbs included ginger, licorice, and poria.
- Soothing herbs, like bupleurum and ligusticum wallichii, that help bronchial irritation.

Through the action of these three categories of herbs, the lungs physically have more space in which to take in more air with each breath. Because what it really comes down to is inflammation. Resprin actually relaxes the lining of the bronchial tubes, allowing more airflow into the lungs.

Increase your lung capacity by almost 40 percent

This is where Tom enters the story. The owner of his company was so amazed with Resprin that he brought it in for Tom to try. He immediately noticed he could breathe more deeply. And he knew he had to share it with others.

Tom started sharing Resprin with people who were having trouble breathing—asthma, COPD, sinus problems—nothing could stand up to Resprin. They were onto something big… so they put it to the test.

Before heading down the road of human trials, Resprin was put through an *in vitro* test in the lab. Normal airway tissue as well as airway tissue from asthma patients was tested. The tissue was exposed to a chemical irritant that is known to spur inflammation. When Resprin was introduced to the tissue, it proved its anti-inflammatory effects by lowering biomarkers of inflammation.

Of course, that wasn't enough for Tom and the rest of the team at Resprin, Inc. He wanted proof that Resprin would work for real people suffering from real breathing problems.

So they commissioned a trial in an independent lab. The trial had three phases, and Resprin proved that it worked almost immediately. During the first phase, participants were given just one dose of Resprin. Even with just that one dose, peak air flow improved nearly 6 percent.

By the third phase, the results were looking even better. Participants took Resprin every day for a month, and by the end of the month, the average improvement in peak air flow was 37 percent. Nearly half of the participants said they felt their energy levels and need for rescue medication were exceptionally improved, and another 28 percent felt they'd seen significant improvement. Most of them said they would keep using Resprin.

Harness the lung-boosting power trusted by marathon runners

Marathon runners are serious about lung capacity. If they can't breathe, they can't run. So it's no surprise that one of the top runners in the world relies on Resprin (though it's labeled as AirAide) to give him an edge.

Kenyan runner Benson Cheruiyot was able to shave a remarkable 2.5 minutes off his personal best marathon time using Resprin. Of course, we're no marathon runners. You're looking for something that will have you taking those deep, life-giving breaths without struggling and wheezing.

Wayne has been singing the praises of Resprin because of its effect on his wife Jeanne. The mainstream hasn't even been able to identify the disease that has been deteriorating her lungs. But Resprin has slowed the deterioration and has helped her to lead a more active life.

Debbie had been looking for a natural alternative to her asthma inhaler. She was skeptical when she received a sample of Resprin. But once she'd taken a few, she found it works just as well as her inhaler, without the risk of side effects.

Sam's had asthma for 15 years and had gotten used to carrying an inhaler with him everywhere he went. Like Debbie, he was skeptical before trying Resprin. Knowing he had his inhaler as a backup, he took Resprin and set out for a workout.

When he stopped to catch his breath at the top of a hill, he noticed something different. He was breathing heavily, sure, but there was no diminished function in breathing. He says he hasn't breathed that well in 15 years, and that he spent the rest of that day walking around, breathing deeply and smiling. When he explained his experience to Tom, he said, "the chains have been cut."

Even if you're not suffering from a serious lung condition, Resprin can help you. Chris was stuck at work with a horrible sinus headache and congestion that left her barely able to breathe. Within minutes of taking Resprin, her headache was completely gone and she could breathe again. She says she always keeps some on hand.

And the makers of Resprin have heard from countless people who swear by it for dealing with colds and allergies.

Ordering information for Resprin is in the Member Source Directory on page 529.

CHAPTER THREE

Clogged Lungs Cleared: Stopping America's 4th Biggest Killer

W hen one of our contacts called us about a product he referred to as "truly bizarre," I thought "How 'out there' can it really be?" After all, we come across some pretty unique and complex stuff almost daily in the course of our research. But in this case, there really is no other word to describe the novel treatment for cystic fibrosis, chronic obstructive pulmonary disease, and other respiratory ailments that he told me about: Bizarre sums it up nicely.

It's a liquid formula of DNA called Mucolyxir that, applied sublingually, helps dissolve airway-blocking mucous. That's right—DNA under your tongue to help you breathe better: See what we mean by bizarre?

But not only does it appear to be safe and effective, it also costs much less than you might expect for something this revolutionary.

Ancient theory meets modern science

One of the primary theories explaining respiratory diseases is that much of the mucous blocking the airways is a result of the immune system's effort to eliminate bacteria from the lungs.

Mucolyxir's developers, John McMichael and Allan Lieberman, took that theory and further hypothesized that such activity, over time, could result in hypersensitivity that would exacerbate the problem of mucous accumulation. To address this problem, they turned to the ancient homeopathic concept of "like cures like."

As you'll see below, much of the mucous build-up involved in respiratory illnesses like cystic fibrosis and chronic obstructive pulmonary disease (COPD) is caused by accumulated DNA. So McMichael and Lieberman chose the "like" cure—DNA—as the basis for their Mucolyxir formula.

DNA therapy interrupts vicious cycle

Inside the lungs, the scenario might go something like this: Bacterial-DNA induces the production of various interleukins (such as IL-8), which are associated with inflammation. The presence of IL-8 sends out a distress signal through your body. In turn, responding immune cells attack and destroy the invaders by engulfing them in mucous. But as the immune cells respond, they spill their own DNA, which is interpreted as an enemy invader in the respiratory environment. This sparks another signal for help, establishing a vicious and continually amplified cycle as the immune cells are repeatedly called into play.

Mucolyxir interrupts this cycle by reducing the production of "signaling" interleukins in order to decrease the production of the protective mucous, which is often more harmful than helpful. It does this in two ways: by regulating anti-DNA activity of the immune system, and by clearing mucous to eliminate matter clogging the airways.

Mucociliary clearance involves the movement of the cilia (the tiny arm-like fibers on the cells lining the bronchial tree), secretion of mucous, and movement of water into and out of epithelial cells. In plain English, that means that the tiny fibers in your lungs are stimulated, causing mucous secretion and movement of water, which, basically, forces you to "cough up" the material clogging your airway. The DNA in Mucolyxir stimulates this process.

The DNA that McMichael and Lieberman used in creating Mucolyxir was extracted from salmon, but it's important to understand that there is no gene transfer with this method of DNA use. In other words, you won't suddenly start showing characteristics of salmon. I spoke to Dr. Lieberman to ask how we can be sure that there's no risk of this happening: After all, you don't need gills or fins.

He explained that Mucolyxir uses a microdose of DNA, meaning that there is not even one full genome present in the product. He pointed out that we eat foreign DNA all the time: When you eat a sardine, you are eating the complete sardine DNA, yet you don't take on any characteristics of a sardine. Fortunately, it just doesn't work that way.

Dr. McMichael noted that, based on his observations, Mucolyxir appears to be "helpful in the treatment of severe respiratory conditions like chronic bronchitis and COPD. People treated with it demonstrate significant improvements in objective parameters such as improved pulmonary function leading to better blood oxygenation efficiency and exercise ability. This product has been formulated to address an unmet medical need that affects a large number of people worldwide."

And that "large number" is growing every day. While cigarette smoke and work environments (such as textile manufacturing and mining) are the most common causes of COPD, it's not just the smokers, miners, and manufacturers at risk. A new generation in respiratory trauma is on the rise, one brought on by irritants like toxic mold found inside-possibly even in your own home. These conditions can lead to cases of asthma and COPD.

While pinning down and eliminating these factors is obviously the best solution, that may not always be possible—especially before the onset of respiratory problems. But the good news is that although the formula was originally developed to treat cystic fibrosis (CF), research also supports Mucolyxir's potential for stimulating an immune response that can protect against or reduce symptoms of asthma and COPD.

Real-world results for conditions from CF to chronic sinusitis

This all still sounds a little like science fiction, but the applications of Mucolyxir are certainly showing real-word results. While it doesn't cure severe respiratory disease, it does make the symptoms more manageable, in turn, improving quality of life. And although there are no controlled clinical trials at this point, there are some remarkable anecdotal accounts.

Consider the case study of 23-year-old twin brothers, both afflicted with cystic fibrosis. Each had a history of hospitalizations for lung clearance and secondary infections diagnosed as being associated with their cystic fibrosis. Each brother began therapy with one or two drops (0.0006 mg/drop) of DNA sublingually per day.

For almost seven years since beginning DNA therapy, neither has been hospitalized. In addition, follow-up evaluations by physicians revealed a 30 to 45 percent increase in airflow in each patient. And that's not all: Forced vital capacity, a common measure of lung capacity, and the extent of mucous clearance in the lungs increased from 60 to 90 percent in each patient.

After approximately one year of therapy, one of the brothers stopped taking the DNA drops. His condition steadily worsened, with increased mucous viscosity, decreased lung capacity, and reduced expectoration. When he resumed taking the DNA drops at the prescribed dose, he immediately improved once again.

Another example of Mucolyxir's potential is that of a 48-year-old woman with chronic sinusitis and bronchitis characterized by chronic head congestion, nasal obstruction, and coughing. She also began treatment with one drop per day of DNA. After just a few days, she noted a dramatic improvement in sinus and chest drainage. Again, when she stopped taking the DNA drops, her condition regressed. Beginning therapy again caused a similar increase in drainage and relief of congestion she'd experienced previously.

Our medical adviser, Dr. Martin Milner, also told us that people with acute or chronic asthma who have excessive mucus production could also be helped by Mucolyxir.

Recommended protocol

When I spoke with Dr. Lieberman, I also asked him to explain what exactly is involved in using Mucolyxir. He told me that it is administered sublingually (under the tongue) in doses of just one drop at a time.

The single drop should be applied on the floor of the mouth, behind the lower teeth, and you should refrain from swallowing for 15 seconds. To avoid dilution, you should also avoid eating or drinking for five minutes after application.

He emphasized that all patients, regardless of diagnosis, are advised to employ the "rush technique" on the first day of using Mucolyxir. This technique involves taking one drop every 15 minutes for one hour. After the first hour, take one drop every hour until bedtime.

On the second and third days of treatment, take one drop four times daily: one after each meal and one before bed. Beginning on day four, use only as needed—more drops on days with severe symptoms, fewer on good days.

Now, what about cost? A formula based on DNA certainly sounds like it would be expensive. But, at about $42, Mucolyxir is actually fairly affordable, especially considering the cost, in terms of potentially dangerous side effects, associated with the mainstream treatments—like bronchodilators, antibiotics, and even lung transplants—currently used for cystic fibrosis and COPD.

The drops are stable whether they're refrigerated or at room temperature, so you can carry them with you, for quick easy access, in your pocket, purse, or briefcase without worry.

Part V

Anti-Aging, Energy, and Weight Loss

CHAPTER ONE

The secret energy-boosting weapon trusted by pro athletes

Few people are in better shape than professional football players. After all, they have teams of experts—from nutritionists to personal trainers—to whip them into shape—and several million reasons to want to stay there. But even with all this ready access to the best resources, sometimes NFL players still run out of steam. You wouldn't know that to look at them though: They keep at it every week and somehow manage to plow through the fatigue. How do they do it? Well, we recently learned one of the ways some players get that extra boost: with an all-natural energy-boosting supplement not many people know about. And if this secret weapon can help pro athletes feel energized, just imagine what it might do for you.

No more short-term "kicks": Create more energy from the start

Most energy-boosting supplements "work" by stimulating the adrenal glands to produce more adrenaline. This does give you a short-term kick, since adrenaline causes your heart to beat faster, sending more blood to your muscles, which then tighten up and make you feel more alert or energized. But "short-term" is the key phrase here. The effects wear off as soon as the supplement passes through your body, and you can end up feeling even more tired than before.

But the product we just learned about, called NT Factor, works by enhancing the actual energy-creating process in your body. And that starts with your mitochondria.

Mitochondria are like microscopic organs inside nearly every cell in the human body. They are responsible for energy production and cellular respiration, a process by which they convert nutrients into energy in the form of *adenosine triphosphate* (ATP). ATP is a nucleotide that serves as cells' primary energy source and is required for RNA synthesis.

Through this process, mitochondria are responsible for creating more than 90 percent of the energy needed to sustain life and support growth in the body. In addition, these tiny structures are also responsible for amino acid synthesis and the breakdown and oxidation of fatty acids. They accomplish this staggering array of tasks using their unique double-membrane structure.

Scientists have devoted entire books to the subject of mitochondrial function, but just from this brief explanation you can see how critical mitochondria are to your health. As we age, our cells function with fewer and fewer mitochondria—and the ones that are left may not do their job as effectively as they once did. If their membranes get damaged, the mitochondria can't function as well—meaning they produce less energy and you wind up feeling run down. So the key to keeping your energy levels at peak performance is to protect your mitochondria from damage. And the key to doing <u>that</u> appears to be phospholipids.

Keeping your energy makers from getting sacked

Phospholipids are fat molecules with one or more phosphate groups attached. They're critical to the efficient structure and function of cell membranes, including the double membranes of mitochondria.

Phospholipids are particularly important to protecting membranes from free radical damage; they are responsible for activating antioxidant enzymes on cell membrane surfaces.

Think of it like this: If each of your cells is its own football team, the mitochondria are the quarterbacks and the phospholipids are the linemen protecting them from getting sacked. So the more phospholipids you have on the job, the better chance your mitochondria have of staying healthy, which translates into more energy for you.

The best food sources of phospholipids are egg yolks and organ meats. But unless you're going to eat large amounts of those foods at every meal, you probably aren't going to get all the phospholipids your cells need through diet alone.

Animal studies have shown that treatment with supplemental phospholipids can improve mitochondrial function and even halt or reverse the damage done by prior mitochondrial dysfunction. In one study, scientists studied the effects of supplemental phospholipid treatment on rats with age-related hearing loss. They found that rats treated for six months with lecithin, a major phospholipid, had "significant preservation of hearing sensitivities" as compared with untreated controls.[1]

Based on the encouraging results of this and other animal and laboratory studies, researchers set out to develop a phospholipid supplement for humans. Today, there are several available, but NT Factor stands out because it has at least three published clinical trials behind it. NT Factor is a proprietary blend of phospholipids, including phosphatidylcholine, glycolipids, and other polyunsaturated phosphatidyl nutrients, along with probiotics like bifido bacterium, L. bacillus, and L-acidophilus.

And all of the research supports its effectiveness against fatigue caused by aging, chronic fatigue syndrome, and even chemotherapy.

"Just make sure I don't run out of this stuff..."

I spoke with Jim Shortt, M.D., a doctor in private practice who recommends NT Factor products to many of his patients, which include some of those members of the NFL I mentioned earlier.

"The players that I treat tell me that after eight weeks of the season, they 'hit a wall' of fatigue," Shortt said. He began using NT Factor about a year ago, and, after a few weeks of treatment, his NFL patients told him, "Don't let me run out of this stuff."

He's also used it with great success in patients with chronic fatigue syndrome. "100 percent of my patients on NT Factor have reported a gradual lessening of fatigue," said Shortt. "It's not overnight, but they slowly feel better."

Reduce fatigue by more than 35 percent in just 12 weeks

But NT Factor isn't just for athletes or people battling chronic fatigue. In one study, researchers assessed the effects of NT Factor on 20 healthy people all over the age of 60. Participants all reported "persistent, intractable fatigue," with conditions consistent with the Piper Fatigue Scale (PFS), the accepted assessment tool for analyzing fatigue conditions, where zero is no fatigue and 10 is severe fatigue. The participants were divided into groups based on their PFS score: Those with scores in the 1-4 range were assigned to the mild fatigue group; scores between 4 and 7 fell into the moderate fatigue range.

The participants took three tablets of NT Factor twice daily for 12 weeks. Blood tests were taken at the beginning of the study, at four and eight weeks, and then again at the end of the study. Then they returned again after 24 weeks for a follow-up assessment.

After just four weeks of treatment, the average fatigue score dropped 20 percent. The scores in the moderate group continued to improve steadily, with a 33 percent reduction at week eight and a 35.5 reduction by week 12. The most improvement was seen in participants with fatigue scores in the moderate to severe range; those in the mild fatigue category were least affected.

The researchers also assessed mitochondrial function throughout this trial through blood testing. After 12 weeks of taking NT Factor, the study participants' cells looked similar to those of healthy young adults' cells. Overall, the scientists concluded that 12 weeks of NT Factor treatment resulted in a 23.7 percent increase in mitochondrial function in the moderately fatigued group.[2]

Another study of healthy adults showed similar results: 34 people with an average age of about 50 had moderate to severe fatigue (scores of 6-10 on the Piper Scale). Participants with PFS scores in the severe range (7-10) took three doses of Propax, a comprehensive supplement containing a full spectrum of vitamins, minerals, and other nutrients, along with NT Factor, daily for four weeks; those who had moderate fatigue, or a PFS score of 6, took two doses per day for four weeks.

After four weeks, the average PFS score had improved 33 percent, going down to 6.1 from the baseline average of 7.9. After eight weeks, it dropped further, to 4.7. Overall, female participants' PFS scores improved 35 percent and men's improved 29 percent.[3]

75 percent of cancer patients get relief from chemo side effects

Researchers also conducted a study in which they assessed the effect of Propax, on cancer patients. A placebo-controlled, double-blind study of 36 patients was run concurrently with an unblinded trial involving 16 patients. All participants were undergoing outpatient chemotherapy for cancer, including cancer of the colon, rectum, pancreas, breast, ovaries, and some types of lung cancer.

In both the blinded and the unblinded arms of the study, both patients and the nurses who cared for them reported significant improvements in the severity of chemotherapy side effects after three months of Propax treatment. In the unblinded study, 81 percent reported overall improvement in quality of life indicators; nurses reported that 68 percent of the participants suffered less chemotherapy-induced toxicity after taking Propax. In the blinded study, 75 percent of the nurses and 63 percent of the patients reported an improvement in side effects overall. Both arms of the study showed particular effectiveness in improving appetite and nausea.[4]

Professional formula now available direct to you

As I said before, there are several products on the market that claim to improve mitochondrial function through phospholipids. But this was the only product I found that had both animal and human trials behind it, published in major medical journals. I spoke with Robert Settinari, M.D., a nutriceutical research consultant and co-author of one of the human trials of Propax, about what makes NT Factor different from the other choices on the market.

Settinari pointed to the probiotics in the NT Factor formula, which can help improve absorption of both the supplemental phospholipids provided in NT Factor, as well as other nutrients. "NT Factor supports the entire biodelivery system," he said. The probiotics support the digestive tract and displace the pathogens which are competing for space. It prepares the digestive tract to absorb nutrients better, and phospholipids are absorbed in the gut."

Whatever the secret, all kinds of people are benefiting from NT Factor, from pro athletes to chronic fatigue syndrome patients. And now it's available direct to you, too.

NT Factor has been available to doctors and other health care professionals for some time. Just recently it became available direct to consumers in two different formulas. The first is Propax, which was used in several of the studies I cited above. As I explained, Propax is a comprehensive mix of NT Factor along with an extensive list of vitamins, minerals, and other nutrients. The dosage is pre-dispensed in packets of four tablets and one softgel capsules; the recommended dosage is one packet three times a day. But while Propax has shown great results, many people interested in NT Factor are already on a comprehensive supplement program and don't want or need all that Propax contains.

Now there's also a new formula available direct to consumers called Mitochondria Ignite, which contains all the power of NT Factor along with a shorter list of additional nutrients: calcium, phosphorus, magnesium, carnitine, creatine, and panetethine. Mitochondria Ignite comes in 300 mg tablets; the recommended dosage is one tablet three times daily. See the Member Source Directory on page 529 for complete ordering information.

Constant, unremitting fatigue can be a sign of serious health problems. If you are feeling tired all the time, and nothing seems to help, be sure to discuss the problem with your doctor to rule out any serious health issues.

If everything checks out, but you're still feeling run down, give your body the extra phospholipids it needs to improve cell membrane efficiency and optimize your mitochondrial function. Those little tiny quarterbacks inside your cells can have a huge impact on how you perform.

CHAPTER TWO

Anti-aging therapy so easy you can do it in your sleep

I t's not just the racing thoughts and worries that keep you lying awake at night when you're stressed. There are actual physiological reactions going on in your body preventing you from falling asleep. Stress causes your body to release adrenal hormones—the same ones responsible for the "fight or flight" response we all have in extreme situations. And now we know that curtailing, or at least reducing, this physiological reaction to stress will not only help relieve your insomnia but it could also help you combat aging.

Insomnia and the hormonal domino effect

Specifically, insomnia has a direct relationship with the hormone cortisol.[1] Dr. Milner, HSI medical adviser, explained to me that cortisol levels are naturally highest in the morning, reduce throughout the day, and are lowest during sleep. But studies suggest that levels of cortisol increase with age. The elevated cortisol level keeps you up and also causes negative changes in hormone activity—such as reducing the production of sex hormones like testosterone, estrogen, and progesterone. Declining levels of these hormones are one of the primary causes of physical and mental aging.

Curbing excess cortisol production and getting a good night's sleep obviously won't reverse the natural, gradual decline of hormones that causes changes like menopause. Yet, it might help to normalize hormones depleted by the natural aging process, such as DHEA. So controlling your cortisol levels just might help you head off some of the other side effects that often accompany aging like memory loss, fatigue, and even weight gain.

Lower stress, better sleep

So combating insomnia by controlling your cortisol levels might be one of the crucial keys to anti-aging. Boosting levels of sleep-supporting substances like serotonin and melatonin will have a further natural relaxing effect. This not only helps you rest easier, but it also combats the stimulating—and aging—effects of cortisol.

We've tracked down two natural formulas that address these factors directly: Seditol and tryptophan. Let's start with the one that targets the main insomnia culprit, cortisol.

87 percent of insomniacs report relief

Seditol was formulated specifically to address excess cortisol in the body, according to Bob Garrison, the CEO of Seditol's manufacturer, Next Pharmaceuticals. It's a blend of two herbal ingredients—magnolia and ziziphus.

I spoke to Garrison, who told me that, like many other supplements, Seditol was born out of unexpected benefits found during human trials. Next has a patented proprietary blend of magnolia, which it originally intended to market solely as a stress reliever. Magnolia bark has traditionally been used as a general anti-anxiety agent, so its benefits typically center on controlling stress and anxiety. But newer claims are emerging that link magnolia's anti-stress benefits with control of cortisol. Magnolia bark is rich in two biphenol compounds, magno-lol and honokiol, which are thought to contribute to the primary anti-stress and cortisol-lowering effects of the plant. These corti-sol-lowering effects go beyond stress relief though, as Next researchers discovered when testing their proprietary extract.

During one study on this blend, they found they were consistently getting feedback not only on reduced anxiety but participants also reported that they had improved sleep. So Next switched gears and developed its magnolia extract as a sleep aid, adding ziziphus—which has been used to induce sleep in traditional Chinese medicine for over 2,000 years—to the mix.

This past August, the results of a small trial on Seditol conducted by an independent research facility in New York showed some impressive results. Participants were asked to try Seditol for 14 days as a nightly supplement. Ultimately, this study highlighted the importance of taking Seditol regularly as a supplement. In other words, Seditol isn't a pill you pop for occasional help with sleeping. Instead, it is a long-term solution to a specific cause of sleeplessness—excess cortisol. The subjects that took Seditol as directed reported the following encouraging results:

- 87 percent said Seditol reduced the fatigue they felt as a result of lack of sleep

- 83 percent said Seditol helped ensure a sound night's sleep

This product's action may be slower than typical over-the-counter sleep aids, but the end result is a natural, gradual change.

The suggested dosage is 365 mg nightly, and you should notice results in one to two weeks, as your cortisol level normalizes.

Seditol is available through various supplement retailers. Check your local health food store to see if they carry it.

Despite bad press, tryptophan is available and safe

One of the key brain chemicals required for sleep is serotonin. Serotonin is produced in the brain by the essential amino acid tryptophan.

So if you're not getting enough tryptophan, you're not making enough serotonin, and odds are, you're not getting enough quality sleep.

You might remember the big scare 15 years ago when tryptophan was linked to an outbreak of eosinophilia myalgia syndrome (EMS), a serious illness characterized by symptoms like muscular and abdominal pain, weakness, mouth ulcers, and skin rash. The FDA enforced an involuntary recall that made splashy headlines, created a panic, and bankrupted many tryptophan suppliers. The fact that the outbreak was later traced to a contaminated batch from a single manufacturer failed to make the same headlines as the original allegations. As a result, many consumers were deprived of tryptophan, despite years of use by millions without incident.

Due to the bad press surrounding the recall, most supplement manufacturers have shied away from producing tryptophan. Even though the FDA never officially banned it, there are very strict guidelines manufacturers must adhere to in order to make and distribute tryptophan. It's a challenge many companies just aren't willing to be subjected to.

But we found one supplier with a tryptophan product, L-Tryptophan, that does meet those purity requirements. In fact, even though it's an oral supplement, it also meets the standards for pharmaceutical-grade intravenous medications. These guidelines are even stricter than those set up for oral medications. You can get this particular tryptophan formula from a company called Vitamin Research Products. For more information, check out the Member Source Directory on page 529.

Absorption of tryptophan is optimized when you take it at least 20 minutes before meals that contain protein or apart from protein completely.[2]

If you're taking prescription antidepressants be sure to consult a physician before trying tryptophan. Like SSRIs, tryptophan also increases the production of serotonin, so combining the two could cause problems.

Reverse age-related sleeplessness and rediscover youthful rest

Now, back to what I was saying earlier about sleep and anti-aging. Researchers say that, particularly for older adults, a good night's sleep may be a natural form of hormone therapy, which has long been touted for its anti-aging benefits.

One study of 149 men ages 16 to 83 found that age-related changes in sleep quality were linked to specific changes in several hormones. As sleep quality and quantity declined, levels of cortisol increased.

In later years, a new sleep pattern emerges in which men get less sleep overall and levels of cortisol go up. These sleep-pattern changes accompany some negative changes in other hormonal activity. Lead researcher Dr. Eve Van Cauter of the University of Chicago concluded that these connections between hormones and shifting sleep patterns suggest that maintaining sleep quality throughout life may have important health benefits.[3,4]

This particular study didn't elaborate on those benefits, but you already know that waking up after a good night's sleep can go a long way in helping you feel better physically and emotionally. And now that this evidence points to rising cortisol levels as the main culprit behind increasing instances of insomnia, it's nice to know that there are some simple, safe, all-natural options for reversing this aspect of aging.

CHAPTER THREE

Harness the power of "young blood" with this Chinese herbal rejuvenator

Mr. Lee walked into Dr. Dexin Yan's office because he was out of options. At only 45 years old, he had been experiencing memory loss, muddled thinking, high blood pressure and cholesterol levels, dizziness, chest pains, buzzing in his ears, numbness in his arms and legs, and purple lips. Five years of prescription drugs had only made his problems worse. Dr. Yan specialized in treating blood and circulatory disorders and was gaining a reputation for his success with difficult cases like Mr. Lee's.

Mr. Lee's blood pressure was 180/110, his pulse was weak, and blood samples showed that his triglycerides were frighteningly high at 1,150 (the normal level is less than 150). Dr. Yan prescribed a specialized herbal formula he'd developed called Vital Cell.

After just 45 days, Mr. Lee reported that all of his previous complaints and symptoms had improved. And the numbers showed it: His blood pressure fell to 170/90, and his triglycerides dropped almost 900 points (to 253).

Teaching old blood cells new tricks

Vital Cell heals the body by going straight to the source of so many aches and pains—the blood. Combining modern science with China's rich herbal tradition, Dr. Yan's groundbreaking formula has helped thousands of patients recover their health and energy by reconditioning blood cells and improving circulation to levels normally seen only in the very young.

When you hear someone mention circulation, you probably think of the heart and major arteries—and for good reason. Circulatory disorders, such as hypertension (high blood pressure) and atherosclerosis (hardening of the arteries) are major risk factors for heart disease, heart attacks, and strokes. But there's more to it than that. With all the attention on the heart and arteries, it's easy to overlook serious health problems affecting the smallest components of the circulatory system—microscopic blood vessels called microcapillaries, where the critical exchange of oxygen and nutrients actually takes place. If blood isn't flowing through this web properly, it can trigger all sorts of health problems—many of which may not seem related to circulation at all.

A number of factors contribute to poor circulation as we age. Arteries and veins become stiff and congested as cholesterol and calcium plaques accumulate and restrict blood flow. Spasms in the smooth muscles surrounding the circulatory arteries and veins can also choke off circulation. These same processes also occur in our microcapillaries, reducing microcirculation and impairing the critical exchange of nutrients and gases in tissues and major organs.

This problem only gets worse as we get older because of changes in the composition and structure of blood cells. As you reach middle age, the blood starts to thicken and congeal as platelets and blood proteins make cells sticky. Plus, the spleen, the organ responsible for removing old, damaged blood cells from circulation, begins to slow down with age, which means new, healthy blood cells are replaced at a sharply reduced rate. And to make matters even worse, as blood cells age, they become stiff and no longer appear round and evenly shaped. This makes it harder for them to pass smoothly through the capillaries. In fact, the angular, jagged shape of the old cells can damage the fragile microcapillaries even further.

Eventually, these age-related changes take their toll on the micro-capillaries, reducing circulation to the tissues and blocking the flow of nutrients and oxygen. Removal of carbon dioxide and other metabolic waste products is also hindered. This leads to a slow build-up of metabolic garbage that can gradually bury the cells in their own waste products. In time, the cells, poisoned by their own metabolic byproducts, begin to waste away and ultimately cease to function altogether.

The combined effect of poor circulation and old blood contributes to a host of symptoms, including deep fatigue, fuzzy thinking, frequent infections, and lowered sex drive—all conditions usually considered just "normal parts of aging." If circulation doesn't improve, it can lead to more serious conditions, such as high blood pressure, heart attacks, strokes, diabetes, and arthritis. But giving your body a fresh supply of healthy blood may target all of these problems and more.

The connection between blood and aging

As a professor and physician, Dr. Yan had received extensive training in both Western and traditional Chinese medicine (TCM). And in Chinese medicine "blood stagnation" is considered to be the primary underlying cause of many conditions characterized by pain. When blood stagnation occurs, the body's internal organs don't receive their normal nutrients, and waste products aren't carried away at a sufficient rate. This stops the organs from performing their functions, resulting in weakness, disease, and aging.

Dr. Yan recognized that the Chinese view of blood stagnation had a strong corollary in Western medicine—especially in the case of diabetes. In diabetes, chronically elevated blood sugar levels damage the microcapillaries and impair blood flow to the retinas, kidneys, and peripheral nerves. Eventually, that can lead to blindness, kidney damage, and potential amputation of limbs.

Basically, diabetes can be thought of as a sped-up form of the typical aging process in the way it relates to blood composition and circulatory disorders.

Noting the similar role circulation plays in aging and in diseases like diabetes led Dr. Yan to theorize that many of the health problems he observed in his older patients might be caused by poor circulation and underlying blood disorders. He believed these problems were damaging vital tissues and organs, just like the damage seen in advanced cases of diabetes.

Dr. Yan joined with other leading medical researchers at the Shanghai Medical Hospital to form a new research team called the Blood Stasis and Aging Research Group. The research group gathered blood samples from both young and elderly volunteers for evaluation. They quickly noticed that blood samples from young adults were thinner and had a brighter red color than the samples from the older adults. Intrigued by this simple visual correlation between blood stagnation and aging, the researchers wanted to test the beneficial effects of a number of natural herbs on blood and microcapillary function.

After eight years of gathering clinical data on microcirculation and evaluating changes in blood flow, Dr. Yan's team arrived at a formula made up of 10 powerful herbs that were shown to restore healthy circulation.

Vital Cell contains astragalus, Atractylodes, San-Qi ginseng, dong-quai, safflower, southern Tsangshu, Lycium Chinense, Codonopsis, red-rooted sage, and Chinese licorice. In addition to their circulation-boosting effects, the ingredients in Vital Cell also support endocrine and central nervous system function and enhance protein metabolism.

By enhancing circulation, nourishing cells, and eliminating waste products, Vital Cell contributes to overall improvements in memory, energy, and health while preventing the onset of a wide range of age-related illnesses.

The key to younger tissues

After numerous animal studies established the safety of the formula, researchers measured the actual effects of Vital Cell on the health of various organ tissues in two groups of 10 rabbits. One group of 10 rabbits received normal food, while the other 10 received food that had been supplemented with Vital Cell. After two years, the researchers gathered tissue samples from the rabbits. They also prepared tissue samples gathered from six-month-old rabbits of the same breed.

The researchers examined samples of tissues from the thymus glands, hearts, lungs, livers, kidneys, spleens, brains, and sex organs. The untreated animals showed all the typical signs of aging: Blood vessel walls were thick, clogged and streaked with plaque, while liver cells were shrunken, misshapen, and full of clotted blood. Sex organs were shriveled and had poor cell structure, and kidney cells were ruptured, essentially reduced to mush.

On the other hand, the animals that had been given Vital Cell barely showed any signs of aging at all. In fact, when the researchers compared the treated rabbits with the young ones, there was virtually no difference between them.

The most notable improvement was in the thymus gland. This gland is the key regulator of the immune system. It usually shrinks dramatically with age, and the loss of thymic tissue is thought to be one of the main reasons for the loss of immune function in the elderly. When the researchers looked at the thymus glands of the old, untreated animals, the signs of aging were clear. They had shrunk to less than one third of the size of the younger animals' glands, and most of the tissue had been replaced with connective tissue and fat cells. By comparison, the thymus glands of the old animals treated with Vital Cell were twice the size of the untreated animals' glands, and the tissue was identical to that in the young animals, with no loss to fatty infiltration or connective tissues.

You <u>can</u> slow down the aging process

With such impressive results in rabbits, the researchers moved on to humans. In the first study, 50 volunteers, ages 50 to 77, received Vital Cell for 30 days, with blood samples gathered at the beginning and end of the test period. Researchers found that Vital Cell had essentially reconditioned the volunteers' blood, restoring its properties to those usually seen in adults in their mid-20s.

A second study showed dramatic improvement in circulation in even the smallest vessels of the body—all the way to the fingernails.

After studying the effects of Vital Cell on elderly patients with circulatory problems, the study authors commented, "From the results reported here, it appears that the Vital Cell formula is not only capable of possibly slowing the aging process, but may also exert beneficial effects on disorders that involve the blood."

In the largest test conducted with Vital Cell, Dr. Yan's team enrolled 150 patients in a clinical study. The test subjects, ranging in age from 55 to 89, each took Vital Cell for one month. At the end of the trial the researchers found significant improvements in many common symptoms of aging, such as the following:

- chest pains
- heart palpitations
- coughing
- shortness of breath
- dizziness
- swelling of the legs and feet
- lack of appetite
- poor mood
- poor skin complexion
- high blood pressure

- decreased capillary microcirculation

- suppressed immunity

The study results indicated that Vital Cell can expand arteries in the brain and lungs, raise T-cell immunity, and promote the synthesis and metabolism of proteins.

The researchers concluded that Vital Cell would offer significant benefits for elderly patients—even those recovering from serious illnesses like coronary heart disease and chronic bronchitis.

Clinical results in the real world

In 1989, after eight years of clinical study on Vital Cell, Dr. Yan was honored at the International Symposium on Geriatrics in Shanghai for his groundbreaking research. Around the same time, Dr. Yan began prescribing his formula to patients across China. Mr. Lee, whom I mentioned earlier, was among those patients, but there are thousands more who have experienced some impressive results.

Some of Dr. Yan's case studies that our contacts at Tango Advanced Nutrition gave us show the wide range of conditions users say Vital Cell has been shown to benefit.

Mr. B., 45, had suffered from debilitating daily headaches for 10 years as a result of severe head injuries he'd suffered in a car accident. By the time Mr. B. went to Dr. Yan, he was taking prescription sedatives three times a day to control his pain. Dr. Yan prescribed Vital Cell and slowly weaned Mr. B. off all sedatives over a three-week period. As his pain subsided, Mr. B. continued to take Vital Cell. After three months he reported that his headaches were gone and that he was pain-free for the first time since his accident.

Mr. W., 37, suffered from severe arterial inflammation and blood clots in his lower right leg, which would occasionally cause him to be paralyzed from the waist down. Even though he sought medical help from many physicians, his condition only got worse. Eventually his toes turned purple and were cold to the touch. After taking Vital Cell for four weeks, Mr. W. reported that his symptoms had disappeared and that he was able to return to work for the first time in a decade.

Mr. C., 68, was admitted to the hospital because of severe chest pain due to advanced atherosclerosis. He was treated with both traditional Chinese and Western medicines, but his pain continued. As Mr. C's condition worsened, Dr. Yan began to administer Vital Cell. Only three days later, Mr. C. reported that his chest pain and the other symptoms had eased. After three months of taking Vital Cell, all of his symptoms disappeared. And for the last five years, he has shown no further sign of illness or symptoms of heart disease.

Mr. Y., 74, suffered from serious cognitive decline. As his condition worsened, he became anxious and confused, and he couldn't sleep. He would forget conversations, dates, places, and names. His gait was unsteady, and he had frequent falls. The family had tried Western medicines but hadn't gotten good results and hoped that traditional Chinese medicine could restore his health. When Dr. Yan first saw him, the patient was absent-minded and talked nonsense to himself. His pulse was weak, his breathing was shallow, and tests revealed that impaired circulation was making his dementia worse. But less than a month after he started taking Vital Cell, all his symptoms disappeared, and he was able to take care of himself again.

Breaking study reveals the power of "young blood"

New research is continuing to uncover the potential healing effects of healthy blood. In fact, 25 years after Dr. Yan began his research, a new study has shown that blood may hold the key to the entire aging process.

The study, published in the Feb. 17, 2005, issue of Nature, reveals that young blood may be the key to health and longevity. In the study, led by Thomas Rando, M.D., Ph.D., associate professor of neurology at the Stanford University School of Medicine, researchers studied specialized stem cells called satellite cells, which are found spread throughout muscle tissue. Satellite cells normally lie dormant until muscle tissues are injured. Then they suddenly come to life and begin building new muscle cells to repair the damage. In older people, these cells are still present, but they don't respond when muscle cells are damaged.

Rando and his group attached old mice to younger ones in a way that allowed the two mice to share a blood supply. Then they induced muscle damage in the older mice. To their amazement, the satellite cells in the old mice suddenly came to life in the presence of the younger blood, and the damaged muscles healed normally. In contrast, when the young mice were injured in the presence of the old blood, their satellite cells failed to respond, and the muscle cells didn't heal.

The group also examined the livers of older mice connected to their younger lab-mates. The cells that help liver tissue regenerate are less active in older animals, but again, the cells responded more efficiently when the livers in older mice were exposed to the younger blood. Clearly, something in the youthful blood was reviving the regenerative cells in the older mice's muscles and livers.

Rondo observed that "We need to consider the possibility that the niche in which stem cells sit (blood) is as important in terms of stem cell aging as the cells themselves."

In other words, it may be the health of the blood surrounding the cells, rather than the cells themselves, that lies at the center of human aging. That means that keeping your blood young and healthy may keep you young and healthy at the same time.

The Chinese anti-aging secret now available in the U.S.

Until recently, Vital Cell was only available in China. Now it's available through limited sources in the United States.

Based on the study results, Vital Cell appears to be mild and non-toxic and may be taken for extended periods of time with virtually no side effects. The recommended dosage is one tablet three times a day.

CHAPTER FOUR

Single formula unlocks the 4 strongest secret weapons of a life-extending diet

The Mediterranean diet has gained nearly universal acceptance as the world's healthiest. Based on centuries of observation, not to mention a truckload of modern research, it's an undisputable fact that people who live in the Mediterranean area and follow the diet have one of the highest life expectancies in the world. This longevity is due at least in part to the remarkably low rates of coronary heart disease, certain cancers, and many other potentially life-threatening diseases residents of this area experience.

But you don't have to completely change the way you eat—or move to the Mediterranean—to receive the health benefits of this diet, including a longer life. In fact, it could be as easy as taking two pills a day.

Although olive oil may be the most famous aspect of the Mediterranean diet, it turns out there are four other elements that are actually more powerful when it comes to promoting good health. Dr. Arnold J. Susser from Great Life Labs took those four elements and put them all in one formula called Botanical Vitality 200+.

These ingredients have been shown to lower blood pressure and cholesterol and to protect against premature aging, Alzheimer's, heart disease, and cancer—just to name a few of the benefits. And two ingredients in particular—red grapes and pomegranates—contain what Susser refers to as "miracle-like molecules."

Uncorking the secret to longevity

The French put their own spin on the Mediterranean diet with what is known as the French paradox—the whole "eat, drink, and be healthy" concept. The French eat a notoriously fatty diet, yet they have an extremely low rate of heart disease. In 1992, investigative scientists found out why. The secret is in the wine.

Studies show that people who drink wine regularly have lower rates of cancer, Alzheimer's, and heart disease.[1] The true benefits of red wine, though, don't come from the alcohol, but from the grapes themselves. Resveratrol, one of the miracle molecules in Botanical Vitality, is a strong antioxidant found in red grapes. Research has shown resveratrol to have a wide variety of benefits:

- **It's good for your heart**. It inhibits blood clotting and helps to prevent bad cholesterol from depositing plaque into the arteries, two of the main problems that lead to heart disease.[2]

- **It promotes balanced hormones**. As a phytoestrogen, resveratrol has all the benefits of estrogen without the harmful effects. As such, it can help prevent diseases like breast cancer, prostate cancer, osteoporosis, and cardiovascular disease.[3]

- **It's an anti-inflammatory** and appears to be a safe, natural COX-2 inhibitor.[4]

- **It has antiaging effects**. Resveratrol has the ability to "turn on" a family of survival genes called sirtuins. When sirtuins are activated, there is an increase in the production of an enzyme that prolongs the time a living cell has to repair DNA genetic material.[5]

Although there hasn't been a study on humans, researchers introduced resveratrol to various plants and animals and found that it tricked each organism into switching on its anti-aging sirtuin gene. Doing so caused the organism's cells to live an average of 70 percent longer.[6]

Heart-healthy benefits that are skin-deep

Another benefit of red grapes is found in the substance that gives all dark colored berries and grapes their color, anthocyanins. Red grapes and mulberries are full of these potent antioxidants. Anthocyanins are extremely powerful protectors of your arteries—stronger than even vitamins C and E. They work by preventing the plaque buildup on your artery walls that can lead to heart disease.[7]

According to Dr. Susser, "Because anthocyanins are vasoprotective, particularly in the microcapillaries, they are valuable to people with circulation-related diseases such as diabetic retinopathy, macular degeneration, cataracts, glaucoma, and varicose veins."[8]

The anthocyanins in red grapes and mulberries could also help treat arthritis and other degenerative joint conditions because of their anti-inflammatory properties.[9]

Power-packed pomegranates

Studies continue to reveal the healing potential of pomegranates. They are a powerful source of antioxidants, they help lower bad cholesterol, they help lower high blood pressure, and they help fight against cancer. In fact, they are even more powerful than green tea and blueberry, cranberry, and orange juices.[10]

One study, published by the European Atherosclerosis Society, showed that after two weeks of consuming pomegranate juice, patients with high blood pressure reported a 5 percent drop in systolic blood pressure, thanks to a 36 percent reduction in angiotensin converting enzyme (ACE). This allows the blood vessels to relax, which lowers blood pressure, increases the supply of blood and oxygen to the heart, and reduces strain on sensitive blood vessels in the brain, heart, and kidneys.[11]

A study published in the June 2004 issue of *Clinical Nutrition* involved patients with carotid artery stenosis, a pre-stroke condition marked by lack of blood flow to the brain due to clogging of the carotid artery. After one year of daily pomegranate juice supplementation, carotid artery swelling went down by as much as 30 percent. Antioxidants increased by 130 percent, and systolic blood pressure was reduced by 21 percent.[12]

The specific "miracle molecules" in pomegranate extract are called hydroxylated polyphenols (which break down into polyphenols and ellagic acid). As Dr. Susser explained, "Hydroxylated polyphenols have shown great promise as powerful antioxidants helping to protect us against premature aging associated with free radical damage."

Ellagic acid has been shown to be effective in both treating and preventing cancer. It treats cancer by binding to carcinogens and initiating apoptosis (programmed cell death). It prevents the disease by binding to healthy DNA and acting as a shield against attacks from carcinogens.[13] Studies show that ellagic acid is even effective in people who are genetically predisposed to the disease.[14]

In addition to fighting cancer, hydroxylated polyphenols also help protect against premature aging by helping fight free radical damage and by preventing the oxidation of bad cholesterol.[15]

Every little bit helps

The remaining compounds in Botanical Vitality all have unique benefits of their own. Quercetin, an additional antioxidant found in red grape skins, has also demonstrated a broad range of therapeutic activity—from antihistamine to anti-inflammatory properties. As an antioxidant, it protects from damage caused by the effects of bad cholesterol. Quercetin is also considered to be a phytoestrogen and was found to inhibit breast cancer cells in one study.[16]

Soy lecithin, an extract from soybean oil, reduces the amount of pure cholesterol in the bloodstream. It's also an essential source of choline, one of the main components of all membranes.[17]

Finally, phytic acid, which comes from rice bran extract, is a natural plant antioxidant. Research has shown that it is the most potent natural iron chelator and that it has strong antibiotic and antioxidant effects. This also makes it anticarcinogenic.[18]

Support for the long haul

Botanical Vitality 200+ decreases arterial plaque buildup, supports healthy circulation allowing better utilization of nutrients for increased energy, supports healthy blood pressure and cholesterol levels, and reduces oxidative damage. With all of these healthful benefits, it is not hard to imagine that it could help you add a few extra years to your life.

If you decide to try Botanical Vitality 200+, you can expect to notice results within one month. Although results do vary, many people say they experience increased mental clarity and an increased energy level.

There are no reported safety issues or contraindications with Botanical Vitality 200+. Recommended dosage is two capsules daily. Susser also encourages you to show the product label to your physician and to always maintain regular medical care if you have a medical condition or are taking any medications.

To find out more about Dr. Susser and Botanical Vitality, go to his website, www.drsusser.com or visit www.greatlife.com.

CHAPTER FIVE

Shrinking that spare tire has never been easier

It seems impossible, doesn't it? Because no matter how much time you spend at the gym or how many dry salads you choke down, it's **still** there. Abdominal fat is the hardest fat to get rid of.

Well, it *was*. Until now.

Participants in a recent 12-week trial whittled their waistlines and shed pounds—while the control group actually gained weight.

The best part? Nobody in the study counted a single calorie!

Because they were taking the <u>first natural product of its kind</u> proven to *shrink* the "impossible-to-lose" visceral fat that builds up in your belly. It's clinically proven to reduce waist circumference and abdominal fat.

We all know that's good for your vanity. But more and more scientists are starting to agree—shrinking that spare tire could actually *save your life*.

Even at a normal weight, hidden fat could kill you

Metabolic Syndrome is a pretty new idea—so new, you might not yet have heard of it. It's a condition in which blood lipids, blood glucose, and blood pressure are poorly controlled. And it's gaining recognition as a major indicator of some pretty frightening diseases. Coronary artery disease, heart attack, diabetes, stroke—even cancer.

It turns out; the strongest indicator of metabolic disease is visceral fat. Not total body fat—I'm talking about the deep body fat that collects around the vital organs in your abdomen, resulting in a large waist circumference (that "spare tire").

Even normal-weight women with increased visceral fat have increased blood pressure, insulin, triglycerides, free fatty acids, oxidized LDL, petin, and increases in inflammatory and cardio disease risk factors.

A study of 387 normal-weight people showed that men with waists measuring 40 inches double their risk of dying prematurely, and women with waists measuring 35 inches were 79 percent more likely to die than women with 28-inch waists.

Brand new research adds another frightening effect to the list. Previous studies have suggested that people with diabetes have a 1.5 times higher chance of experiencing dementia than people who don't have diabetes. In this study, people with high blood sugar performed poorly in three cognitive tasks. Researchers concluded that higher blood sugar levels are associated with lower cognitive function.[1]

Researchers first recognized the link between visceral fat and Metabolic Syndrome when, in a preliminary study, visceral fat was surgically removed from aging rodents. The rats' insulin levels were reduced to those of young rats. There were dramatic results even with rats genetically predisposed to develop diabetes—removing visceral fat delayed the onset.

There is good news—even **modest** reductions in visceral fat can help reverse the effects of Metabolic Syndrome. Vitamin Research Products (VRP) has the solution with a new supplement over 10 years in the making. It's called Glabrinex, and it's proven to shrink that spare tire.

No more belly fat—break it down before it has a chance to collect

Researchers at VRP screened hundreds of food ingredients before finding the perfect one for Glabrinex. And so, out of something that's been consumed for over 4,000 years—black licorice—comes the latest and greatest in the battle of the bulge.

Licorice root contains a flavonoid called glabridin. In addition to containing antioxidants and demonstrating blood-sugar-lowering properties, it's this flavonoid that's been shown to decrease deadly visceral fat.

It does this in several ways. Glabridin increases the activity of enzymes responsible for the breakdown of fat tissue. It also stimulates the metabolism of fatty acids in the liver—effectively increasing your body's fat-burning ability.

It lowers the level of plasma and liver triglycerides—the main constituents of fat. This puts the brakes on your body's fat-forming process. As if this weren't enough, it also produces a positive signaling effect on DNA, changing the way visceral fat cells mature.

Animal studies and human clinical trials have both demonstrated that glabridin can reduce the amount of visceral fat, helping to eliminate the biggest cause of Metabolic Syndrome.

Banish that impossible-to-lose fat without a single sit-up

In several studies on both animals and humans, the effects have been stunning. Glabridin has been proven to:

- reduce body weight
- reduce waist circumference

- reduce abdominal fat

- help control blood glucose

- suppress the formation of visceral fat and shrink visceral fat deposits

In one study, obese rats fed a high-fat diet were treated with licorice-root extract. Even on that high-fat diet, the extract significantly decreased the weight of the rats' abdominal fat tissue.[2]

A similar study, in which diabetic mice were fed a high-fat diet, further demonstrated the extract's effect on fat. It significantly decreased body-weight gain, weight of abdominal fat tissue, and blood sugar levels as compared with the control group.[3]

Yet another study on obese mice fed a high-fat diet took it a bit further—glabridin actually shrank abdominal fat cells and improved the fatty state of liver cells.[4]

In one human trial, researchers found that 900 mg of glabridin per day resulted in significant decreases in body weight and body mass index (BMI) after just four weeks. Patients on 900 mg per day also lost visceral fat after eight weeks.

While results were most impressive at 900 mg, that same test showed significant decreases in fat mass when patients took 300, 600, or 900 mg per day.

Another clinical trial demonstrated the effectiveness of glabridin at 300 mg per day. All subjects in the trial were moderately overweight, with BMIs between 24 and 30 (the designation of "overweight" is 25-29.9).

Subjects on a placebo gained weight—an average of over 2 pounds per week—while those taking glabridin lost weight. Interestingly enough, the study was conducted during the Thanksgiving and Christmas season—and participants weren't required to change their eating habits. They also weren't required to exercise.

Over the course of 12 weeks, over a quarter of the participants taking glabridin lost 2 pounds or more. Their BMIs were also significantly reduced.

Researchers determined that the change in participants' body weight was specifically due to a reduction in body fat. Though glabridin showed impressive effect without any lifestyle changes, researchers speculate that it could be even more effective when paired with mild dietary restriction and/or physical activity.[5]

The flavonoid has also been shown to exhibit direct anti-inflammatory activity and cardiovascular protective functions. Additionally, it inhibits the re-uptake of serotonin, so it may help combat mild to moderate depression.

Clinical safety testing proved that Glabrinex is safe even up to 1200 mg/day.[6] If you want to take the 900 mg per day I mentioned above, the chief science officer at VRP recommends taking four soft gels before breakfast and five before dinner. Of course, you can stick to taking the suggested dose of 300 mg per day, since that was proven effective.

Get ready to start tightening that belt

The chief science officer at VRP is a Glabrinex user himself—he's seen results taking 300mg/day. I heard about another man who started seeing results after six weeks on 300mg/day. After eight weeks, he had dropped 10 percent of his body fat and one belt notch. Since then, he's taken the belt down another notch!

Glabrinex is not a quick-loss diet pill. It's about changing your body composition, finally getting rid of the deep-seated visceral fat that puts your life at risk. This might result in only a 5-10 percent loss of body weight, but will do wonders for your health.

Ordering information for Glabrinex is in the Member Source Directory on page 529.

CHAPTER SIX

Ancient apple takes anti-aging technology into the future

"It's visibly erasing my crow's feet, and there were no bags under my eyes when I woke up. And it worked so fast—I saw a noticeable difference within the first week… and it wasn't even a regular week, I was traveling, which usually makes my eyes worse."

That glowing endorsement comes from Jenny T…. and she isn't easy to impress with new products. Still, she bought this revolutionary anti-aging product as soon as I told her about it. "I really love this product," she told me. "I ordered more last night."

With the hundreds of anti-aging beauty products on the market—ranging in price from dime store to diamond ring—it takes something pretty special to interest HSI. And the CSI (Cosmeceutical Sciences Institute) line has just that: a wide range of products with scientifically proven ingredients—including an extremely rare, natural wrinkle eraser that plays a starring role in CSI Anti-Aging Fruit Stem Cell Serum—the very product that Jenny was raving about.

Believe it or not, this anti-aging wonder serum all starts with a Swiss apple with incredible anti-aging properties. And this now-rare apple—there are only three trees remaining—brings us one of the most powerful wrinkle removers ever seen outside of the operating room.

The Uttwiler Spätlauber apple tree was cultivated a few hundred years ago because of the amazingly long storage properties of its apples—a very important issue back before they had refrigerators. Sure, the apples didn't taste great, but they remained fresh and vibrant and unwrinkled months longer than other apples did.

When modern scientists tried to figure out what kept these rare fruits fresh, they stumbled upon their secret: especially long-living stem cells.

Everything starts with stem cells. And, basically, stem cells have two major functions: They can replenish and renew themselves (repairing injured tissue, for example), and they can generate differentiated cells (meaning they start out as blank slates, and can become any kind of cell necessary).

Your skin, being the largest organ in your body, has special stem cell needs. That's because skin cells shed constantly, and need to be replenished continuously. But as we age, that turnover process slows down. When that happens, skin cells die off more quickly than they can be replaced... and that can make your skin start to look older, fast.

Enter Mibelle Biochemistry—a company that found natural way to make your skin look years younger. Their scientists created a unique technology that revolves around plant stem cells—a technology that's been shown to have exciting applications for more beautiful, younger looking skin. And that's where the Uttwiler Spätlauber comes in.

Rare Swiss apple extract visibly reduces crows feet—by 15 percent—in just 28 days

The secret to cell longevity appeared to be hidden in the extraordinarily long-lasting—but rare—Uttwiler Spätlauber apple. So scientists came up with a way to take a tiny stem cell sample from the plant, and

Avoid The Paraben Problem with CSI Products

Most of the personal care products available today—from anti-aging skincare products to underarm deodorants—contain powerful antimicrobial preservatives called parabens. In theory, this is a good thing, as these preservatives help keep products from spoiling and becoming contaminated. But they come with a very big downside: cancer.

A few years ago, a group of British researchers found that 18 out of 20 breast cancer tumours contained intact parabens. What does that mean? The researchers believed that the parabens didn't get there through the digestive system where they would have been broken down, but instead were absorbed directly into the skin in their original form. Basically, they entered with full-strength, causing maximum damage.

Luckily, parabens are very easy to spot in ingredients labels… and therefore very easy to avoid. The most commonly used forms are:

- Methylparaben
- Ethylparaben
- p-Propylparaben
- Isobutylparaben
- n-Butylparaben
- Benzylparaben

At least they aren't cleverly disguised names that would make them nearly impossible for consumers to detect!

You'll find these potentially toxic chemicals in literally hundreds of skincare products, from drugstore brands (like Olay Regeneriste) to high-end and department store brands (like Estee Lauder).But you won't find them in any CSI products—not now, not ever.

grow more in the lab.

The researchers at Mibelle used that process with this apple—and they set out to prove their theory that this unique fruit extract could produce an anti-aging effect on human cells.

When Mibelle Biochemistry tested their PhytoCellTec™ Malus Domestica cream against crow's feet, the results were simply beautiful. During the four-week trial, the 20 subjects saw their wrinkles begin to fade away after applying the cream just twice a day to their crow's feet.

And while the difference was visibly noticeable to the participants, it was also scientifically measured using the PRIMOS system (a standardized three-dimensional, high-resolution method used for measuring wrinkle depth). After just two weeks, wrinkle depth was reduced by 8 percent... and by the end of the study—just 28 days—wrinkle depth decreased by a full 15 percent.

In addition to that, the cream was shown to boost human stem cell production *in vitro*. In the lab, PhytoCellTec™ Malus Domestica was added to a culture of human stem cells (derived from umbilical cords), and the number of stem cells increased by 80 percent. Not only that, adding the apple extract also appeared to protect those stem cells from ultraviolet (UV) light.

The researchers decided to test the extract's protection factor to see just how well it could shield your skin. So they hit the cultured stem cells with UV light, just like your skin gets exposed to it every time you go outside. The cells in plain growth medium (the control cells) didn't fare so well—almost half of them died.

But the protected cells, the ones shielded by fruit extract, experienced only a miniscule loss... less than 10 percent. The researchers conclusion: PhytoCellTec Malus Domestica appears to protect stem cells from damaging UV light.

In addition to the apple stem cell cultures, CSI Anti-Aging Fruit Stem Cell Serum contains hyaluronic acid and chondrus crispus extract (from seaweed)—both of which bring their own unique skin-beautifying properties to the formula.

Hyaluronic acid brings more wrinkle-reducing power to the serum

Hyaluronic acid (HA) may be now be a staple among anti-aging creams, but it wasn't nearly so common when HSI first wrote about it back in 2002. Since then, HA has become a shining star in the anti-aging industry, backed by an impressive body of evidence.

It's really no surprise that many anti-aging compounds contain this crucial skin-smoothing ingredient. HA is a naturally-occurring chemical in your body—with more than half of that supply (56 percent to be exact) found in your skin. And one of its main functions is to keep your skin hydrated and supple.

But as we age, our HA stores decline... so much that by age 60, many of us have none left in our skin at all! Luckily, applying HA to your skin can make up for that loss. It can help your skin retain more moisture, improving elasticity and helping diminish the formation of wrinkles... perhaps even minimizing their appearance.

Specifically, HA keeps moisture in your skin, and acts as a lubricant between your skin's connective tissues. Your natural supply dwindles with as you get older, though, and that can contribute to the visible signs of aging. But simply applying HA to your skin topically can make all the difference—and there's plenty of science to prove it.

- One study found that HA helps your skin retain the perfect amount of water in its connective tissue, improving your skin's elasticity (and loss of elasticity is a major contributor to the appearance of wrinkles)

- Another study found that most people lose ALL of the natural

HA in their skin by age 60, and that may explain the outward signs of aging (like wrinkles and sagging skin)

- Anecdotal evidence shows that topically applied HA may slow down premature skin aging, including damage that's caused by UV radiation

The HA adds another dimension of wrinkle-reduction to the formula, along with a generous helping of added moisture for your skin. But the serum's benefits don't end there…

Chondrus crispus brings power-packed nutrients to the formula

Chondrus crispus is a red seaweed that is found exclusively in the waters off the Atlantic coast. Also known as Irish sea moss, Carragheen, and Pearl moss, this briny ocean delicacy comes jam-packed with vitamins, minerals, and amino acids—all of which can benefit your skin.

This nutrient-rich seaweed can help nourish your skin with its wide variety of healthful constituents, including an abundance of beneficial mineral salts:

- iodine
- iron
- manganese
- phosphorous
- sodium
- zinc
- mucilage
- amino acids
- vitamin K
- vitamin B2
- bromine
- calcium
- magnesium
- potassium
- copper
- selenium
- carrageenans
- beta carotene
- folic acid

Chondrus crispus extract is very versatile, and it's used in a broad range of products, from creamy foods (like puddings and yogurts) to facial moisturizers and eye gels. It acts as a thickening agent, giving anti-aging potions their creamy textures, and quite a bit more. It can help moisturize and soften your skin, and it's gentle enough to apply to the sensitive area around your eyes without causing irritation... unlike cheaper, synthetic thickeners used in lower-quality products.

The seaweed extract used in CSI Anti-Aging Fruit Stem Cell Serum is specially designed to contain substantially more seaweed than water, maximizing the nutrient content... which means more nourishment for your skin. And the natural pH of the extract also minimizes the risk of irritation.

This skin-smoothing (and soothing) combination of ingredients comes together to bring you more radiant, younger-looking skin... and fewer wrinkles. By simply applying a tiny amount of this serum to your skin just twice daily, you can get rid of wrinkles around your eyes—and help combat the clock by helping protect the longevity of your skin's stem cells.

CSI Anti-Aging Fruit Stem Cell Serum is just one of the high-quality natural anti-aging products in the CSI line, a collection of cosmetics that offers some very distinct advantages—not the least of which is affordability. The products are formulated with the highest-quality ingredients, contain no synthetic preservatives, artificial colors or fragrances. These cosmetics are also 100 percent paraben-free, which (as explained in the sidebar above) may help you avoid a higher risk of certain types of cancer.

Ordering information for CSI Anti-Aging Fruit Stem Cell Serum is in the Member Source Directory on page 529.

CHAPTER SEVEN

Who wouldn't want 52 percent more energy: What the "Goldilocks Effect" can do for fatigue and your immune system

W e wade through so much dense science every day that when someone came to us recently and wanted to talk about Goldilocks, it was a welcome change of pace. But you'd be surprised just how closely related science and Goldilocks really are—especially when it comes to your energy levels.

Remember her unwavering dedication to finding things that were "just right" for her needs? Well, the new product HSI recently learned about takes this lesson to heart, and, as a result, provides significant relief of fatigue in over 90 percent of the people who try it.

It's called COBAT and it was originally developed by cancer researchers. Unlike toxic chemotherapies that are designed to destroy cancer cells, COBAT, a combination of two amino acids, taurine and beta-alanine, is a type of immunotherapy and is designed to stimulate the patient's immune system into anti-cancer activity. This can be a risky proposition for the patient: Sometimes stimulating the immune system can create other problems, such as allergic reactions or autoimmune disorders. But, in this case, the researchers found that COBAT didn't simply stimulate the immune system, it normalized it. It's actually an immune modulator.

Another way to describe COBAT's effect is "adaptogenic." An adaptogen is a substance that the body uses as it is needed. Instead of having one specific effect, adaptogens allow the body to adapt to various conditions, bringing it into a state of normalcy. For example, an adaptogenic substance that helps regulate temperature wouldn't be limited to making you either hot or cold but would cool you when you're too warm and warm you when you're too cold. COBAT seems to have this kind of effect on the immune system.

Not your average energy booster

And it's these immune-regulating effects that make COBAT so different from other energy boosters.

To combat fatigue, most people choose some type of stimulant, whether it's caffeine, an herbal supplement, or sugar. Those inclined to natural products might buy herbal stimulants, long-distance truck drivers and late-studying students favor mild over-the-counter stimulants, and some folks take their chances by abusing legal or illegal drugs. Overall, Americans spend over $100 billion dollars a year on "pick-me-ups."

But all of these substances generally address one or more of the same mechanisms to alleviate fatigue. They stimulate the central nervous system, which increases blood pressure and heart rate; they stimulate the endocrine system to produce more adrenaline, which, in turn, stimulates the central nervous system; they elevate blood sugar; and/or they alter brain chemistry. These approaches do yield short-term results but often have long-term side effects. They stress the body and can eventually lead to a variety of illnesses-and, ironically, increased fatigue.

COBAT, on the other hand, goes directly to the cause of fatigue: irregularities in your immune system. Of course, that begs the million-dollar question:

What does the immune system have to do with fatigue?

Fatigue can seem to result from a number of causes: blood sugar disorders, chronic infections, allergies, and toxicity. But all of these affect, or are affected by, a group of chemicals called cytokines. Cytokines are proteins produced by various types of white blood cells that make up the immune system. They act as messengers between the cells, enabling them to work together. Cytokines also stimulate cells to produce other cytokines, resulting in "cytokine cascades." Cancer researchers studying the immune system have long known that an increase in certain cytokines can cause a "cytokine syndrome" of fatigue, fever, brain fog, muscle pain, and depression.

At the 38th annual meeting of the American Academy of Environmental Medicine in 2003, Aristo Vodjani, Ph.D., of ImmunoScience Laboratories, presented studies on 2,500 patients with chronic fatigue syndrome, fibromyalgia, and Gulf War Syndrome—all fatiguing illnesses. Dr. Vodjani showed that these patient groups exhibited surprising similarities in cytokine patterns. It appeared that the body, in trying to protect itself from infection and other stressors, established a cytokine pattern associated with lower energy and pain. While it's obviously critical to deal with underlying infections and stressors, it also makes sense to consider balancing the cytokines directly.

This is where Goldilocks comes into the story

Not too many. Not too few. Just the right amount of cytokines.

According to research done at the University of Maryland, COBAT increases the production of some cytokines and decreases others, and this alters existing cytokine patterns that apparently are a major cause of fatigue.

Floyd Taub, M.D., one of the chief investigators, described this as the "Goldilocks effect": Not too much, not too little, but just the right balance of cytokines.

Another member of the research team, Thomas M. Dunn, M.D., noted that COBAT's key effect might be the change in calcium flux it induces. Calcium flux, the movement of calcium ions in a cell, is the primary activation signal for immune cells that leads to an amplifying cascade of immune stimulation under the appropriate conditions.

Safety proven in homeopathic trials

COBAT is basically a combination of the amino acids taurine and beta-alanine. (COBAT is short for the chemical name "carbobenzoxy beta-alanine- taurine.") Taurine and beta-alanine perform numerous biological functions. Taurine helps regulate the heartbeat, maintain cell membrane stability, and prevent brain cell overactivity. Beta-alanine is a constituent of vitamin B5 (pantothenic acid) and coenzyme A, both of which play important roles in various metabolic reactions.

COBAT is similar to garlic, alpha-lipoic acid, MSM, and N-acetyl cysteine in that it contains a sulfur compound. However, while these substances and amino acids are usually administered in doses of up to a gram or more, COBAT's therapeutic dosage is measured in billionths of a gram. To get to those tiny dosage amounts, COBAT is prepared in the same way as homeopathic preparations, diluting it by a factor of 10 six times ("6X" in homeopathic nomenclature).

These miniscule amounts are one reason COBAT is considered nontoxic and extraordinarily safe. One animal study found that rats tolerated 2,000 mg of COBAT per kilogram of body weight for 14 days with no adverse effects. The normally prescribed dosage of COBAT is 1 billion times lower than this level. Other animal studies found no signs of toxicity, no increase in mortality, and no abnormal findings when COBAT was administered at thousands and millions of times the prescribed dosage.

In March of 2001, 39 normal volunteers completed the first homeopathic proving trial for COBAT. In this case, the term "normal" means random, in that the volunteers were not chosen because they had specific conditions, as was done for other trials.

The study was conducted by David Riley, M.D., associate clinical professor at the University of New Mexico School of Medicine, editor in chief of the peer-reviewed journal *Alternative Therapies in Health and Medicine*, and co-founder of the Integrative Medicine Institute. The volunteers were given one or two drops of COBAT in 6X or 8X strengths for at least one month.

In this double-blind trial, 92 percent of the patients given COBAT reported significant reductions in fatigue, versus 26 percent of the patients given a placebo. A few volunteers felt better in minutes, the majority felt a difference in days, and a few not at all.

Dr. Riley told me that in all of the trials similar to this one that he's been involved with, "COBAT produced the strongest effects." Another measure of how significant these results are came from Dr. Taub, who verified the significance of these results, saying that "standard allopathic treatments for fatigue are effective less than half of the time." But, as mentioned before, those positive effects come complete with a variety of side effects and compromises—unlike COBAT.

Trials show a number of other benefits

Reduced fatigue was not the only benefit found in the homeopathic trial. Other symptoms addressed by COBAT in this study included appetite abnormalities, coughs and colds, headaches, digestive problems, uterine fibroids, headaches and muscle aches, neurological problems, and premenstrual syndrome (PMS).

One patient, a 55-year-old female with lung cancer, entered the study for fatigue and allergies. In addition to less fatigue and less frequent and severe allergy symptoms, she reported that COBAT helped with her recovery from chemotherapy by helping to maintain her appetite and weight.

In a trial held in 2002, all but one of 16 patients diagnosed with cancer, hepatitis C, or chronic fatigue syndrome reported significant improvements. COBAT was four to 10 times more effective than conventional drug therapies in reducing fatigue in CFS patients. The rest of the subjects reported an average 52 percent improvement in their energy levels. There were no other interventions or changes in diet and activities, and about half of the improvement was noted within four to 10 weeks.

Again, patients reported positive effects on other health complaints, citing improvement in memory, and decreases in depression, headaches, allergies, pain, and gastrointestinal symptoms. Several patients also entered the trial with elevated liver enzymes, a sign of liver disease. All of their readings decreased to normal during the trial.

Effective against mild fatigue in healthier people

Normally, we should experience fatigue only as a sign that it's time to go to sleep, after extraordinary physical or mental exertion, or when we have serious health conditions, like the patients in the studies outlined above. These days, however, fatigue affects many of us even when we seem to be in otherwise good health. Everyone wants more energy, and COBAT appears to be unequaled in its effectiveness, safety, and ancillary benefits.

So after all the formal results were in, Stephen Levine, president of the Allergy Research Group, was curious about how COBAT would work on people who are generally healthy but describe themselves as having "mild" fatigue. He recruited a few friends and co-workers to try COBAT. These anecdotal comments don't compare to the scientific evidence, of course, but they are interesting.

A co-worker with fibromyalgia said that after five days on COBAT, she "awoke feeling like a completely different person." Her twin sister, who has chronic pain from an unsuccessful shoulder operation, said "after two weeks, I started waking up feeling refreshed and had a better ability to concentrate." A menopausal woman noted that COBAT "decreased brain fog and increased my mental clarity… I slept soundly and awoke refreshed and relaxed." And one person (lucky enough to have no health complaints), said "COBAT… creates no buzz or edginess, yet it provides energy for both physical and mental work. It allowed me to stop drinking caffeinated coffee for the first time in my adult life."

Where to get COBAT and how to use it

COBAT is sold under the brand name Taurox 6X. While the full dose is 12 drops daily, many of the test participants gained full benefits with less. In fact, the label suggests trying "half or even fewer drops." If you do, you can stretch a half-ounce bottle into more than a one-month supply.

Dr. Levine told me that "each patient should determine his or her best dose—the fewest drops that produce the desired benefit without any symptoms." He went on to comment that patients who start with the 6X who get headaches or find themselves with "too much energy" should use fewer drops.

The manufacturer warns that Taurox 6X should not be taken with immunosuppressive agents, or by patients who have had an organ transplant. People with autoimmune diseases should consult with their doctors before using it.

Because of a lack of testing, Taurox 6X is not recommended for pregnant or nursing women or children under 15.

Taurox does run on the expensive side: The 6X preparation averages about $50 for 13.5 ml. (See the Member Source Directory on page 529 for complete ordering information.) But keep in mind that, as an adaptogen, odds are it might help improve other aspects of your health too, by regulating your immune system's cytokine levels. In other words, Taurox could go a long way in helping you reach your own personal "just right." Goldilocks would be proud.

CHAPTER EIGHT

An anti-aging breakthrough that will change the way you think about taking supplements forever!

When world-renowned physician and author Dr. Mitchell Ghen was asked to create a revolutionary anti-aging supplement, his agreement had a few conditions.

It had to be spectacular, it had to be like nothing else out there, and it had to be good enough for clinical use without the headache of sorting through countless bottles.

So he opened up his own medicine cabinet and took a look at all the nutrients he was taking every day… and the wheels started turning.

What if he could put all of those anti-aging miracles into one bottle? It was a major undertaking, to be sure—to put every single nutrient you need to fight the ravages of time into one product?

But if anyone was up for the challenge, it was Dr. Ghen. With 29 years of experience under his belt, he knew exactly what the formula needed.

So he identified four essential areas in which he feels the battle against aging is fought—free radicals, inflammation, hyperviscosity, and mitochondrial DNA (don't worry, I'll explain all of these later).

By addressing those four areas (and by throwing in a ton of other nutrients the body needs to keep running smoothly), he ended up creating the first truly serious, head-to-toe, everything-you-need anti-aging powerhouse: RegeneCell.

It packs absolutely everything you need to arm your body against aging—in *one scoop a day*. And there's just one place you can get it… again, more on that later.

First, let's break down those areas of aging.

Antioxidant superstars "seek and destroy" free radicals

If you've been reading the *Members Alert* for a while now, free radicals are nothing new to you. The free-radical theory of aging is based on the idea that highly reactive substances (free radicals) damage the body's cells and speed up the aging process.[1]

It's been shown that antioxidants can chemically prevent this damage. This may help prevent disease and protect our bodies against the signs of aging.

Dr. Ghen estimates that the average person gets only about 1,200 ORAC units of antioxidants per day, but researchers estimate we need more like 3,000 – 5,000 to really do the job. You'd have to eat at least 10-12 servings of fruits and vegetables to get that. And let's be honest: How many of us are really eating that much fruit?

RegeneCell is chock-full of antioxidants ready to fight those free radicals. Vitamin C, for example, is one of the most potent antioxidants in human blood, and research suggests it plays a major role in protecting against damage caused by oxidative stress.[2]

It's needed for tissue growth and repair, proper adrenal-gland function, immune function, and collagen formation. When pollution wreaks havoc on your body, vitamin C can help protect you from the effects.[3]

You've heard time and again that green tea is good for you. Its antioxidant power has been demonstrated in quite a few studies. In one recent study, subjects were exposed to benzene, a chemical that induces the formation of free radicals at the same time it reduces the activity of antioxidant enzymes, leaving the body with less protective power. One group drank six cups of green tea per day for six months—the tea was able to cut most of the toxic effects of benzene. It also increased antioxidant-enzyme activity in red blood cells.[4]

The man behind the formula

Dr. Mitchell Ghen has 29 years of experience in anti-aging and holistic and integrative medicine. He is the co-author of three textbooks: The Advanced Guide to Longevity Medicine, The Ghen and Raines Guide to Pharmaceutical Compounding, and the Anti-Aging Physicians' Handbook of Compounding Pharmaceuticals.

In addition, he has authored dozens of articles in peer-reviewed journals. He has been a host and guest on hundreds of radio and television programs, where he has been featured as an expert in alternative health.

Dr. Ghen, in addition to being a physician, holds a Master's Degree in Biomechanical Trauma and has a Ph.D. in nutrition and psychoneuroimmunology. He is an international lecturer on topics about oral and IV nutrition and stem-cell transplantation.

"Dr. Ghen is among the top 20 anti-aging/regenerative medicine clinicians in the world practicing this new science today," according to Ron Klatz, M.D. President of the A4M, representing 22,000 physicians and scientists from 100 countries who know aging is no longer inevitable.

The antioxidant punch provided by RegeneCell is rounded out by beta-carotene, vitamin E, carnosine, and a handful of other powerful free-radical scavengers.

Keep inflammation in check

Almost everything that can go wrong as we age can be linked to inflammation. Sure, inflammation is a normal and healthy response to damage—it's how you know your body is working to heal itself—but the trick is to keep it from getting out of hand.

Dr. Ghen has packed RegeneCell with the top nutrients for promoting a healthy inflammatory response. Among them is curcumin, which he says is among the best substances known to man for this purpose. If you're a curry fan, you've had your share of curcumin—it's a compound found in turmeric. Turmeric has been traditionally used for ages in Chinese and Ayurvedic medicine as an anti-inflammatory.

Curcumin actually offers greater protection against certain free radicals than vitamins C and E. In addition to its antioxidant activity, curcumin can help support joint health. It also has been shown to help keep blood flowing smoothly and to promote a healthy inflammatory response.[5]

Curcumin is joined by several other substances that can help keep your body's inflammation response healthy and productive. Quercetin, a flavonol derived from plants, has recently been shown to help manage pro-inflammatory signaling *in vitro*.[6] Royal jelly, which is secreted by honeybees for the development of the queen bee, has been found to have antioxidant and anti-inflammatory properties.[7]

Feed every system in your body with free-flowing blood

As we age, our blood actually becomes more viscous—this causes sluggish blood flow and means less oxygen gets where it's needed. Our bodies start to make more fibrin, a protein involved in blood clotting, which can make circulation slow.

This hyperviscosity is actually linked to many health concerns our bodies face as we age. Think about it—if all of your body systems need oxygen to survive, what happens when you cut back on that supply? Studies have shown a rise in blood viscosity with age and a decreased blood flow to the brain.[8]

So, if blood flow is so important to our bodies' functions, how do we keep our minds sharp, our hearts pumping, and everything else working in tip-top condition?

Did you really think Dr. Ghen wouldn't include his answer in RegeneCell?

For that answer, he once again turned to something he was taking every day—nattokinase.

It's an enzyme inside natto, a traditional Japanese food made from boiled and fermented soybeans. The Japanese have consumed natto for centuries.

Culinary use aside, nattokinase has drawn much interest in the scientific community for its ability to aid in the breakdown of fibrin. This helps keep blood from getting too viscous.

Nattokinase has actually been reported to have about four times the activity of plasmin, a natural bodily enzyme that plays a role in healthy dissolution of clots.[9]

A clinical trial in China found that nattokinase was able to promote healthy blood flow. This trial was conducted on a very small group—four men—and it's unclear how much nattokinase they consumed, but it does contribute to the growing body of research proclaiming the benefits of nattokinase.[10]

Nattokinase's effect on blood viscosity could even have effects on the entire body, including helping keep the heart healthy—and RegeneCell packs even more power when it comes to helping keep your heart pumping and your blood flowing.

In addition to vitamin E, magnesium, and flavonoids, RegeneCell contains CoQ10, well-known for its heart-healthy action.

Keep your "cellular power plants" churning out energy

I promised I would explain mitochondrial DNA—and why it's so important to take care of as we age. Mitochondria are in most of the cells of your body, and they are sort of like little power plants. They make energy for cells, in addition to being involved in controlling cell death and growth.

Mitochondria make energy by creating adenosine triphosphate (ATP), which stores and transports chemical energy within cells for metabolism. It's continuously recycled, and a healthy body turns over its own weight in ATP each day.

Keeping the mitochondria healthy could be the key to winning the battle against aging, as mitochondrial DNA can be damaged by oxidative stress.[11]

A study in mice suggested that mitochondrial DNA mutations can actually lead to premature aging.[12]

The answer to this, Dr. Ghen believes, lies primarily in D-ribose. It's a kind of sugar that's actually a fundamental building block of ATP. Studies have shown that ribose supplementation can help enhance energy levels in the heart and may support the body's antioxidant defenses.[13]

Other ingredients in RegeneCell can support the action of D-ribose. Magnesium is critical to the activity of ATP. And acetyl-L-carnitine is an amino acid that helps transport substances across the membrane of mitochondria—this plays a role in energy production within the brain.[14]

From your bones to your brain to your immune system—RegeneCell has it covered

The four areas I just told you about make up the backbone of the

RegeneCell formula—but the power doesn't end there. RegeneCell truly contains everything you may need to address every system of your body.

It can help your bones stay strong thanks to vitamin D and calcium, both shown in many studies to benefit bone density.[15,16] Bones can also get a lift from magnesium and zinc.

Want to keep your mind sharp as a tack? Research at the Linus Pauling Micronutrient Research Center at Oregon State University estimates that 10-15 percent of people over 60 are deficient in vitamin B12. Such a deficiency can lead to decline in brain function.[17]

RegeneCell contains B12, as well as boron. People deprived of boron actually showed poorer performance in assessments of attention and short-term memory.[18]

Another brain-booster featured in RegeneCell is acetyl-L-carnitine (ALC). This amino acid has been shown to have a positive effect on cognitive and memory function. It's thought that it may help enhance energy metabolism in the brain, benefiting cognitive function.[19]

Several trials have demonstrated its positive effect, including one small study in which 30 subjects showed statistically significant improvements in memory and verbal fluency after taking 2 g. of ALC every day for three months.[20]

Certain aspects of the immune response change as we age. And that's where probiotics come in. They enhance the beneficial bacteria in the gut and have been speculated to help keep your immune system in top condition. Probiotics may enhance gut-barrier function, which promotes a healthy balance of beneficial bacteria.

Vitamin E and selenium can also contribute to helping keep your immune system running at the top of its game.

Of course, all of these benefits mean nothing if your body can't access them. And that's why RegeneCell packs nutrients especially geared toward your digestive health.

Improved digestion means
you get all you can out of RegeneCell

The digestive support offered by RegeneCell actually helps increase the digestibility of the other nutrients in the formula.

Fibersol-2™ is a digestion-resistant maltodextrin made from corn starch. It consists of 90 percent dietary fiber. In addition to this fiber, RegeneCell provides digestive enzymes that promote good digestion and enhance the absorption of nutrients. They've been shown to help in the management of occasional bloating, stomachache, and nausea.[21]

Arabinogalactans, from larch-tree extract, are considered prebiotics. These are substances that are fermented in the colon by probiotic organisms. They've been shown to help stimulate the growth of these beneficial bacteria. Because of the way they're structured, arabinogalactans are fermented at a slower rate than other carbohydrates and may actually contribute to a larger increase in probiotic population.

There's so much more I could say about RegeneCell—there is something here to optimize your body's systems and help arm every one in the fight against aging. You'd probably have to take 20 pills a day to get close to the benefits of this revolutionary supplement. With RegeneCell, all it takes is a scoop of powder mixed into a glass of water.

Now, I want to warn you—when you turn to the Member Source Directory on page 529 for ordering information, you might be hit with a bit of "sticker shock." RegeneCell is not cheap. But when you consider all that you're getting out of it (and the rows and rows of bottles it will replace), I think you'll find it's a bargain.

Please note: HSI doesn't accept fees from outside companies for editorial coverage. However, NorthStar Nutritionals is one of HSI's dietary supplement affiliate companies. Even though we would never recommend any product we don't believe in, you should know about that relationship when deciding whether to try their products.

CHAPTER NINE

Replenish your body's supply of this natural moisturizer and say goodbye to wrinkles and joint pain

The promotional material reads like an Oil of Olay commercial: "Reduce wrinkles and visible signs of aging" with a dietary supplement used by the porcelain-skinned beauties of Japan. Yes, natural medicine—that wholesome realm of herbalists, naturopaths, and health nuts—has gone "glam" and produced a "cosmaceutical."

But heck, if natural medicine can generate products that boost the immune system, lower cholesterol, and ease hypertension, why can't it formulate products that combat wrinkles too?

A new wave of supplements containing hyaluronic acid—a complex carbohydrate that has been described as "nature's moisturizer"—are purporting to nurture smoother, younger skin. And anecdotal evidence suggests they may also support more limber, less painful joints. Further, some limited clinical experience indicates that hyaluronic acid supplements prevent bruising and accelerate wound healing—a property that benefits diabetics in particular.

But overwhelmingly, HA is a beauty supplement. Over the years at the HSI Symposia, we've met some of the youngest 70-, 80-, and 90-year-olds you can imagine. And since a lot of you let us know that you want to look as young as you feel, we decided to digress from our usual roster of stories about hardened arteries, cancer threats, and liver disease, and devote a few pages to the pursuit of youth—naturally.

The key here is *naturally*. There are plenty of ways to get rid of wrinkles, but whether those products and procedures are safe is another issue entirely. The newest trend involves injecting the toxic substance (an FDA-approved toxic substance, but toxic nonetheless) Botox, into the face. Despite the obvious dangers associated with injecting poison into the body, women around the country have started to abandon Tupperware and bridge parties for Botox parties. We kid you not. Women are inviting friends over to have a strain of the botulism virus, which literally paralyzes the muscles, injected below their eyes, around their mouths, anywhere they have wrinkles—all while munching on chips and salsa and gossiping about the neighbor's affair. We were, quite frankly, very disturbed by this trend and decided to explore a natural alternative. We found one in hyaluronic acid (HA).

When was the last time someone told you how "Toki" you look?

There is actually some science and research to demonstrate that hyaluronic acid can help you look younger. To get to the science, we had to get past a lot of the cosmetic-counter-style marketing lingo. But we just can't move on without sharing a taste of it. Toki, for example, is a multiple-ingredient beauty supplement that includes HA. In Japanese, *Toki* means "skin of a porcelain doll," writes the product's previous North American distributor, Lane Labs. "The highest compliment a woman can receive in Japan is that she is looking Toki."

Nobody said beauty comes easily. To understand how HA can foster younger skin (and produce a few other health benefits) you first have to understand how your skin, joints, and soft tissue function at a cellular level. It's a little complicated. One senior educator with a formulating company told us that she has a particularly difficult time educating sellers about her HA supplement simply because the science behind HA is so much more complicated than the science behind a vitamin or herbal formula. So we've tried to make the science a little more digestible.

Hyaluronic acid is a gel that is found in soft tissue throughout your body. Its function is to lubricate and cushion tissue whether that tissue is part of your skin, joints, eyes, cartilage, blood vessels, heart valves, whatever. It accomplishes that function in a couple of ways:

- HA is a major component of your extracellular matrix (the liquid between your cells). There, HA retains water, hydrates your cells, and provides a medium to carry nutrients to cells and waste away from them. In short, it keeps your cells healthy and resilient.

- HA is also a primary constituent of synovial fluid (the liquid that fills each joint cavity). There, it serves as a shock-absorber for your knees, ankles, elbows, etc. HA also serves as the primary source of nutrients for your cartilage. (Cartilage isn't connected to the blood system, consequently it can't get nutrients from the blood stream.)

- HA supports the formation and maintenance of collagen. As the principal protein in human skin, bone, cartilage, tendons, and connective tissue, healthy collagen levels are critical to skin, joint, and bone health.

- Finally, HA contains glucosamine—a carbohydrate that supports joint health and has become an effective supplement for many osteoarthritis sufferers. (In fact, it's so common you can probably find it right next to the aspirin in your grocery store.)

HA's impact on your skin is obvious, keeping it smooth and moisturized. It also helps your skin resist and repair bruises and cuts by helping cells move to new tissue sites. In less obvious ways, HA provides exactly the same benefit to joints, eyes, and other parts of your body.

As we age, however, our bodies produce less HA. Production starts to lag around age 20. By 40, diminished supplies of HA leave us with those aches, pains, and wrinkles we've always thought were "unavoidable parts of aging." So all we have to do is supplement our HA levels, right? Unlike many of the natural remedies you've read about here, it just wasn't that easy with HA. But today it's possible, thanks to some new advances.

HA supplements: Two decades in the making thanks to two big challenges

Mainstream medicine began studying and using hyaluronic acid 20 years ago. It developed a few products to heal wounds, burns, sores, and surgical incisions, to speed recovery from eye surgery, and to ease the symptoms of advanced osteoarthritis. But researchers ran into two problems when they started developing HA treatments. First, it doesn't last long in the body (so you have to take it frequently). Second, in their natural state, HA molecules are so large that they can't pass through the intestinal tract and into the blood stream. In other words, raw HA cannot be effective when taken orally.

Consequently, HA hasn't yielded many convenient treatment options. Osteoarthritis sufferers, for example, have gotten substantial relief from HA treatment.

(HA provided better pain relief than naproxen in one study.[1]) However, the regimen involves getting injections in the joint (usually the knee) five times a week. Not surprisingly, the pain and inflammation caused by the treatment was sometimes as severe as the pain and inflammation caused by the disease!

Mini molecules offer big benefits

Alternative medicine researchers, however, claim they can now access the benefits of hyaluronic acid through a dietary supplement. Deanne Dolnick, an educator with Soft Gel Technologies in California, says researchers have found a way to reduce the size of HA molecules so that they can pass through the lining of the digestive system and deliver potent HA to the blood stream.

"There are scientists in Japan who have patented an enzyme-cleaving technique," Dolnick says. "What they have done is they have made hyaluronic acid into smaller polymers so that it's a smaller version of the original without chemically altering it. It functions in the body just as hyaluronic acid would." Right now, the evidence showing that HA can be effective as an oral supplement is limited. But some does exist.

Wounds heal 5 days faster

In one test, researchers anesthetized lab rats and gave them each identical skin wounds. The animals were divided into three groups: One group received 3,000 mg/kg of oral HA daily (in the form of Injuv™ supplements), the second group received an oral placebo daily, the third group received daily topical doses of a commercial wound-healing ointment. Researchers measured the wounds each day for ten days and concluded that oral HA dramatically reduced healing time. Rats fed HA healed within 13 days—five days faster than placebo-fed rats. In addition, the HA delivered almost as much benefit as the commercial wound-healing ointment. Rats treated with the ointment took 10.6 days to heal.[2]

Over 80 percent of study participants report "great improvement"

Healing wounds on rats was a promising start. But researchers still needed to determine if HA could improve the skin of creatures that aren't covered in fur. So researchers at Ohtsuma University in Japan conducted a small trial with humans. They monitored the impact of oral HA on 96 women, aged 22 to 65. Every day for 45 days, the subjects consumed six capsules of Injuv. Each capsule contained 6.3 mg of hyaluronic acid, for a total daily dose of 37.8 mg. More than 80 percent of the women reported "great improvement" in skin moisture, smoothness, and firmness on their faces, hands, elbows, knees, and heels. More than 70 percent noticed significant relief from stiff shoulders and joints.

According to Dolnick, hyaluronic acid has not triggered any adverse side effects in people using Soft Gel's HA supplement. (Extracted from roosters' combs, the product could theoretically trigger allergic reactions in people sensitive to chicken or eggs. But so far, none have been reported.) The product has also passed an oral toxicity study in which 10 rats (five male and five female) were given 5050 mg/kg daily for four days. The high dose triggered diarrhea in some animals, but no other side effects. Researchers found no abnormalities when they later euthanized and autopsied the animals.[3]

Wrinkle reduction in a lemon-flavored drink

Obviously, some results posted from skin care studies are inevitably subjective. When it comes to determining how dry a person's skin feels, researchers often must rely on the impressions of the test subjects. But researchers can measure changes in wrinkles and other visible skin conditions. Lane Labs, conducted a small scale human trial of Toki—that all-natural secret of Japan's porcelain-skinned beauties—and obtained some impressive results.

Toki is a different kind of supplement. Sold in powder form, Toki is mixed with cold water to create a drink that tastes like generously sweetened lemonade, and contains several ingredients that can promote skin and joint health—hyaluronic acid, collagen, calcium, vitamin C, glucosamine, and seaweed extract.

Iron out wrinkles in as little as two weeks

Researchers asked 38 women ages 35 to 65 to take Toki for eight weeks (three times a day for the first two weeks to achieve a "loading dose," then twice a day for the remaining six weeks). Each woman's face was examined and photographed at the beginning of the study, focusing particularly on wrinkles, puffiness, and sagging around the eyes. Researchers re-examined each woman every two weeks for the duration of the study. They documented significant reduction of wrinkles and other signs of facial aging after just two weeks of supplementation, and dramatic improvement by the end of the study. Through a series of blood tests, they also determined that participants' blood collagen levels actually increased an average of 114 percent after 30 days of supplementing with Toki.

One-third of the women experienced mild to moderate side effects from the treatment (primarily itching and gastrointestinal upset). However, those conditions disappeared quickly and did not prompt any women to discontinue the supplement. After all, remember, women are injecting poison into their faces to get similar results. So what's a little gas or scratching?

Laugh lines might not be all you lose…

The women in Lane Labs' study also reported one unexpected effect. They lost weight. On average, each participant lost two pounds during the study, although some women dropped as much as seven pounds. "We're not promoting it as a weight-loss product," says Jennifer Nissen, N.D., Lane Labs' manager of nutritional research. She suspects Toki's collagen content was responsible for the incidental weight loss. "Collagen is a protein and protein helps level out your blood sugar, decreasing blood sugar crashes and sugar cravings. Protein is also filling, so if women drink it before a meal, they may eat less."

Beauty…at a price

Regardless of whether it's new and alternative, Toki holds true to one old adage: Beauty doesn't come cheap. A box containing 60 packets of Toki sells for $175 plus shipping. That means younger skin is going to cost you roughly $200 a month (and closer to $300 in the first month when the recommended dosage is higher). But then again, Botox treatments start at about $300 per injection. And a small bottle

(1.7 ounces) of Clinique's "anti-aging serum" will set you back more than $50. Any way you look at it, the fountain of youth comes with a steep price tag.

Please refer to the Member Source Directory to find out how to order this product.

CHAPTER TEN

Flirting with perfection: Open the floodgates to the youth elixir in your blood

There's a hormone in your body; the primary function of which is to make you beautiful and strong.

It's no joke! In fact, this hormone has the ability to make you so stunningly strong and vital that as soon as the bodybuilding industry got wind of it, it began researching ways to enhance its production!

This hormone is called, simply, growth hormone (GH). Despite its simple name, GH does a lot more than stimulate growth. It causes tissue to grow and stored energy (fat) to be consumed.

The problem is, however, that nature played a cruel trick on us. As we age, our bodies make less and less of this magic chemical!

When you were a preteen, growth hormone stimulated your skeletal growth. In your teens and early 20s, it reduced stored fat and increased muscle and tissue mass. Sadly, when you hit your mid 20s, GH production started to slow…and it continues to slow to this day.

But you can still tap into it…and turn your body into a youth machine designed to tone you down to your most trim, energetic, and healthy form.

Before we tell you about the different ways to stimulate GH production—including through the use of a new, safe, and powerful GH-stimulating supplement—we want to warn you about the GH stimulants on the market that are, in fact, dangerous.

As we mentioned before, such a powerful youth- and beauty-enhancing chemical is of obvious interest to athletes and bodybuilders. The sports market provided much of the motivation for early research and experimentation with growth hormone. Anabolic steroids have been abused for years by people interested in bodybuilding to enhance their athletic performance. But the effects of overuse of artificial substances have often been tragic. Another GH stimulant, synthetic human growth hormone, has been available since 1986. Though it is not nearly as dangerous as anabolic steroids, it has been linked to heart disease, and some forms can actually cause antibodies that combat growth hormone.

But here's a simple, safe strategy for stepping up your body's GH production.

- **Eat more cereal grains, nuts, and seeds**. Although these foods contain less arginine than do meat, potatoes, and milk, they also contain less of the amino acids that compete with arginine to cross the brain-blood barrier where they can act on the hypothalamus.

- **Supplement your diet with liquid potassium**. Researchers have discovered a correlation between a reduction in growth hormone and the reduction of dietary potassium. Although you can restore your body's potassium levels by eating natural, whole foods (which have more potassium than sodium), rather than processed foods (which almost always have more sodium than potassium), this is often easier said than done. Liquid potassium tonics are available in health stores.

- **Snack often**…as long as you are snacking on low-sugar, health-ful foods! This will keep your blood-sugar level stable. Main-taining stable blood-sugar levels keep your pancreas from producing excess insulin. When there's too much insulin in your blood, your body reacts by producing a chemical called somatostatin. Somatostatin suppresses insulin release…but it also suppresses GH release! This is also a good reason to avoid sugary sweets (especially before bedtime): <u>High sugar snacks prevent the release of GH!</u>

- **If you enjoy exercising, be sure to avoid eating at least two hours before you begin**. To make the best of the small, exercise-induced release of GH, your blood-sugar level must be stable.

- **Make sure you don't eat (again, especially high-sugar foods) within two hours of sleep**: In adults, <u>the largest daily secretion of GH begins about an hour after the onset of deep sleep</u>.

- **Take the dietary amino acid arginine**. As stated before, it has been shown to act on the hypothalamus, which produces a growth-hormone-releasing hormone (GHRH).

HSI Panelist Dr. Allan Spreen told us that arginine is one of the best-known stimulants of the formation of growth hormone by the human body.

As he pointed out, "The injectable HGH (human growth hor-mone) is risky, as it causes the body to make less of its own, while arginine is the antithesis of that—it causes the body to make *more* of its own. Growth hormone is a wonderful 'youth agent,' and we make less as we age. The effects of rejuvenating the body (its skin, muscles, energy, what-have-you) apparently have been shown to extend to the immune system also."

This safe, proven plan can help you <u>reverse aging</u>, <u>eliminate obesity</u>, and even, according to some experts, convert your body to the Tarzan or Jane musculature into your seventh, eighth, ninth, and even 10th decades!

An important aside

You're probably already familiar with your body's needs for the essential fatty acids found in olive oil and fatty fish, such as salmon and mackerel. Your body needs these fats in order to maintain good heart health, to keep your cells properly lubricated, and to transport the fat-soluble vitamins, A, D, E, and K. Essential fatty acids make up a major part of the membranes surrounding all cells. Unsaturated fats help your body handle saturated ones. A small amount of fat is an important aspect of healthful dieting.

CHAPTER ELEVEN

Nature's surprising fat fighter: You knew it was good for you... now find out how it helps you lose weight fast!

In a recent obesity study, a group of rats was given a choice of the usual fare of American supermarket snack foods. Remarkably, the animals chose biscuits, chocolates, and marshmallows over regular nutritionally balanced chow.

In 60 days, these ravenous creatures gained an average of 78 g... which, for a rat, is a lot.

Yes, even a rat can be seduced by foods that are fast, simple, and stimulating.

No one is immune to the temptations of 20th-century, fast-food cuisine. But these foods are not only high in fat and calories and almost devoid of any real nutrition, but also lacking a crucial fat-fighting nutrient—one that you simply cannot afford to be without.

Overcoming the pitfalls of our modern, fat-promoting culture can be as simple as adding to your diet this naturally occurring nutrient that is fat-free, cholesterol-free, calorie-free…and almost completely missing in popular supermarket junk foods: fiber.

It may not be new and exciting… but it IS radical…and it works!

You see, we are bombarded with foods that have been processed so extensively that they are virtually devoid of fiber. Eighty percent of the food we consume in this country is processed. The more the product is refined, the more fiber is removed.

This remarkable nutrient naturally blocks the absorption of fat!

When healthy adults are fed equal amounts of fat in the forms of whole peanuts, peanut butter, and peanut oil, more fat is absorbed from the peanut oil than from the peanut butter, and more from the peanut butter than from the whole peanuts. Why? Fiber blocks the absorption of fat—and hence calories—in the intestines.

The greater your fiber consumption, the higher your caloric waste. Fiber causes a true alteration in digestion and in the absorption of fat. Part of the fat becomes "associated" with fiber, so that it is unavailable for digestion and increases fat excretion.

What's more, when you consume enough fiber, both your small and large intestines contain more watery material. When your bowels are full, you do not feel empty. You stop eating.

What happens when you remove fiber from your foods?

Quite simply, you gain weight much more easily. Here's why.

There's an enzyme in your fat tissue that has the primary function of protecting you from starvation. As soon as any weight loss takes place, this enzyme sends a message to your brain to increase your caloric intake. (Like it or not, this is how our bodies have been responding across the centuries; a reponse more suitable to an age long before the availability of 4,000 foods in your 24-hour supermarket.)

Now, when you eat a natural, high-carbohydrate food that's been stripped of fiber…you're dumping too much sugar into your blood, causing the production of too much insulin.

Too much insulin <u>initiates communication between this enzyme and your brain</u>! In other words, when you eat foods devoid of fiber, you are essentially sending the message "I'm starving!" to your brain, setting in motion the chain of events that leads to slowed calorie burning and more stubborn fat-storage mechanisms.

As you can see, fiber is critical to maintaining a healthy weight.

But how can you get enough fiber in your diet—the <u>40 to 60 g required for weight control</u>—when you get only 6 grams of fiber in five heads of lettuce? 2 grams of fiber in an apple? Very little fiber in leafy greens? You can't!

Even worse, if you dine out often, or don't have time to buy and prepare fresh, fiber-rich foods on a regular basis, you'll never meet your daily requirement through your diet.

But you can manage a high-fiber intake without making major adjustments to your usual eating regimen.

Fiber supplements contain naturally occurring plant fiber. The formulas are derived from plants that are basically old-fashioned foods but are cloaked in late-20th-century technology.

Note these advantages of fiber supplementation in powder form:

- Grinding fiber into very fine particles makes it more readily digestible.

- Fiber supplements slow digestion, a very beneficial metabolic advantage.

- A high-quality fiber supplement offers standardized pectin, otherwise available only through the consumption of fruits, which may be off-limits to those with blood-sugar problems or those who eat out more than at home.

- Different types of fibers vary in function, and supplements contain a greater variety than you would ordinarily get on your dinner plate even if you chose natural foods as your meal choices.

Taking a fiber supplement on a regular basis assures an ongoing weight-loss advantage on two counts. First, it makes you feel full, which helps control your food consumption. Second, it adds no calories! With supplementation, you can manage a high-fiber intake without adding significant calories—a double whammy to those extra pounds!

It can't be overstated: Fiber is the only component in your daily diet that contains no calories, no fat, and no cholesterol!

An ancient health and beauty secret revived

Two thousand years ago, Hippocrates encouraged high-fiber diets. Fifteen years ago, Denis Burkitt came to this country from England and Africa to share his knowledge about fiber. No one seems to have paid much attention to either of these men of renown.

But the Health Sciences Institute wants you to be fully aware that the addition of a fiber supplement is in your best health interest and is a highly effective way to help lose weight safely and naturally.

There are a few good fiber supplements available. (A good supplement has a blend of natural fibers.) Among them are the following:

- gums, especially guar gum, which moderates sugar absorption better than any other fiber
- psyllium seed husk, which will have a beneficial effect on your glycemic index, your body's response to sugar, and also has great bulking activity
- pectin, mentioned above

Start your fiber supplementation slowly. Work up very gradually to 3 level teaspoons in at least 12 ounces of water. The more water you drink, the better. After two weeks, take the mix twice a day. If necessary, take it three times a day.

It's not necessary to spend a small fortune on fiber, though. You can get a perfectly good fiber supplement containing the above ingredients at your local health-food store.

CHAPTER TWELVE

Erase debilitating pain and fatigue by recharging your cells' batteries

Low energy is probably the No. 1 complaint I hear from my patients. But in many cases, the underlying problem may be more serious than "just getting older." It can actually reflect reduced energy in the cells, much like a battery wearing down and needing to be recharged. And the key to boosting cellular energy is to provide the cells with the fuel they need to function at peak performance, the enzyme adenosine triphosphate (ATP). How? With a simple five-carbon sugar found in every cell of the body called D-ribose, or simply "ribose," the cellular battery recharger.

Ribose's main function is to regulate the production of ATP—the major source of energy for all your cells. This action makes it useful for all sorts of conditions, including heart disease, congestive heart failure, and fibromyalgia. It's even good for supplying extra energy for workouts, and restoring energy after sustained exertion.

Ribose can be made naturally in the body, but it's a slow process limited by several enzymes that are lacking in heart and muscle cells. There are no foods containing ribose in any substantial amounts. Still, under normal circumstances getting enough ribose isn't a problem.

But when the heart or our muscles are challenged from stress or lack of oxygen for any number of reasons, they need an extra ribose boost to restore ATP levels.

The problem, until recently, was that the manufacturing processes for making ribose were so expensive that supplements just weren't a practical—or even feasible—solution for many people. Now, though, there is new technology for ribose production, and the resulting formula, called Corvalen M, offers simple solutions for many people who just didn't have options before.

Two weeks of treatment erases debilitating pain and fatigue

Take fibromyalgia for example. It's often difficult both to diagnose and to treat.

Until now, there have been few tools to help these patients. However, we've found that ribose can provide significant improvement, as seen in the following case study published last year in the journal *Pharmacotherapy*.[1]

At 37, Kris, a veterinary surgeon and researcher at a major university, became so debilitated from fibromyalgia she had to give up her practice.

But then she joined a clinical study on fibromyalgia and began taking 5 grams of ribose two times per day (10 g per day). Within a week, she felt better. Within two weeks, she was back at work in the operating room.

Over the course of the following month, she continued to improve. After a month, however, Kris stopped her treatment. Ten days later, she was totally debilitated again and could no longer perform surgery. So she began ribose treatment for a second time, again with dramatically positive results, and has remained symptom-free as long as she takes the supplement regularly.

While there's no official explanation as to why ribose is so effective for fibromyalgia, it could go back to its roots in ATP production. People with fibromyalgia have lower levels of ATP and a reduced capacity to make ATP in their muscles.[2] The effect of ribose on the production of ATP may be the link to reducing the strain in affected muscles and allowing patients to return to their previously active lifestyles.

There are other nutrients that, like ribose, are necessary for ATP production. One is malic acid, which also helps to combat fibro-myalgia's chronic muscle soreness. I have been recommending it along with magnesium to my fibromyalgia patients for years with relatively good success. But adding ribose has sparked even better results. Corvalen M, mentioned earlier, combines all three nutrients into one powdered formula, lending a much-needed touch of simplicity to this complicated disease.

Ribose gets to the heart of the matter

I've seen similarly remarkable results in people with heart problems. Heart disease, heart attack, heart surgery, and organ transplants can all lead to restricted blood flow, called ischemia in which your cells don't get the oxygen they need to properly burn ATP for energy.

In addition, individuals who are on inotropic drugs to make the heart beat harder then have an <u>additional</u> strain on the heart's energy production.

So it is especially important that patients with congestive heart failure, chronic coronary artery disease, or cardiomyopathy take extra ribose to offset their energy-draining effects.

Research shows that supplementation with ribose can offset this energy drain without interfering with the effects of any other medication the person might be taking.

Side-effect free at 12 times the standard dose

One of the best parts of the ribose story is that, despite it being so powerful, it has almost no side effects, with thousands of patients having taken ribose in doses up to 60 g per day.

How can we be so sure that ribose is safe? Well, first, ribose is made naturally by the body and works with the body's own chemistry. Glucose, the main sugar of the body, is converted to ribose in the cells. Corvalen M contains Bioenergy RIBOSE™, which is chemically identical to the ribose made by the body from glucose. Second, the amount of ribose recommended for supplementation is very small: only about 5 grams one to three times per day. And finally, there's virtually no chance of over-supplementation: Your body safely eliminates what it doesn't need. The only warning I give patients is that it may cause over-stimulation if taken too close to bedtime. In that case, I recommend that they take it earlier in the day, i.e. not past 4 p.m.

How much ribose should you take?

No matter what end of the health spectrum you're on, ribose may help restore energy levels. To keep cellular ATP levels at their highest, ribose should be taken daily.

Maintenance doses of 1 to 5 grams per day should be enough to maintain normal ATP levels. Corvalen M comes in a powder form than can be mixed with water: 5 grams is about 1 teaspoonful of the powder.

If you're concerned about your cardiovascular health, you may want to take more—perhaps 5 to 10 g per day. However, you should try the lower dosage first and increase as needed. For fibro-myalgia sufferers, I recommend 5 grams two or three times daily. For you athletes: To supercharge your workout and recovery, take 5 grams before and afterwards.

Although ribose is a sugar, for those of you watching their carbohydrate intake, including diabetics, ribose does not act like glucose in raising blood sugar. In fact, it causes a brief dip in glucose, which then normalizes.

So whether you have fibromyalgia, cardiac problems, low energy, or simply want to enhance your workouts, you can recharge your cellular batteries with Corvalen M's special combination ribose formula.

Hyla Cass, M.D., is Assistant Clinical Professor at UCLA School of Medicine and author of several books including Natural Highs: *Supplements, Nutrition and Mind-Body Techniques* (with Patrick Holford) and *8 Weeks to Vibrant Health: A Woman's Take-Charge Program to Correct Imbalances, Reclaim Energy, and Restore Well-Being*. She also serves on the board of Vitamin Relief USA, which provides daily nutritional supplements to at-risk children across the country. For more information see www.drcass.com.

CHAPTER THIRTEEN

Turn back the clock with nature's new fountain of youth— Six times stronger than the anti-aging secrets of the stars

Imagine if the fountain of youth really existed. Imagine if you could wash yourself in its healing waters and walk away feeling and looking like you were in your prime again. What if you didn't have to worry about cancer, hypertension, or other age-related diseases?

Just think about it…would you live your life differently? Would you spend more time visiting friends, outdoors, or at the beach? Would you get started on all those projects around the house that you never have the energy for? Would you lead a more active love life, take up a new hobby, change careers, or just play with your grandchildren on the floor once in a while?

This doesn't have to be just a fantasy. You can now slow, halt, and even reverse the effects of aging on your body. Health Sciences Institute has recently uncovered what could be the most powerful anti-aging supplement ever developed. This breakthrough has been proven to literally reverse the body's aging process by rebuilding old, damaged cells. With this powerful, life-changing panacea you can:

- Protect your cells from degenerative ailments like heart disease, MS, and Parkinson's disease
- Improve chronic age-related conditions like arthritis and osteo-porosis
- Wipe away wrinkles and liver spots
- Feel an overwhelming sense of well-being throughout the day
- Regain muscle mass and mobility in your limbs
- Improve the luster and vitality of your hair, nails, and skin
- Sleep through the night and wake up feeling alert and energized
- Boost your immune system

Ultra H-3 promises all this and more. It's the next generation of an anti-aging formula developed in Romania almost 50 years ago and heralded by the TV show 60 Minutes back in 1972. The difference is, Ultra H-3 is six times stronger 15 times longer than the original Romanian formula...and it lasts.

This cutting-edge compound has been developed by a distinguished think-tank of scientists and researchers—including HSI panelist, acclaimed author, and nutritional expert, Ann Louise Gittleman, N.D., C.N.S, M.S. It's just been patented in the United States, so there aren't many clinical studies yet. However, the initial results collected by Gittleman and her associates are so astonishing, we wanted to tell you about it immediately so you don't have to wait years for Mike Wallace to get wind of it.

The Romanian anti-aging miracle similar to an ingredient every dentist uses

The story of Ultra H-3 actually begins almost 100 years ago in Austria. Procaine—the primary active ingredient in Ultra H-3—was first discovered in 1905 by biochemist Dr. Alfred Einhorn while he was looking for a non-toxic, non-addictive anesthetic. At the time, cocaine was primarily used, but its negative characteristics were becoming apparent and its use was going to be outlawed. Procaine (very similar to novocaine) became a safe alternative anesthetic.

Nearly 50 years later in 1949, Dr. Ana Aslan of the National Geriatric Institute in Bucharest, Romania, discovered Procaine's anti-aging properties virtually by accident. Familiar with its anesthetic properties, Dr. Aslan began to inject her elderly arthritis patients with Procaine. To her surprise, not only did her patients experience decreased pain and increased mobility, they also began to experience overwhelming physical and mental improvements.

Dr. Aslan called her new discovery GH-3 and began a massive series of clinical trials that studied the effects of Procaine on 15,000 patients between ages 38 and 62. The study included over 400 doctors and 154 clinics, and at that point may have been the largest double-blind trial ever undertaken.

Procaine repairs the damage of old age, toxins, and disease from the inside out

By the time most of us reach 30, our bodies stop reproducing cells at the rate they once did. We literally lose more cells than we gain. And the cell membranes begin to erode and don't absorb nutrients as efficiently. New scientific evidence even suggests that many degenerative diseases—such as cancer, MS, and Parkinson's—are manifestations of damage to these cell membranes.[1]

Dr. Aslan and her research team found that Procaine works by penetrating old or damaged cell membranes and repairing the erosion caused by old age, disease, toxins, food additives, and stress. Bathed in this powerful elixir, cells in the body are then able to receive nutrients and vitamins and expel toxins effectively. This makes for a healthier—and younger—body, from the inside out.

In 1956, Dr. Aslan presented her findings to the European Congress for Gerontology meeting in Karlsruhe, West Germany. While her claims were initially met with skepticism, Aslan's astonishing conclusions could not be ignored for long:

- Close to 70 percent of GH-3 patients never contracted a disease
- Overall, the death rate in the GH-3 group was more than 5 times lower than the placebo group over 3 years
- Patients were less prone to infectious diseases and seasonal influenza
- Reduction of sick days off work by almost 40 percent
- Joint mobility improved in 56 percent of cases2

While not a cure to any single disease, GH-3 was proven to target and improve many common chronic diseases and conditions including:

- Acne
- Arthritis
- Decreased sex drive
- Dementia
- Depression
- Emphysema
- Excessive cholesterol
- Failing memory
- Heart disease
- Hodgkin's disease
- Hypertension
- Lethargy

- Lethargy
- Liver spots
- Migraine headaches
- Multiple sclerosis
- Osteoporosis
- Parkinson's disease
- Peptic ulcers
- Poor circulation
- Rheumatism
- Sickle cell anemia
- Sleep disorder
- Varicose veins

60 Minutes uncovers Dick Clark's anti-aging secret

During most of the 1960s, GH-3 fought its way through U.S. federal regulations. Then in 1972, Mike Wallace of 60 Minutes did an investigative piece on this underground anti-aging formula and much of the western world finally took notice. Since it was first developed, over 100 million people in more than 70 countries have used Dr. Aslan's formula. Hundreds of thousands of people were treated with GH-3 at her Romanian clinic, including many leaders from around the world, such as Mao Tse-Tung, Charles de Gaulle, Ho Chi Minh, Winston Churchill, and John F. Kennedy. Even many Hollywood stars—including Dick Clark, the Gabor sisters, Marlene Dietrich, Charlie Chaplin, Lillian Gish, Lena Horne, Charles Bronson, Kirk Douglas, and Greta Garbo. All traveled to Romania for Dr. Aslan's GH-3 treatments.

Next generation formula issix times stronger than the GH-3—and without the downside

While Dr. Aslan's results were extraordinary, her Procaine formula has its limitations—its beneficial effects wore off too quickly and the market was (and is) flooded by cheap and ineffective imitations. But now, through the HSI network, you and other members are among the very first in the United States to hear about Ultra H-3, the new and improved Procaine compound.

According to Gittleman, "Ultra H-3 is the most advanced and only patented Procaine formula ever developed. It's so powerful, many people respond to it within the first three days. I have actually had to reduce my dosage to half a pill because it's so powerful."

The secret to the new formula lies in the purification process. Ultra H-3 is run through a highly complex filtering process—making it 100 percent bioavailable. That means all the Procaine nutrients can be absorbed into the blood stream. Otherwise, Procaine leaves the body too quickly, providing only temporary relief.

Ultra H-3 actually lasts 15 times longer and is 6 times stronger than Dr. Aslan's formula, which only delivered 15 percent of the nutrients and costs thousands of dollars to administer.

According to Gittleman, "Ultra H-3 is a potent anti-aging supplement that keeps you feeling energized all day long. We have an enormous number of success stories from people who've felt relief from arthritis, depression, and lowered libido, and other chronic ailments associated with aging. We have even seen a return of some patients' original hair color. But most of all, you feel this overwhelming sense of well being." Gittleman added, "It's almost like an adaptogenic herb—it seems to provide whatever your body needs."

Ultra H-3 is all-natural, and you don't have to go to Romania to get it

Like the original formula, Ultra H-3 is a completely natural substance, and you don't need a prescription. It comes in pill form and should be taken once or twice daily (six to eight hours apart) with a glass of water, one hour before or two hours after eating. For most people, taking Ultra H-3 twice a day on an empty stomach for three months gets the best results.

Ultra H-3 can be taken with other vitamins and supplements. In fact, your regular supplements may be absorbed more efficiently while taking it.

Through Health Sciences Institute's cutting-edge network of alternative doctors and researchers, members like you can be the first to benefit from this anti-aging breakthrough, and you don't have to travel to Romania to do so. If you want a powerful, all-natural way to slow, halt, and even reverse the aging process—you need to give Ultra H-3 a try. To find out what the "fountain of youth" can do for you refer to the Member Source Directory at the back of this book.

Part VI

Osteoporosis

CHAPTER ONE

Build bone density and heal fractures in half the time with the Chinese tradeshow secret

When you see a "made in China" sticker, it's usually on the bottom of some sort of novelty gift: fuzzy bulldog bobble heads, cookie jars that play "C Is for Cookie"—things like that. And those are the types of products that Kate Ross has been traveling back and forth to China for 20 years to buy. She had a successful wholesale business specializing in gifts, and many of the items she sold came from tradeshows she attended in China. Ross usually stuck to the gift-type items featured at the shows, but she told me she was always intrigued by the myriad of other things available— especially the herbal remedies. She didn't really explore this area of the Chinese market until a series of coincidences convinced her to at least check it out.

One day, out of the blue, she received a fax inviting her to a trade-show in China specifically for herbal- medicine products. She was curious but didn't think too much of it. Then she received an e-mail from the hotel in China where she usually stayed, inviting her to this same tradeshow. Next, the airline sent an invitation for discounted plane tickets to the area. And with this series of pushes, she left for China and the tradeshow for Chinese herbal-medicine products.

From there, Ross' curiosity evolved into a brand new business venture: bringing a 3,000-year-old bone health formula to America, where it could fill the void left by the inadequate, even dangerous, conventional bone-building drugs we've had to rely on for so long.

And when I say it boosts bone health, I'm not just talking about osteoporosis: The reports I read claim that this remedy can actually heal bone fractures in as little as three weeks—literally half the usual healing time.

Common bone builder used in Chinese hospital makes its U.S. debut

It wasn't long after she arrived at the show that Ross found the ancient bone-building formula: While it's new to this country, the formula Ross discovered on her trip to China has been used there for centuries. It's also routinely used in many of China's most prestigious hospitals. Clinical trials in these hospitals yielded such remarkable results that it has become commonplace.

The formula, marketed under the name Osteoking, includes astralagus root, Asian ginseng root, safflower, tienchi ginseng root, Eucommia bark, tangerine peel, and purified water. Even taken individually, these ingredients each have their own benefits, yet combined in the manner and ratios found in Osteoking, they appear to have a more specialized bone-building action.

Osteoking targets the most important organ for maintaining bone health

A lot of the material and research discussing bone health from a Traditional Chinese Medicine (TCM) point of view talks about the importance of kidney health. Ross explained to me that in TCM the kidney is the vital Qi (life force) organ. This piqued my curiosity, so I searched for a modernized explanation.

Healthy kidneys convert a hormone called calcitriol to its active form of vitamin D. Calcitriol lets your body absorb calcium from the food you eat or standard calcium supplements. When your kidneys are not working well, they start to make less calcitriol—so even if you eat calcium, your body can't absorb it. That's when your parathyroid hormone (PTH) kicks in to make sure you always have enough calcium in your blood. PTH is produced by several small, bean-like parathyroid glands in your neck whose "job" is to tell your bones to release calcium into your bloodstream. Over time, this process can actually weaken your bones.

Understanding this important link, it makes sense that some of Osteoking's individual ingredients—astragalus, ginseng, and Eucommia bark—are known for their tonic effects on the kidneys. But Osteoking also has more direct effects on bone formation.

To get a better idea of how it works, it helps to know more about the actual structure of your bones and how they're made.

Two types of bone cells are involved in the bone-building process: osteoclasts and osteoblasts. The osteoclasts trigger bone resorption—which means to lose substance. In other words, they're the cells that break down existing bone to make way for new bone.

After the osteoclasts do their work, the osteoblasts trigger the bone-building that's necessary to replace the bone that has been resorbed. From childhood until around age 30, the osteoblasts work harder than the osteoclasts, which means more bone is built than is resorbed. Around age 30, you reach your peak bone mass—the time when your bones are as dense as they will ever be. Then the balance begins to shift.

For a while, the osteoclasts and the osteoblasts work pretty evenly, but around age 50, the osteoclasts (the resorbers) begin to outpace the osteoblast (the builders), which means more bone is resorbed than is newly made. This is what causes bone density to decrease.

Boosting basic bone-building functions

One of the studies I found on Osteoking, done by Kunming Medical College's Department of Orthopedics, demonstrated Osteoking's ability to increase bone health. Researchers studied three groups of rabbits: one group received no treatment, one received a "saline/model" treatment, and the remaining group received Osteoking. In the no-treatment group, researchers noted that the rabbits' bone cells were normal. In the saline/model group, the bone tissue deteriorated and even showed some bleeding. But in the Osteoking group, more osteoblasts, osteoclasts, neonatal bone cells, and cortex were seen, along with calcium salt deposits. The bone in the saline/model group was also soft and easily cut, while the Oseteoking groups bone was dense and hard to cut.[1]

Cut your time in a cast in half

I spoke with Steven Hathaway, who works for the company producing Osteoking. He started taking it after he was diagnosed with a condition called osteopenia, a loss of bone density that can lead to osteoporosis. He'd been taking Osteoking for about five weeks when he found out just how well it really works. As he recalled, on December 14, 2004, he went up into his attic to bring down his parka for the winter. He turned to come down the stairs, now blinded by the huge parka, and just as he was stepping down onto the landing with the full force of his weight, he stumbled on one of the household hazards many of us face every day—shoes.

He severely turned his ankle on a pair of shoes left on the landing. Immediately, the swelling began, and by the next morning, he was off to the hospital for X-rays. He'd suffered torn ligaments and a fractured fibula in his left ankle. The doctor put him in a cast, which limited his mobility and was just plain uncomfortable.

Hathaway was told he would need to wear the cast for the standard six weeks. But after just two weeks, he began insisting that the doctor do another X-ray so the cast could be removed. They reached a compromise: At three weeks, the X-rays were repeated—and the cast came off. That's half the standard healing time for fractures.

To confirm Hathaway's account, I was able to read a letter from his doctor stating, "This is very impressive since normally it takes about six weeks of healing time in a cast for this type of injury and you healed in half the time."

Bone density improves in only six months

Another Osteoking success story happened to Helene Y. She had been fighting osteoporosis for about four years and was taking lots of calcium supplements and walking every day to try to keep it from getting any worse. Yet, in July 2003, she broke her hip and underwent hip replacement surgery.

A November 25, 2003 bone scan highlighted her fears—her bone density was getting worse. She'd heard about Osteoking and decided to start taking it.

What happened next amazed everyone. As Helene recounts, "Six months later, on May 25, 2004, I had another bone scan done by my doctor, and the results of the test were stunning. The scan showed an increase in bone density of 8.8 percent after only six months." Helene's doctor said he "was very impressed and surprised to see such a significant gain in bone density in such a short period of time."

I spoke to Hathaway about Helene's case. He admitted that he couldn't rule out that the dramatic increase in bone density could have been due to discrepancies in the machines used to do the screenings.

So he asked the president and chief scientific officer of Sutton Medical Services to evaluate the results of both bone scans considering the variability of the machines. He used a different method of analyzing Helene's before-and-after bone health called a T-score assessment. Overall, Helene had an improvement in five out of six T-scores, putting any doubts about her progress to rest.

The testimonials are great—and promising. Of course, they're all from Osteoking's distributor, which obviously has more to gain in sharing good feedback than bad. But I was also able to turn up results from several human clinical trials that appear to back up the good reports.

95 percent improved fracture healing

I got a copy of the final report on the treatment of 60 cases of traumatic fracture with Osteoking from the Department of Orthopedics at the Hospital of Traditional Chinese Medicine in Kunming City. Researchers compared the results of patients taking Osteoking to a control group using a different remedy called Wudidang. The clinical evaluation showed that Osteoking reduced swelling by 95 percent and improved fracture healing by over 98 percent. It also appeared to be 98 percent effective as an analgesic.[2]

In another study, done at the Department of Orthopedics in the 59th Central Hospital of the People's Liberation Army (PLA) in China, researchers studied the effects of Osteoking in 60 people, all with traumatic fractures documented by X-rays. The fractures were caused by various events in various bones, so we can get a good idea of how many types of fracture can be affected.

Study subjects in the Osteoking group took 25 ml of Osteoking every other day for 12 days. The control group subjects took four capsules of a formula called Yushangling three times per day for 24 days.

At the end of the study, the researchers concluded that "the efficiency rates of analgesic, repercussion, and fracture union of the Osteoking group were more significant than those of the Yushangling capsule group. The Osteoking formula demonstrates improved effects on the union of fractures. It could shorten the time required for such a union to occur."[3]

Starting in March 1998, the Kunming Medical College began to study Osteoking's ability to combat bone necrosis. Necrosis basically means your bone is eroding or slowly dying.

Researchers administered the suggested dosage of Osteoking (25 ml every other day taken at bedtime) to subjects needing treatment for necrosis of the hip. The duration of treatment varied depending on the state of illness of each subject, ranging from 180 days to 720 days, and was combined with a course of exercise.

Of these cases, 51 subjects had necrosis in both hips and 25 had necrosis in just one hip, which makes for a grand total of 127 hips that the researchers evaluated. Among the 127 hips, 105 showed good results from the treatment. And it seems that only three of the 15 severe cases went on to receive hip replacement operations. While not all subjects experienced these results, after half a year to one year taking Osteoking, many showed "repair and changes around the necrosis region."[4]

The price of purity

Osteoking comes in one-month supplies. Since it's a liquid formula and is packaged in individual doses, it is a little more expensive than most supplements—about $118 for a one-month supply. But part of the cost also goes toward ensuring the product's safety and purity.

Both safety/toxicity studies I read showed Osteoking to be a pure, non-toxic, natural product. The manufacturer, Crystal Natural Pharmaceutical Corp., explained that, to test the safety of Osteoking, laboratory animals were given 540 times the normal dose, and the animals still continued to grow in size, strength, vigor, and health—with no apparent ill effects. However, you should know that it is not recommended for use by pregnant women, those with mental disease, glaucoma, or anyone suffering from heart, lung or kidney failure, or excessive bleeding.

The recommended dose is one bottle (25 ml) every other day. In the human studies, Osteoking was taken at bedtime—your body's natural regeneration period. And for best results, it is recommended that you take it for at least one month.

CHAPTER TWO

Reverse osteoporosis AND erase osteoarthritis with a single pill

When it comes to 'bad bones,' there are a lot of drugs and supplements out there—but none of them can actually fix what's wrong.

That's why Jerry Stine of ZyCal Bioceuticals was practically doing cartwheels when he came across a product that actually makes a difference... a product that helps your body grow new bone right where it's needed. And that's practically a miracle, but the benefits don't end there. This bone-building dynamo can actually improve the quality of your bones and joints, making the pain of osteoarthritis and the dangers of osteoporosis things of the past.

If you know anyone who doesn't have either osteoporosis or osteoarthritis, consider them very lucky—as lucky as a lottery winner. Because there's only a very slight chance that you won't get hit with at least one of the two once you get to a certain age.

The statistics alone can make your bones ache.

- Nearly 27 million Americans are affected by osteoarthritis (OA), including about one-third of Americans over age 65

- About 10 million Americans have osteoporosis... and around 8 million of those are women

- Osteoporosis causes at least 1.5 million fractures every year... including more than 300,000 hip fractures

- Almost 25 percent of people 50 and older who've fractured a hip will die within one year of the break

- Neither mainstream medicine nor nutritional supplements have successfully *fixed* the problem...

Until now.

Now, thanks to Stine's work with this remarkable product, you can actually turn osteoporosis around and create healthy new bones... and eliminate osteoarthritis pain by creating new cartilage, which is crucial for optimal joint health.

A complete bone-boosting game plan

At ZyCal Bioceuticals, they focus on the aging process... and how to stop, stall, and reverse it. It's all they do, and they won't even consider a product that doesn't tackle a fundamental aspect of aging.

Bone problems—like osteoarthritis and osteoporosis—are absolutely age-related. As we get older, the key mechanisms that build bone and cartilage slow down dramatically.

At the same time, though, your old bone removal system keeps running full speed ahead—a process called resorption. For that, special cells called osteoclasts travel through your bones looking for any pieces that need renewal. When they find one, the osteoclasts dissolve that piece, leaving an empty space.

When your body works at peak capacity, those spaces get filled in by another type of specialized cells called osteoblasts. Unfortunately, this process works less efficiently as we get older—so old bone is removed faster than new bone can replace it.

The common 'answers' to this problem are slowing down resorption (with drugs like Fosamax), and taking bone-strengthening supplements like calcium and vitamin D. But these solutions work around the real problem… not on it.

Ostinol helps your body grow new bone and cartilage

No other product on the market turns on the stem cell process of growing new bone and cartilage. Some drugs and supplements may help the process once it's started, but they can't make bone regrowth happen on their own because they don't contain BMPs (bone morphogenetic proteins)… the key component of *Ostinol*™.

BMPs are biologically active proteins—they actually stimulate your cells, putting them back to work. These unique proteins actually turn on the chemical signals that trigger the healing process in your bone tissue, telling your cells to start growing bone and cartilage. On top of that, BMPs have shown anti-inflammatory effects, a very important part of treating both osteoarthritis and osteoporosis.

And when you use Ostinol™ in combination with the right joint support supplements—watch out! The BMPs work together with things like calcium, vitamin D, glucosamine, and chondroitin… helping you build good quality bone.

In fact, it can even be used together with bone resorption-slowing drugs, for better results than you'd see with the drugs alone.

What's more—there doesn't appear to be any downside. Stine's clinical experience with Ostinol™ shows that the supplement is well-

---

You might be losing bone… without even knowing it

You may be one of the estimated 18 million Americans have osteopenia—low bone mass—even if you don't know it. In the early stages, bone loss causes no noticeable symptoms, but it does make your bones weaker, setting the stage for full-blown osteoporosis.

tolerated. In fact, none of his patients have reported any negative effects. Rather, he's seen many positive outcomes… even in highly unlikely situations.

BMPs are proven effective and safe

Stine isn't the only medical professional who's used BMPs successfully. There are forty years of research and twenty years of clinical experience behind the Ostinol™ formula—it's safety and efficacy are very well-established. In fact, there have been thousands of studies done on how BMPs work to form, fix, and stabilize bone and cartilage.

And since the 90s, BMPs have become a standard for use in bone surgeries. There, a liquid extract is poured directly on to the bone to kickstart healing… with an excellent success and safety record.

More recently, BMPs have been studied in connection with osteoarthritis by ZyCal Bioceuticals, Inc. (Osteoarthritis gets all the study funding because results are more obvious and come much quicker.) Here's what their two in-house OA studies found:

The pilot study focused on six patients with mild to moderate joint pain and stiffness, who were otherwise in good health. This small group of patients completed the Visual Analog Scale (VAS) questionnaires of pain and stiffness, at the study's outset. They all were given one tablet of Chondrinol® (a combination of Ostinol™, glucosamine and chondroitin), three times daily. And by the end of just one week, these subjects reported better than 50 percent reduction in pain and stiffness.

The encouraging (and very quick!) results from the pilot study prompted a larger and more elaborate follow-up. The second study (which is currently being submitted for medical review and publication in a major medical journal) was a Phase II, prospective, multi-center, open-label clinical trial. The twenty-three subjects all suffered from physician-documented moderate to severe cases of osteoarthritis, and no other serious ailments. Each completed the VAS questionnaire at the start of the trial.

These patients were all given Chondrinol® daily (1 tablet, three times a day), and after just one week, the group reported an average 27 percent decline in pain and stiffness. And by the end of the fourth week, they reported…

- 55 percent reduction in pain
- 59 percent drop in pain frequency
- 44 percent increased ability to participate in recreational activities
- 38 percent increase in strength

"Whatever your son is giving you, stay on it!"

And while no studies have yet been conducted on Ostinol's impact on osteoporosis (though some of its components have been studied), some success stories have been reported. Like the case of a 64-year-old woman (whose name has been omitted to preserve her privacy) with severe osteoporosis.

Her case was advanced and very difficult—her spinal DEXA scans showed 25 percent bone loss from 2004 to 2007. Still, she did not want to take pharmaceutical drugs, holding out hope for a natural remedy. Luckily, her son was a chiropractic physician, and he knew about Ostinol.

He put his mother on a regimen of Pro-Stiminol® (a combination kit of Ostinol™ and Tricalcidin-3®, a blend of organic calciums), one

---

Slowing down resorption can be a very bad thing

In theory, drugs that slow down bone loss sound like a good thing—but they're not. When you stop your body from clearing out old bone cells, it doesn't make your bones stronger or healthier. In fact, leaving old bone tissue in place can cause very serious side effects—like bone death (a.k.a. osteonecrosis) and severe infections.

tablet per day. After a year of using the supplement, her bone loss rate slowed by 25 percent… but she still wasn't regrowing bone.

So he had her take an Ostinol™ tablet in addition to her daily Pro-Stiminol®—and that brought on remarkable results. After six months on the new regimen, tests showed that her bone loss had stopped completely… and that her bone density had actually increased by 10 percent.

Her regular doctor was very impressed with the outcome. He told her, "Whatever your son is giving you, stay on it!"

The tip of the iceberg

While you don't need a consultation to buy Ostinol™ from ZyCal Bioceuticals, Stine says most people would benefit from talking with one of their medical professionals.

"Osteoporosis, and to a lesser extent osteoarthritis, are what I call 'tip of the iceberg' conditions," Stine told me. That's because losing bone density may be just the surface issue, complicated by something deeper—there are a wide variety of metabolic disorders and other serious health conditions that can set the stage for osteoporosis:

- Hormonal imbalance
- Cortisol regulation issues
- Blood sugar and insulin resistance problems
- Any inflammatory condition
- Low grade infections (like periodontal disease)
- GI disorders (including food sensitivities)
- Thyroid problems (especially if you take synthetic thyroid medication, like Synthroid)

With a more complete picture of your overall health, Stine and the other professionals at ZyCal Bioceuticals can develop a customized program that addresses your unique situation. They can also track your progress—osteoporosis takes a very long time to correct, two years or more, and it can seem like nothing is happening. That's why he recommends periodic testing using a special urine test that can measure your bone resorption rate, letting you see the improvement.

And while Ostinol™ is busy helping new bone grow, your body may require additional support to make sure that bone is of the highest quality. Stine may recommend some joint support products, a custom calcium/vitamin D blend… or tell you that what you're already taking can do the trick.

The standard dose of Ostinol™ is one tablet per day, but Stine told me that sometimes two a day may be necessary to get the job done.

You'll find ordering information for Ostinol™ in the Member Source Directory on page 529.

CHAPTER THREE

Addressing bone density is not enough... Breakthrough reverses osteoporosis by actually rebuilding bone

If you're approaching or past menopause, you're probably already paying a lot of attention to your bones and your risk of osteoporosis. And you're probably doing everything right—well, everything we knew was right before the newest bone-health breakthrough hit the scene.

Let's run down the list:

- Weight-bearing exercise? Check.
- A healthy diet? Check.
- Calcium-regulating supplements (like Tango's Osteophase, recommended several years ago in the *Members Alert*—see the December 2004 issue in the archive at www.hsionline.com)? Check.

These can all go a long way toward boosting your bone density.

For some time now, osteoporosis has been defined by low bone-mineral content (low bone density). So drugs treating osteoporosis have been developed to preserve the mineral content of bones.

But it turns out that boosting your bone density is only half the picture—in fact, if you're mineralizing your bones without addressing the underlying structure, you could actually be *increasing* your risk of fracture.

Thankfully, this new breakthrough supports the whole spectrum of bone health—by actually helping to rebuild the very structure of your bones. And it's the very first supplement of its kind to do so.

HSI medical adviser Dr. Martin Milner brought this one to me, saying "I have never seen a natural-medicine product better developed to specifically address the underlying limitations preventing bone re-modeling and osteoporosis reversal."

Why just increase density when you can actually rebuild bone?

The strength of your bones is about more than density—it's about the integrity of the bones' architecture—the bone matrix. In fact, after the age of 50, the bone matrix declines before bone density, leaving bones weak and fracture-prone.

And the continued strength of that matrix comes from a process called bone remodeling. Bone is living tissue that is constantly being broken down and rebuilt. Osteoclast cells remove old and damaged bone tissue, then osteoblasts and osteocytes create a new bone ma-trix—the web-like architecture of bone. This matrix incorporates min-erals to give bone its density and hardness. The process ensures your bones' structural integrity. This reduces your risks of fractures and os-teoporosis.

During your younger years, the remodeling process leans toward bone formation, increasing bone growth until peak bone mass is reached around age 30. In your mid-thirties, the rate of removal of weak bone starts to exceed that of new bone formation, meaning that you're slowly losing bone over time. The bone matrix (sort of the frame the bone is built upon) weakens. If you're taking supplements to mineralize and increase bone density, this hardening of partially formed or incomplete bone matrix means your chances of fracture are greater.

Once you hit menopause, lower levels of estrogen and progesterone start to affect the process of bone remodeling. Bone tissue starts to go through the turnover process at a higher rate—increasing fracture risk by decreasing matrix quality without having much effect on density.

Inflammatory agents that increase resorption (the breakdown of old bone cells) and suppress bone formation are no longer kept in check by estrogen. Because of this, you could actually lose up to 20 percent of your bone mass in the first five to seven years after the onset of menopause.

Up until now, women have been increasing bone density with calcium and vitamin D supplements. But this does nothing for the remodeling of the bone matrix. Fortifying a weak matrix doesn't change the matrix itself—meaning bones are still weak despite your best efforts.

This is where Ostera comes in.

Rev up your body's bone-building cells

Recently, there's been a shift. The new thinking is that certain body chemicals—scientists call them "biochemical markers"—tell us more about a woman's osteoporosis risk. Bone density tests only measure 20 percent of the skeleton, but these biomarkers show what's going on with the whole thing, as well as with the bone remodeling process. They hint at turnover rate, formation of bone, resorption of bone, and formation of new bone.

The level of the hormone osteocalcin (OC) is especially telling. This hormone controls the deposit of new bone. As osteoclasts destroy old bone, OC is released into the bloodstream. The more OC in the bloodstream, the faster the turnover of bone—and the higher your risk of fracture.

While Dr. Milner told me it's too soon to verify bone remodeling in his practice (Ostera is just that new!), a clinical trial, the results of which were published earlier this year, proves how well it works by examining the biomarkers associated with bone remodeling.

In the trial, 77 postmenopausal women—45 with Metabolic Syndrome and 32 who were generally healthy—participated. Both the trial group and the control group were instructed to follow a Mediterranean diet and exercise aerobically 150 minutes per week. Both groups did those things, but while the trial group also took Ostera twice daily. None of the subjects took calcium supplements or a multivitamin that might have contained calcium and/or vitamin D during the 14-week trial period.

At the beginning of the trial, both groups had elevated OC levels, indicating an increase in bone turnover rate and an increased risk for osteoporosis. At the end of the trial, the levels had gone up by 16.4 percent in the control group. The trial group, however, saw a significant decrease of 31 percent. Among women with Metabolic Syndrome, the increase in the control group was even higher (22.6 percent), but the trial group saw the same decrease as the women without Metabolic Syndrome.

The other biomarkers associated with bone remodeling and osteoporosis showed impressive results. P1NP, a marker of bone formation, significantly increased with use of Ostera, and significantly decreased in the control group. And IGF-1, a marker for vertebral fracture risk in postmenopausal women, increased significantly with Ostera (by 21.2 percent), which means they faced lower risk of fracture. The control group saw a decrease of 13.1 percent. An increase in IGF-1 in women with low estrogen is very impressive.

Serum vitamin D went up by 16.2 percent in the test group and decreased by 14.6 percent in the control group over the course of the trial.

As part of the trial, researchers also looked at estrogen levels. They found that these levels didn't change on an observable level, meaning that the positive effects on the bone-remodeling-related biomarkers didn't have anything to do with estrogen—it was all due to Ostera.

Overall, researchers concluded that a combination of the low-glycemic Mediterranean diet, exercise, and Ostera positively affected bone remodeling in postmenopausal women with low estrogen levels. They suggest that you could gain even more positive results with mineralization support and weight-bearing exercise.[1]

Four bone-boosting powerhouse ingredients in one formula

The benefits of Ostera come from a quartet of natural agents that are proven bone savers.

Rho iso-alpha acids (RIAA), derived from hops, modulate substances involved in bone degradation. Inhibition of these substances has been shown to promote bone formation and prevent the inflammation that accelerates bone loss.

Berberine acts in a similar way. It inhibits the activity of osteo-clasts, the cells that take part in the breakdown of bone tissue. It's also been suggested that berberine can positively influence the formation of osteoblasts, cells that build up bone tissue.

Then there's vitamin D, which you know for going hand-in-hand with calcium. In addition to helping the body absorb calcium for mineralization of bone, it also plays a role in regulating bone turnover. Low vitamin D intake has been linked to increased fracture risk and increased rates of bone loss.

Finally, vitamin K plays a major role in the metabolism of bone proteins that are central to bone quality, integrity, and support of overall bone mass. Regular intake of vitamin K has been linked with increased bone mineral density; it also has been shown to have a positive effect on bone remodeling.

The vitamin K in Ostera may interact with a common blood thinner, Coumadin(wayfaring sodium). If you are taking this medication, contact your physician before starting on Ostera. Too much vitamin K in a high-dark-green-leafy-vegetable diet and/or from supplementation can excessively thicken blood. If you have a tendency toward forming blood clots or need to thin your blood for other reasons such as coronary artery disease, contact your physician before taking Ostera.

It's an all-natural formula without serious adverse effects. Combined, the four components in Ostera help your body actually rebuild bone, instead of just increasing the density of bone that is already there.

Ordering information for Ostera is in the Member Source Directory on page 529.

CHAPTER FOUR

The milk-less secret to preventing osteoporosis

In October 2004, the U.S. Surgeon General released the first-ever report on bone health—and the news wasn't good. Apparently, by 2020, half of all Americans over age 50 will be at risk for low bone density and osteoporosis. But this dire warning did come with a silver lining: The risk will only increase that much if no one takes any immediate action to protect her bones.

No problem—we can all handle taking action. It's figuring out what action to take that can present a challenge. Of course, there are the prescription drugs like Fosamax, designed to build bone mass, and the dairy industry still clings to its claim that milk builds strong bones.

But osteoporosis drugs come with their own risks like nausea, altered sense of taste, and bone or joint pain. And milk just doesn't cut it in terms of bone health: In fact, studies show it's not the best source of calcium, the most crucial bone-health nutrient, and it doesn't actually protect against fractures or other bone problems.

You may have already made the switch over to calcium supplements to protect yourself from bone loss and osteoporosis. The key to keeping your bones strong and healthy is to regulate the calcium in your body.

And now there's an all-natural product that can help you do that.

It's called Osteophase, and preliminary studies show that it can reduce the loss of calcium, increase bone density, and increase bone remodeling.

Calcium regulating superstars
that will save your bones

Osteophase is the first nutritional supplement that reliably regulates calcium homeostasis to rebuild skeletal bone and resolve calcium overload.

It's a marine-based formula made from oyster shell lining combined with 21 different amino acids, iron, zinc, and three specific herbs—stragalus, Angelica sinensis root, and Coix seeds.

The inner lining of the oyster shell contains biologically active proteins and enzymes that are responsible for stimulating the formation of the hard outer shell from available calcium. The manufacturers of Osteophase developed a method of extracting these bioactive ingredients from the shell lining, along with calcium from the actual shell.

When they're combined with the three herbs in the formula, the active components of the oyster shell lining help regulate the functions of calcium in the body, pulling it out of soft tissues where it can cause damage, and re-directing it into the bones to strengthen them.

Research has shown that Astragalus extracts inhibit bone loss in rats that have had their ovaries removed. This could indicate that it may be a good bone-protecting alternative for post-menopausal women who were counting on hormone replacement therapy for this purpose.

Angelica sinensis is frequently used as the main ingredient in herbal prescriptions for bone injuries. One study found that Angelica stimulated synthesis of a substance called OPC-1, which is a crucial part of bone formation.

Coix seeds help counteract the degeneration of bone and cartilage.

For once you need even less than the "experts" recommend

The dose of Osteophase used in the clinical evaluation in China contained less than 125 mg per day of calcium. This level of calcium intake is actually far below the 1,000 mg of daily supplementation recommended by U.S. health authorities to protect against bone loss. But despite the lower level of calcium, the researchers found that Osteophase reduced the loss of calcium by up to 69 percent, increased bone density by 27 percent, and increased bone remodeling by 100 percent.

These results support the notion that Osteophase achieves its results by regulating the amount of calcium in the body—not by increasing it.

So even though the U.S. government probably won't add it to its list of ways to head off the burgeoning epidemic of osteoporosis and bone loss, it certainly looks as if Osteophase might be one of the best tools for taking that "immediate action" the Surgeon General recommended. See the Member Source Directory on page 529 for ordering information.

Part VII

Diabetes

CHAPTER ONE

Blood sugar buster three times more effective than top-selling diabetes drugs

A lmost as soon as it was introduced, the success stories started flooding in. Sugar levels were falling, pounds were plummeting, and blood pressure was sinking. All thanks to an herbal powerhouse called Syntra5™ (formerly known as Diatroxal).

But the word-of-mouth wasn't enough for the scientists behind this diabetes beater. So it was put to the test in a randomized, double-blind, placebo-controlled trial—the gold standard of scientific testing.

It turned out to be an **all-out assault** on diabetes. Fasting blood sugar dropped a shocking 107 points. Triglycerides fell by an impressive 20 percent. LDL cholesterol tumbled by more than 34 percent. And total cholesterol dropped over 29 percent.

If that weren't enough, participants in the trial lost an average of nearly 10 pounds—without changing eating or exercise habits.

And those were the results after only 90 days.

It all adds up to one undeniable fact—no other product, pharmaceutical or natural, created to treat diabetes has been shown to be even one half as effective as Syntra5™.

A formula so powerful, one company was willing to lay it all on the line to prove it

It's true. Even the top-selling diabetes drugs only drop blood glucose levels by <u>at most</u> 36.6 points. That makes Syntra5™ three times more effective—without the side effects of those drugs.

It's hard to believe it took a major gamble to get this powerful diabetes thrasher the attention it deserves. The story starts about 10 years ago, when Ken Hampshire, the co-founder of Syntratech, the group that developed Syntra5™, met Dr. Vern Cherewatenko, the author of *The Diabetes Cure*.

Dr. Cherewatenko had turned to Ken for help formulating and manufacturing a new product for type 2 diabetes. Together, they created Ultimate HCA, one of the first safe and effective solutions for type 2 diabetes.

Ken knew it was good, but he thought it could be even better. So when, three years later, Dr. Cherewatenko turned his attention to another project, Ken started scouring scientific journals.

In reviewing 20 years of research, he started seeing the same herbal extracts come up again and again—extracts that were able to lower insulin resistance in the body. Extracts that no other companies had seemed to notice.

These extracts were expertly combined to become Syntra5™. When it was introduced, the testimonials started pouring in. But for Ken, that wasn't enough. He wanted verifiable evidence that it was working.

Now, clinical trials are expensive. Too many companies with wonderful products simply can't afford to prove their effectiveness. So Ken commissioned a small study to see how Syntra5™ fared. Though there were only 17 participants, the results were very positive—so positive, in fact, that Ken decided to lay it all on the line.

Syntratech is a small company. So it was a big deal when the team there decided to put their entire marketing budget into a large-scale, randomized, placebo-controlled human clinical trial conducted at an independent lab. If Syntra5™ wasn't proven effective, they would be positively ruined.

But, as you already know—it worked. In fact, the results went beyond even their greatest expectations.

Top-selling diabetes drugs just can't touch it

When it comes to fasting blood glucose, a level below 100 mg/dL is considered normal or healthy and 100-125 mg/dL is considered pre-diabetic (and brings with it increased risk of cardiovascular disease). A count of 126 mg/dL, measured on two different days, is indicative of diabetes.

And of course, that means big health risks. Damage to the eyes, kidneys, blood vessels, heart, and nerves, as well as cognitive decline and even dementia, are all linked to diabetes.

All of the participants in the trial had chronic uncontrolled blood glucose, with fasting blood glucose counts between 160 mg/dL and 225 mg/dL.

In only 90 days, Syntra5™ brought those numbers down, on average, a whopping 107 points. Every participant taking it saw his or her fasting blood glucose drop to within the normal, healthy range.

If you're watching your blood sugar levels, you're also paying attention to your two-hour glucose level. This should be below 140 mg/dL. A count between 140 and 200 mg/dL indicates impaired glucose tolerance, and a level over 200 mg/dL goes hand in hand with diabetes.

Over the course of the trial, participants taking Syntra5™ experienced a 54.55 percent decrease in two-hour glucose levels. For participants taking the placebo, the level rose an average of just over 4 percent.

A third test measures the average amount of glucose in the blood over the 2-3 months prior to the test. It does this by measuring the concentration of hemoglobin A1c, or glycated hemoglobin. A 1 percent change in A1c reflects a change of about 30 mg/dL in average blood glucose level.

When blood was drawn from participants taking Syntra5™ at the end of the trial, A1c levels had dropped from an average concentration of 7.7 percent to an average of 4.66 percent—a highly significant 3 percent drop. All of the subjects in the active group had their A1c levels drop to 5 percent or below.

Now, Syntra5™'s effect on blood glucose levels would be impressive on its own. But this herbal formula had more in store for the trial participants.

Triglycerides, a type of fat within the bloodstream, decreased an average of over 20 percent in participants taking Diaxtroxal. With placebo, there was an average increase of 6.6 percent.

Cholesterol levels were also positively affected by Syntra5™. In the active group, participants' LDL cholesterol was lowered by over 34 percent, and their total cholesterol went down by 29 percent.

Syntra5™ demonstrated action on blood pressure as well. Over the course of the 90 days, participants taking Syntra5™ were rewarded with an average 25 percent drop in systolic pressure, 5 percent diastolic.

Then there was the weight loss. Prior to the trial, most of the participants had already been trying to control their blood sugar levels with diet and exercise. But they weren't having much luck. The researchers conducting the trial told the participants not to make any changes in diet, exercise or water intake.

Even without making such changes, the participants in the Syntra5™

group lost an average of almost 10 pounds. They expressed no changes in hunger or appetite, and no changes in cravings for sweets.

Of course, all of these numbers are meaningful. But they become even more important when paired with how the participants *felt* during the course of the trial.

Only two weeks in, 25 percent of the people in the active group said they felt better than they had in years. After one month, half of them reported having more energy.

Of course, the overall result of the test, reported by the researchers, was that Syntra5™ is a very safe and effective product for the management of diabetes.[1]

When the results of the study went through the peer-review process, it was noted that Syntra5™ beat the heck out of the leading diabetes drugs.

The seven leading pharmaceutical drugs for diabetes lower A1c less than 1 percent, and none of them are able to lower it to a level below 7 percent. Put simply, Syntra5™ produced more than a three-fold greater decrease in A1c than pharmaceuticals.

And when it comes to fasting blood glucose, pharmaceutical products can't touch Syntra5™. The most fasting blood glucose drops with the top-selling diabetes drugs is 36.6 mg/dL. In the Syntra5™ trial, the average was an amazing 107 points. This great an effect was previously unheard of.[2]

20 years' worth of research
boiled down into one breakthrough blend

When I talked to Ken, I asked him to tell me what he considered the "super stars" among the herbal extracts that make up Syntra5™. He didn't have to think long.

Back when he was scouring 20 years' worth of research, he saw two substances come up more than any others.

Hydroxycitric acid (HCA) and Gymnema sylvestre extract work in a number of ways to improve glucose metabolism. While there are quite a few studies on these components, two provide a good example of their effect.

In a 2004 animal study conducted at Georgetown University, HCA was found effective and safe as a weight-loss agent. It was also shown to inhibit the enzyme that controls the synthesis of fatty acids, cholesterol, and triglycerides. The effects were dramatic after a period of only eight weeks.[3]

In another study (also conducted at Georgetown) combining HCA with chromium (which is also in Diaxtroxal) and gymnema sylvestre extract, total cholesterol was lowered 9.5 percent and LDL cholesterol was lowered 19 percent, while HDL cholesterol went up by 22.1 percent. Triglyercides dropped by 20.5 percent.[4]

These two ingredients are joined by ten other active ingredients, all painstakingly researched by Ken. And what he *didn't* include is almost as important.

In many popular natural products used to treat diabetes, you'll see the same ingredients pop up over and over. Ingredients like alpha lipoic acid and CoQ-10 were not included in Syntra5™ because Ken just wasn't seeing the evidence that they work. Rather than following the trend set by other companies, he has created a completely new formula. And the evidence speaks for itself.

Drop blood sugar, pounds, and blood pressure in one easy step

A while ago, I mentioned that when Syntra5™ was introduced, the testimonials started pouring in. Well, they haven't stopped. I was given pages and pages of them, and promised more if I needed them. I'll share just a few.

Charles in Arizona didn't want to take drugs to control his blood sugar, so he went in search of a natural option. An Internet search led him to Syntra5™, and he decided to take a chance. After just a couple of weeks, his energy returned and he had started losing weight.

His blood sugar had started in the high 300s, but plunged to the high 90s. He says he's very satisfied, but jokes that "the drug companies are probably not happy with Syntra5™ because their bank accounts are smaller."

Lynn in New Mexico wanted another option when her doctor presented her with a month's supply of Avandia. She never even broke the seal—instead, she found Syntra5™.

Just over three months later, she had dropped 20 pounds and four inches in her waist. Her blood sugar had gone down from 182 to 111. At her last checkup, her blood pressure was 110/80. Her doctor was amazed, and told her to just keep on doing what she'd been doing.

Mike in Minnesota has also been singing the praises of Syntra5™. His blood sugar has gone from 180 to under 120 and he's feeling a lot more energetic these days. He unexpectedly lost 10 pounds and "would highly recommend this product to anyone."

Ordering information for Syntra5™ is in the Member Source Directory on page 529.

CHAPTER TWO

Forget willpower: Overcome sugar addiction in 21 days with a natural herb

I f it's ever happened to you, you know it's something far beyond will-power. Maybe you're driving home from work, maybe you're reading a gripping murder mystery. But all of a sudden your thoughts turn to a leftover piece of cake in the fridge. You're not even hungry and you *know* you don't need the extra calories, but you literally cannot stop thinking about it. Finally, you get to the fridge, fork in hand, and you give in. It isn't a lack of willpower that got you, it's a full-fledged addiction.

The same brain receptors that can lead to drug and nicotine addictions also let you become addicted to sugar.[1]

Understanding that it's *not* personal weakness, but a true physical addiction, is the first step to overcoming the cravings. Let's be honest: It's not easy to give up sugar. Cravings—physical and mental can dominate your thoughts. Quitting "cold turkey" sometimes works to curb cravings, but that can backfire. Avoiding sweets can lead to such an uncontrollable craving for sugar that you "give in" just once—and end up bingeing. And then the cycle continues.

Pavlov's dogs hold one key
to beating your habit

Research shows that certain activities or habits (like sitting down to that mystery novel) may be compelling you to eat sugary foods. This goes back to the studies done by Pavlov. We all remember the story of how he conditioned dogs to salivate when a bell rang by ringing a bell whenever they were fed. Eventually, the dogs began to salivate just from the sound of the bell—food was no longer required.

Your sugar habit may have a similar psychological connection. You may crave sugar because of certain surroundings, smells, sounds, or circumstances.[2] If, for example, you always eat a candy bar when you go to the movies, then viewing a film on your VCR may stimulate the same cravings. This sort of behavior pattern becomes an even bigger problem when the frequency of the activity increases: You probably watch movies at home more often than you do at the theater. If you give in to your sugar cravings each time you pop a video into the VCR, you'll significantly increase your sugar intake.

Eating sweets fuels cancer growth

One of the most devastating side effects of sugar consumption is accelerated cancer growth. Seventy years ago, Otto Warburg, Ph.D., won the Nobel Prize in medicine when he discovered that cancer cells use glucose (sugar) for growth. All cells have a requirement for glucose, but cancer cells have a much greater need. In fact, they're unable to multiply rapidly without it.

Besides fueling cancer growth, other health problems may be linked to eating too much sugar. In addition to causing obesity, excess sugar intake can lead to diabetes, encourage an overgrowth of pathogenic intestinal flora, aggravate gout, and cause or exacerbate panic attacks, hyperactivity, and depression. Not to mention what it does to your teeth!

"Just for the taste of it" puts you back at the beginning

For some people, changing their behavior is all that's needed to stop eating sugar. But, if you crave sugar because you're dependent on it or are physically addicted to it, environmental and behavioral changes probably won't halt the incessant cravings. And it's important to note that switching over to artificial sweeteners won't help.

It's the sweet *taste* that generates the release of addiction-building brain chemicals. According to Dr. Bart Hoebel, a neuroscience addiction researcher at Princeton University, the surge of dopamine and opioids—brain chemicals that "drive" the addiction process—occurs regardless of the number of calories in the sweetening agent.[3]

Dr. Hoebel's animal research indicates that rats experiencing sugar withdrawal displayed symptoms such as teeth-chattering, anxiety, and "high-pitched crying." These are classic displays of withdrawal from an addictive substance, although Dr. Hoebel claimed they were milder than those suffering from drug withdrawal.

If your sugar cravings are linked to dependence or addiction, you should expect to go through some withdrawal if you don't eat or drink something sweet when your body signals a need. Again, the symptoms of sugar withdrawal are similar to those of drug withdrawal, though not as severe.

Don't "tell" your brain that you're eating sugar

To break the endless cycle of sugar cravings, you have to address your <u>physical</u> requirement for a "hit" of something sweet as well as the <u>behavior</u> that automatically makes you reach for something sweet— even if you don't crave it at that moment.

There are different taste buds on your tongue. In order for you to taste something, it must touch the appropriate taste receptor, or bud, on your tongue. When the taste bud receives its "signal," it sends an impulse to the brain—and you know what flavor you're eating. If you eat something sweet but your tongue doesn't perceive it, it won't send the appropriate signal to your brain.[4]

Gymnema sylvestre, an herb well known by diabetics for reducing high blood-sugar levels, can prevent you from tasting sugar. When gymnema comes in contact with the taste buds on your tongue, it "binds" with the ones that receive the signal for sweet flavors and blocks the taste of sweet things from being perceived by your tongue.[5] Since your tongue doesn't know it's eating something sweet, it won't signal your brain's receptors to release opioids and dopamine.

Although the brain secretions of opioids and dopamine have been prevented, the chemistry of your brain has not been altered.[6] But it does mean you're defeating the cycle of physical addiction by stopping sweet flavors from "communicating" with your taste buds. It also means your brain's addiction receptors are not receiving a sugar fix. This may send you into some form of withdrawal.

Chew your way beyond the craving

Gymnema is available in capsule form at most health food stores.

CHAPTER THREE

Cutting-edge sugar research may revolutionize your health

Scientists predict that the next great frontier of research will center on sugar, of all things. And their findings are likely to change the way the world thinks about medicine and health.

It's already changing the way some forward-thinking doctors approach many diseases—not to mention general preventive care. And after reading this, it may change the way you approach your own health, too.

The next health frontier

Now that the human genome project is nearing completion, many scientists predict that the next big research initiative will focus on *glycobiology*, the study of the role of sugars in all living things. In fact, some believe that "the sugar code" is even more complex than the genome, and may have an even more significant impact on the worlds of science and medicine.

HSI Medical Advisor Martin Milner N.D. clued us in to the research being done to break the sugar code. "Glyconutrition is a new flourishing area of nutritional research," says Milner. "We are finding glyconutrient deficiencies associated with a large range of diseases."

That's no exaggeration. In my research for this article, I found glycobiology mentioned in relation to everything from skin aging to rheumatoid arthritis to cancer. That may seem like a stretch, but when you begin to understand just what these sugar complexes are responsible for, you can see how a deficiency in any one of them can wreak havoc with your health—and how correcting those deficiencies can help relieve—and prevent—a whole host of problems.

Essential sugars may be more vital than fatty acids or proteins

Research over the past decade or so has shown us that there are essential fatty acids and essential proteins (amino acids); now we're just beginning to understand that there are essential sugars, called monosaccharides, as well. Specifically, the basic eight are: glucose, galactose, fucose, mannose, xylose, n-acetyl-neuraminic acid (NANA), n-acetyl-glucosamine and n-acetyl-galactosamine. These individual sugars also function as building blocks to build a virtually innumerable variety of complex molecules called *glycans*, *glycoforms*, or simply sugar chains.

There are two ways that these sugar chains impact our health. The first we touched on in the April 2003 issue, when we told members about Xlear, a xylose-based nasal spray that clears lingering bacteria from the nose. Xlear is an example of sugar's anti-adhesive properties; literally, these sugars can prevent viruses and bacteria from adhering to cells by taking up all their receptor sites. If the virus or bacteria can't bind to a cell, they can't make you sick; it's as simple as that. Turns out other sugar chains can work in similar ways to bind up all sorts of viruses and bacteria in other parts of the body. In fact, pharmaceutical companies are focusing a lot of attention these days on developing anti-adhesive drugs to treat a wide range of conditions.

But there's another more complex role that these sugar chains play in the body. Glycans form a sugar coat around every single cell in the body, as well as filling up the spaces in between cells. They act as a sort of information super highway for the body, regulating communication both within the cell and between that cell and other cells, as well as other critical physiological processes.[1]

Breaking the sugar code

Unlike the building of DNA, RNA, or proteins, glycan synthesis doesn't follow a template that churns out identical copies over and over again. Instead, the monosaccharides can combine with each other in almost innumerable ways.

That's why so many scientists refer to glycobiology as "the sugar code." Each of these combinations is like a complex code, sending a specific message to a specific target, whether it be another cell, substances within the same cell, a circulation hormone or protein, even an invading bacteria or virus. These sugar chains play a vital role in nearly every physiological process known to man: immune system response, tissue regeneration, cell replication and growth—the list goes on and on.

This staggering capacity for variation is both glycans' strength and weakness. On one hand, according to scientists, "the potential... exceeds that of nucleic acids or proteins."[2] But on the other hand, one tiny misstep in the complex glycan construction process and things can go horribly awry.

You can't get enough from food alone

Unfortunately, there's a lot of opportunity for things to go wrong. You see, of the eight basic monosaccharides needed to build these complex glycans, most people only get enough of the first two, glucose and galactose. You may get a little bit of the other six here and there in your diet, but modern agricultural methods, processing and chemical contamination have all but erased them from our food supply.

Think of it in the same way you think of the vitamins and minerals your body needs to stay healthy: In today's environment, it's nearly impossible to get all the vitamins you need from your food alone. And while the body manages to function without supplemental vitamins, operating under these conditions takes its toll, opening the door for disease.

It's the same with these essential sugars. When forced to, the body is able to synthesize the missing monosaccharides it needs to build these complex glycoforms. But the conversion process diverts energy and attention from more urgent needs in the body—and increases the risk of critical errors in process.

Think how one little letter can completely change the meaning of a word, or how one pencil stroke can change one letter into another. It's the same way with cellular communications. In building these complex glycan codes, just one little error can completely change the meaning.

Dr. Milner explains it this way, "If one cell intends to communicate to another cell that it is a *F*R*I*E*N*D*, yet the molecular structure says that it is a *F*I*E*N*D* due to an imperfect conversion that resulted in a missing 'link,' then that cell will be destroyed, although it is a perfectly healthy and normal cell." And, as you can imagine, that one small miscommunication can lead to big problems.

Sugar's role in aging, autoimmune disease, even cancer

While much research still needs to be done to completely break the sugar code, there is already a large body of evidence supporting the idea that providing supplementary monosaccharides to the body can improve cellular communication and impact a whole host of conditions—from things as seemingly minor as skin aging and bacterial infection to debilitating illnesses like muscular dystrophy, atherosclerosis, Alzheimer's disease, and Parkinson's disease.[3-6]

Numerous studies also show how various monosaccharides and sugar chains play a role in autoimmune diseases. For example, studies have shown that rheumatoid arthritis patients have an abnormally high volume of Immunoglobin G molecules that lack galactose.[7] In addition, RA patients' glycoproteins demonstrate an abnormal uptake of fucose, another essential monosaccharide.[8] People with lupus show a deficiency in mannose.[9] And multiple sclerosis (MS) patients have demonstrated abnormal xylose absorption and excretion levels.[10]

More research has shown that cancer cells contains different glycan structures than normal cells, structures that may promote cancer progression. Glycans on cancer cells may promote metastasis by helping cancer cells bind to tissues, and may promote cancer cell *angiogenesis*, the development of blood vessels, which helps cancer grow and spread.[11]

As you can see from this extensive and wide-ranging list, there are vast implications of this new field of study. Just last year, MIT Technology Review included glycomics in its list of "10 Emerging Technologies That Will Change the World." Pharmaceutical companies are busily working to try to create synthetic versions of these essential glycans in their laboratories. The pharmaceutical companies, of course, need a synthetic version to get their patents—and their profits.

But remember, all of these essential sugars exist in their original, pure—un-patentable—forms in nature. That means you don't have to wait while dozens of scientists complete decades of research to document every last detail of the sugar code. And you don't have to wait for a prescription to be available to treat an existing condition.

Glyconutrients save patient from "death's door"

Dr. Milner has just started using a glyconutritional supplement in his practice that provides all eight essential monosaccharides. After just a few months, he's already seen results in a patient with a chronic skin condition called *folliculitis*, inflammation of the hair follicles. He's currently using it in a patient with an inflammatory joint condition similar to arthritis. And he's in the preliminary stages of planning a clinical trial in conjunction with the National College of Naturopathic Medicine to assess glyconutrient supplementation's effectiveness against a whole range of conditions.

Dr. Milner learned about this glyconutrient therapy from a patient of his, James Macfarlane, who used the approach himself when an accident caused second and third degree burns over nearly 30 percent of his body. I spoke to James and heard his amazing story firsthand.

When he was first taken to the hospital after the accident, doctors told him he would need massive doses of antibiotics to prevent infection, and skin grafts in order to heal normally. They also told him he'd be in the hospital for at least two weeks. After treating himself with glyconutrients, Macfarlane says he was able to leave the hospital in under a week, without any antibiotics or skin grafts. Today, he says, the skin has healed without scarring and looks completely normal.

James then referred me to Michael Schlachter, M.D., a board-certified internist in Las Vegas, who uses glyconutrient therapy with his patients.

Dr. Schlachter has used glyconutritional therapy on patients with amyotrophic lateral sclerosis (also known as ALS or Lou Gehrig's disease), asthma, and cardiomyopathy. But his most compelling story involves a patient he saw in a Las Vegas area hospital suffering with streptococcal toxic shock syndrome. (While toxic shock used to be associated primarily with tampon use, doctors now know that this blood borne infection, caused by the streptococcal or staphylococcus bacterium, can strike anyone.)

Dr. Schlachter told me that when he encountered the patient, "He was literally at death's door." After several weeks battling his sickness at home, then several days of hospitalization and aggressive treatment with antibiotics, the patient was deteriorating rapidly and experiencing multi-organ failure. Dr. Schlachter stepped in and asked the family for permission to treat with glyconutritionals. They agreed, and according to Dr. Schlachter, just a few hours after he administered a large dose of glyconutrients through the patient's feeding tube, the patient's condition began improving.

Have you taken your multi-glycan today?

Dr. Schlachter is convinced that glyconutrients saved this man's life, and that they can do the same for many others. "The whole premise of glycobiology, it's so simple, it's sickening that most doctors don't get it," says Schlachter. "I believe glyconutrients should be used as a broad spectrum preventative therapy."

Many doctors, including Dr. Milner, agree. Just as a daily multi-vitamin has reached mainstream acceptance, glyconutrition proponents believe that someday even conventional medicine will recognize the benefits of a daily "multi-glycan." By taking a daily multi-glycan supplement, we may be able to prevent a vast number of communication errors between cells that lead to depleted immune defenses, allergic reactions, and even deadly disease.

But, like I said, you don't have to wait until the mainstream catches up. Through Mannatech, HSI Members can now get the same glyconutrient formula that Dr. Milner and Dr. Schlachter use with their patients.

Provide your body with the glyconutrients it's missing

It's called Ambrotose, and it's a blend of essential monosaccharides, all derived from natural sources. Ambrotose contains glyconutrients from the larch tree, the aloe vera plant, the Indian sumac tree, the astragalus shrub, the bacteria *xanthomonas campestris*, the acacia shrub, and even seashells—all combined to provide the building-block sugars our bodies need.

Ambrotose is available in both capsules and powder form. Dr. Milner recommends one to two capsules two times a day or 1/2 teaspoon of the powder dissolved in juice or water and taken twice daily.

The Ambrotose glyconutrient complex is also available in another formula, combined with a blend of antioxidants for even more benefits. The Ambrotose AO formula contains the same glyconutrients in the regular formula, as well as antioxidants like vitamin E, quercetin, grape skin extract, green tea extract and Australian bush plum.

Forward-thinking scientists and doctors championed the "radical" cause of vitamin supplementation for decades before the mainstream accepted its benefits. No doubt glyconutrient supplementation will encounter similar obstacles.

But you don't have to wait until they get on board, or until some drug company comes up with a synthetic derivative. Make glyconutrients part of your daily preventative program now, and you can be enjoying the benefits long before it ends up on every grocery store shelf.

CHAPTER FOUR

The battle is won: Maintain healthy blood sugar, once and for all

No matter how hard you try, you're losing the battle with blood sugar. You worry soon your levels will creep out of the normal range. Eating flavorless food and dealing with the dreaded treadmill aren't helping enough. And you're afraid that some of the consequences you've heard about might just happen to you.

Unless you find a way to maintain healthy blood sugar levels within the normal range. Fast.

Luckily, you may be able to do just that, with an extraordinary product from one of the most innovative (and controversial) doctors I've ever come across.

And this product is a true solution, one that addresses more than just maintaining healthy blood glucose levels—it can also help protect your body from the effects of excess sugar. That sounds like an impossible task, especially for a natural product, but this formula (with more than half a century of science to back it up) combined with a healthy diet and exercise, may just be able to accomplish the impossible.

Three sugar-busting ingredients are all you need

I've been searching for a solid, effective blood sugar product all year—with no luck, which is why you haven't seen one in your *Members Alert*. Until now.

It took medical maverick William Campbell Douglass II, M.D. to come up with the ultimate blood sugar maintenance formula—a formula that contains just three sugar-busting ingredients. And while Dr. Douglass could have included more in the mix, well, he just wouldn't. Because stuffing the formula with more ingredients 'would just make you take more pills and cost you more money.' (I'm paraphrasing here—Dr. Douglass uses much more colorful language.)

Bottom line: His formula contains "everything you need, and nothing you don't."

And when you learn more about the trio of sugar-managing nutrients he chose, you'll see why GlucoComplete is indeed the perfect choice for helping keep blood glucose under control.

But this formula doesn't stop there. Not only can GlucoComplete help you keep your blood glucose levels under control, it may also help protect the cells of your kidneys, heart, nerves and eyes from the ravages of excess blood sugar.

Hidden solution helps protect you from the effects of high blood sugar

When you battle with blood sugar spikes, all of your cells are surrounded by blood that contains too much glucose. And while many cells can just ignore that extra sugar—keeping their internal glucose levels normal—some just can't. Those cells end up with too much internal sugar, and that's where some truly devastating problems start.

Excess sugar inside a cell creates something called reactive oxidative species (ROS). This leads to oxidative stress, which damages and ages your cells and surrounding tissues.

But it turns out there may be a way to teach your cells exactly how to handle that excess sugar and keep them healthy. In fact, the Japanese uncovered this solution way back in the 1950s, and European doctors have been prescribing it for decades. So why aren't we using this solution by the bucket in the good ol' U.S.A.? According to Dr. Douglass, it's all about the money.

See, the patent on this solution has expired—and no patent means no big payday for Big Pharma. But it also means a highly effective way for you to manage your blood sugar, naturally and safely.

The solution is benfotiamine, a special form of thiamine (also known as vitamin B1). What makes this vitamin different from standard thiamine is the way your body processes it: benfotiamine is fat-soluble, which means that your body can absorb and use more of this essential nutrient than its regular water-soluble form (that passes through your system before it has a chance to work).

And just a small amount of benfotiamine can help keep extra glucose from damaging your cells… and has been shown through *in vitro* studies to also help protect organs and tissues struggling to handle excess blood sugar.

Your cells can't handle sugar without thiamine

Though you hardly ever hear about it, your body needs thiamine—especially if you have to fight to keep your blood sugar under control. It plays a key part in carbohydrate metabolism within every cell of your body, and that's the process that helps your cells handle sugar.

So having adequate levels of thiamine in your body can help protect your cells from the oxidative damage that can be brought on by blood sugar spikes.

Here's the problem: virtually all thiamine supplements are water-soluble, so your body breaks them down too fast and they pass through too quickly to really help.

Benfotiamine solves that problem.

Because of its special structure, this form of thiamine gets absorbed much better by your body than typical thiamine supplements.[1] That gives benfotiamine more time to work with your cells, helping them manage glucose much more effectively. While the research is still pre-liminary (meaning we need human studies to confirm the results), ben-fotiamine seems to act by allowing thiamine to boost the activity of cer-tain enzymes including transketolase. Transketolase helps your cells use up glucose properly, instead of letting it hang around to cause trouble.[2]

When transketolase levels go up, your cells have an easier time han-dling excess glucose, a critical step for maintaining healthy blood sugar levels. But benfotiamine doesn't stop there. By redirecting glucose away from damaging pathways, benfotiamine could help protect your kid-neys, eyes, nerves and heart cells from damage caused by excess sugar.

You see, excess glucose in cells can actually cause a chemical reac-tion between glucose and proteins that create AGEs (advanced gly-cation end products). What are they? AGEs literally age your body prematurely. Benfotiamine appears to enhance the activity of certain enzymes which halt the chemical reaction that forms AGEs, sending any excess glucose on a safer pathway—one that avoids, and maybe even helps, repair your cells.[3]

And there's plenty of research to back that up.

Study after study shows just how protective benfotiamine can be

This super nutrient does all the work of essential vitamin B1, only more and better. There are many studies that demonstrate its amazing ability to help protect against the effects of blood sugar spikes, but we'll just look at the highlights.

First, when researchers reviewed benfotiamine studies, they found that this nutrient appears to stop sugar-induced oxidative damage in its tracks. It does that by calming the harmful effects of elevated glucose levels.[4,5] Specifically, *in vitro* studies have shown that this nutrient may actually protect endothelial cells (special cells that line the inside of those blood vessels) from the effects of high blood sugar.[6] That's important because those special cells play a part in forming healthy blood vessels.

But benfotiamine's protection isn't limited to blood vessels. An *in vitro* study found that it could also help protect your eyes, and that could make all the difference in preserving your vision. It turns out that benfotiamine may help keep cells of the retina (a critical part of eyesight!) from dying off after exposure to high blood glucose levels.[7,8]

And an animal study found that three potential damage-causing biochemical pathways, which are activated by elevated blood sugar levels, had been "normalized" in benfotiamine-treated lab rats. This was most clear in the animals' eyes: their retinas were similar to normal retinas. A microscopic examination revealed that the retinas of the benfotiamine-treated animals had been protected from the effects of high blood sugar.[9]

On top of that, another *in vitro* study found that benfotiamine contributed strong antioxidant properties in kidney cells.[10] And then there are the benefits it can bring to your heart cells (which also needs protection from spikes in glucose levels)…

- Animal studies show that benfotiamine supports cardiovascular health.[11]

- One animal study found that a two-week regimen of benfotiamine improved heart function in mice.[12]

- Researchers also found that benfotiamine treatment helped reduce oxidative stress and helped maintain proper calcium levels in the hearts of mice—and the heart simply can not beat properly when calcium levels aren't well-regulated.[13]

So benfotiamine can help keep your nerves, heart, kidneys and other vital organs healthy by reducing oxidative stress caused by blood sugar spikes. But what it doesn't seem to do is actually help maintain healthy blood glucose levels. Which brings us to the second critical ingredient in Dr. Douglass' GlucoComplete formula.

Apple pie surprise astonishes researchers with its insulin-boosting powers

No blood sugar formula would be complete without an ingredient that actually worked to help support healthy blood glucose levels— and that's why Dr. Douglass included cinnamon, but not just any cinnamon, as you'll learn in a moment.

Cinnamon first came to light as a potential blood sugar manager more than a decade ago. And like many natural remedies, this one was discovered by accident.

When I talked to USDA scientist Dr. Richard Anderson, he told me just how he stumbled upon this sugar-busting spice. He'd been studying the link between low-chromium diets and high blood sugar (more about chromium in a minute), and discovered what turned out to be a revolutionary find. As part of the study, he had to come up with tasty chromium-free foods... and that got apple pie on the menu. Surprisingly, the apple pie sent insulin activity through the roof. After finding that apples couldn't be the reason, they looked at the cinnamon, and changed the world of blood sugar management forever.

"When you improve insulin function, you improve many things," Dr. Anderson told me. He explained that components of cinnamon have been shown in *in vitro* studies to actually inhibit the kinase enzymes, which are thought to decrease the activity of insulin receptors. Inhibiting these enzymes, in turn, may increase your body's insulin sensitivity, which can help support healthy blood sugar levels.

Cinnamon can help increase insulin activity to help keep blood sugar levels under tight control

Let's start with the facts. Cinnamon can help:

- Support insulin activity
- Boost cell receptor sensitivity, which helps your cells metabolize sugar better
- Decrease fasting blood sugar levels (up to 29 percent in one study!)
- Maintain healthy blood pressure

One of the most important things cinnamon can do is help your body use its own insulin to manage blood sugar more effectively, and it does that in two ways. First, unique compounds called type-A polymers can boost insulin activity. One *in vitro* study found that these polymers increased insulin activity twenty times—that's 2000 percent![14]

Then, an animal study[15] found that cinnamon extract increased the sensitivity of the cell receptors that handle sugar metabolism. In this three-week study, rats were given either 30 mg or 300 mg (per kg of body weight) of cinnamon extract or placebo every day. Then the rats got glucose and insulin IVs so the researchers could follow their insulin response. The rats in the 300 mg/kg group saw a 33 percent increase in cell receptor activation—meaning that the cinnamon extract helped improve the way their bodies handled glucose.

And a randomized, placebo-controlled human study[16] uncovered even more benefits. This 60-day trial, which included 60 subjects divided into six different treatment groups, found that the subjects in the cinnamon groups saw healthier cholesterol and triglyceride levels after 40 days (a very good side effect!). On top of that, the people in the cinnamon groups saw substantial improvements in their fasting blood sugar levels—decreases between 18 percent and 29 percent. The capper: Those lower blood sugar levels stuck even twenty days after they stopped taking the cinnamon (this was the lowest-dose—gram of cinnamon per day—group only).

Cinnulin PF can help knock down fasting blood sugar levels… and much more

Cinnulin PF is a special proprietary cinnamon extract that has been shown to have a very powerful effect on blood sugar: boosting glucose metabolism to maintain healthy blood glucose levels, along with some other very beneficial effects—and that's why Dr. Douglass decided to include this unique cinnamon extract in his formula.

In one small twelve-week human trial[17], researchers discovered subjects that were given a 500 mg daily dose of Cinnulin PF for 12 weeks reduced their fasting blood sugar levels by 8.4 percent, a very substantial decrease. On top of that, the subjects in the Cinnulin PF group also saw a 3.8 percent decrease in systolic blood pressure and an improvement in their body composition—less overall body fat!

With just Cinnulin PF and benfotiamine on your side, you could start seeing some pretty substantial changes in the way your body handles blood sugar and insulin. But Dr. Douglass knew there was one more ingredient to add—one that no sugar management formula should be without.

Chromium—you can't make 'glucose tolerance factor' without it

A little earlier, we mentioned chromium in passing, but this essential mineral deserves its own glowing review. Scientists have known since the 1950s that chromium plays a role in blood sugar management. In fact, your body can't make a substance called 'glucose tolerance factor' without it. And, as you can guess from the name, your body can't properly manage glucose without enough glucose tolerance factor.

The most power comes from the chromium picolinate form—so, of course, that's the form Dr. Douglass added to GlucoComplete.

What kind of power are we talking about? Take a look.

- Chromium works by increasing the number of insulin receptors in the body, also improving their performance.[18]

- A 2009 placebo-controlled human study found that 46 percent of subjects in the chromium picolinate group (taking 1,000 mcg daily for 24 weeks) showed "improved insulin sensitivity".[19]

- A 1998 review (conducted by Dr. Richard Anderson—the apple pie guy) found that chromium boosted glucose tolerance in nine studies and promoted healthy cholesterol levels in five studies.[20]

- A 2005 animal study found that chromium picolinate appeared to promote healthy kidney function in mice with elevated blood sugar levels.[21]

- Researchers saw a definitive reduction in blood glucose levels in one 1997 human study, when subjects were given 1,000 mcg of chromium daily for four months.[22]

GlucoComplete can help keep your blood sugar in balance

With these three sugar-busting ingredients, GlucoComplete contains everything you need—and nothing you don't—to help your body keep blood glucose under control.

The manufacturer recommends taking one capsule, two times per day, on an empty stomach. For optimal effectiveness, it's best to take GlucoComplete about thirty minutes before meals.

You can find ordering information for GlucoComplete in the Member Source Directory on page 529.

Please note: HSI doesn't accept fees from outside companies for editorial coverage. However, Real Advantage Nutrients is one of HSI's dietary supplement affiliate companies. Even though we would never recommend any product we don't believe in, you should know about that relationship when deciding whether to try their products.

CHAPTER FIVE

Dodge the sugar bullet— and double your chances of beating this leading killer

For years, HSI Panelist Jon Barron had resisted suggestions that he devise an approach for battling diabetes. His reluctance, he told me, stemmed from his belief that using formulas to manage the symptoms of diabetes without dealing with the underlying causes ultimately fails. The responsible approach, he thought, was to help people optimize the health of the organs in the body that control blood sugar levels—not to treat the symptoms after people had the disease.

But the realities of the American diet finally changed his mind, and he began to look at botanicals that could actually accomplish both things simultaneously, help control blood sugar levels and help rebuild the organs that control those levels—not just in diabetics and pre-diabetics, but in anyone eating a less than perfect diet.

A number of herbs, including milk thistle, bitter melon, ginseng, and aloe, are used to control blood sugar. Ayurvedic medicine offers more than 44 different herbal therapies and formulas for diabetes. Both fenugreek and gymnema, for example, come from this tradition. And these two have been the subject of 30 different studies of varying degrees of scientific rigor in Indian and Western literature. Only two did not favor the treatment being tested.

After investigating a number of botanicals, Barron settled on four. The first two come from the Ayurvedic tradition and the third from Japan. There is extensive research, including clinical trials, on these three. The fourth, nopal cactus, has a folk tradition in the American Southwest and Mexico; research on it is promising, but not as extensive as the others.

It's worth noting that several of these botanicals also impact high blood pressure and abnormal blood lipid levels, both characteristics of pre-diabetes, as well as blood sugar levels. Evidence suggests that one even regenerates cells in the pancreas, which, in turn, facilitates healthier insulin levels.

Blood sugar levels plummet by 30 percent with one herb

Seeds from fenugreek plants (*Trigonella foenum-gracum*) have long been used in India, Africa, and the Middle East to treat gastrointestinal problems, gout, wounds, hyperlipidemia, and diabetes. Clinical research dating back to 1939 suggests that fenugreek helps normalize how the body absorbs and uses glucose. The seeds contain a rare type of fiber that forms a gel inside the stomach, reducing its ability to absorb sugar and fat. The gel also makes the stomach feel full faster and longer, promoting weight loss.

On average, participants in fenugreek clinical trials have seen their fasting blood sugar drop by 30 percent, their sugar levels after eating drop 20 to 35 percent, and their hemoglobin A1C drop by 12 percent. (The A1C test is an index of diabetes severity that measures the average amount of sugar molecules that have attached to red blood cells.) In one study, participants experienced a 54 percent drop in urinary glucose levels.[1]

Other clinical trials have shown that fenugreek can reduce total cholesterol, LDL and triglyceride levels, particularly in individuals suffering from coronary artery disease and type 2 diabetes.[2,3] In short, it may help diabetics reduce both their blood sugar and blood lipid levels.

However, the news isn't all good. To get those effects, some study participants had to take large amounts-as much as 100 g a day-of a herb that tastes acutely bitter and makes for foul smelling sweat and urine. In addition, fenugreek can trigger some side effects, specifically cramping, diarrhea, flatulence and other gastrointestinal disorders. But a recently developed extract eliminates some side effects (specifically, the taste and odor) and concentrates the active ingredient, making smaller doses possible. Fenugreek, however, is still contraindicated in some circumstances. Because of its high fiber content, it can alter your absorption of other medications (such as anticoagulants, MAO inhibitors, and hypoglycemic medications) and change their effectiveness.

Herbal "sugar killer" makes sweets hit a sour note

A woody vine used in Indian medicine for over 2,000 years, gymnema sylvestre is commonly known as the "sugar destroyer." A peptide found in the plant blocks certain receptor sites on our taste buds and eventually makes sugar taste, well, not sweet.[4] But gymnema does more to ease diabetes symptoms than quell our sugar cravings.

Gymnemic acid (a key active ingredient) fills sugar receptor sites in the intestine, too, making them unavailable to ingested sugars. If the sugar you eat doesn't get digested, it doesn't filter into your bloodstream. Clinical research also indicates that gymnema regenerates beta cells in the pancreas (which are involved in insulin production), stimulates the release of increased amounts of insulin, and increases the permeability of cells so that they absorb more insulin.[5]

Several clinical studies have measured gymnema's effect on both type 1 and type 2 diabetes. Type 1 diabetics who took 400 mg for 6 to 30 months saw their blood sugar levels drop 52.6 percent on average.[6] Most participants in an 18-month study achieved such significant and consistent blood sugar decreases that they were able to reduce their medication. Five participants were able to discontinue insulin use entirely and maintain healthy blood sugar levels by taking only 400 mg of gymnema sylvestre extract daily.[7]

To date, no one has reported experiencing adverse side effects from the herb, and it is not contraindicated for any condition. No tests, however, have been conducted to determine whether it can be safely taken by pregnant women.

Ancient blood sugar controlling secret also drops blood pressure and cholesterol

You've probably never heard of konjac mannan (I know I hadn't before I started researching this article), but it's been used as a food remedy for over 1,000 years in Japan. And it's also been tested in a number of clinical trials. In a 65-day trial, 72 patients with adult-onset diabetes who took konjac saw their fasting blood sugar levels drop an average of 51.8 percent and their levels after eating drop 84.6 percent.[8] In an eight-week trial, pre-diabetics reported improvements in their blood sugar and cholesterol levels. On average, their total cholesterol dropped by 12.4 percent, LDL levels dropped by 22 percent, and LDL/HDL ratios fell by 22.2 percent.[9]

Other benefits have been reported for konjac. Patients with type 2 diabetes also suffering from high cholesterol and high blood pressure experienced an average drop in their systolic blood pressure of 6.9 percent after supplementing with konjac mannan.[10] Twenty obese individuals who took konjac for eight weeks lost an average of 5.5 pounds even though they were explicitly told not to change their diet or exercise routines. They also experienced significant reductions in their LDL and total cholesterol levels.[11]

At the University of Toronto, researchers concluded that konjac mannan extract is two to four times more effective than pectin, psyllium, guar, oats, and other fibers at reducing cholesterol. It also proved to be equally effective as statin drugs at lowering LDL cholesterol and as some conventional diabetic agents, such as Acarbose, at controlling blood sugar levels.[12]

Fiber-rich Indian remedy solves prickly problem of sugar/fat conversion

Leaves from the nopal cactus, commonly known as the prickly pear cactus, have long been regarded as health food by native peoples in Mexico and southwestern United States. There's not a lot of clinical research into the botanical's medicinal benefits, but anecdotal evidence and several small studies suggest that eating nopal leaves with a meal can help contain and even reduce serum glucose levels.[13] Individuals with type 2 diabetes have experienced a 10 to 20 percent reduction in blood sugar levels after eating nopal. Researchers aren't certain how nopal lowers blood sugar, but they suggest that its rich fiber content inhibits the absorption of glucose in the intestinal tract.

A larger body of research indicates that nopal can reduce both cholesterol and triglyceride levels.[14] Researchers have suggested that it accomplishes this by eliminating excess bile acids (which eventually turn into cholesterol) and by inhibiting the conversion of blood sugar into fat.

This four-in-one solution kicks sugar and fat metabolism into overdrive

These four botanicals make up what Jon Barron refers to as his "sugar, lipid metabolic enhancement formula," officially called Glucotor. It's designed to offset the impact of high-sugar, high-fat foods. In pre-diabetics and non-diabetics, it can help promote healthier blood sugar and cholesterol levels...and a healthier weight. Jon told me he takes it himself on occasion and avoids the sleepiness that follows a few hours after indulging in a meal that's a little too rich or too sweet.

For diabetics, Glucotor may have even bigger ramifications. Although the formula hasn't undergone clinical trials, one physician has tested it in his family practice in Evansville, Indiana, on diabetic patients. According to Barron, "It produced results that the doctors have not seen before, even with hard core drugs," including dramatic changes in blood sugar levels.

Patients find fast diabetes and hypertension relief— without prescription drugs

To find out more, I called Anthony Hall, M.D., the physician in Indiana. It turns out that he's in training to be a naturopathic doctor, and he was happy to provide information on the 15 patients who agreed to take the formula.

Three of them, he told me, dropped out of the trial due to digestive problems caused by the product. (The formula can stimulate large, urgent bowel movements, so people just starting the supplement may want to take only half of the standard daily dose and give their digestive systems a chance to adjust.)

He monitored the effect of Glucotor on his patients' blood sugar, blood pressure, and cholesterol levels, and cautions that, if you're on medication to control any of those levels, you absolutely should consult with your doctor before trying Glucotor and arrange to have your levels checked regularly.

One of Dr. Hall's patients was a 56-year-old woman who had been on varying doses of insulin and oral hypoglycemics since she was diagnosed with diabetes in 1993. Before she began taking Glucotor, her hemoglobin A1C level was 9.0. (A reading of 9 indicates severe diabetes, while 6 or less indicates a healthy, non-diabetic condition.) Over the course of taking Glucotor for six weeks, she discontinued her insulin and Metformin (the generic form of Glucophage, one of the most common prescription drugs used to treat diabetes) and reduced her oral hypoglycemic from 8 mg to 2 mg per day. At the end of the trial, a second test showed her A1C level had fallen to 5.7, a healthy, non-diabetic level.

During our conversation, Dr. Hall also told me how surprised he was to see dramatic changes in blood lipid levels in some of his Glucotor patients. One man's total cholesterol dropped from 297 to 210 and his triglycerides from 580 to 506 after four weeks of taking the supplement. Another patient, a woman this time, had a 23.5 percent reduction in her total cholesterol, a 32 percent drop in her LDL level, and an 18 percent drop in her triglycerides. After 5.5 weeks of taking Glucotor, her blood pressure dropped from 140/96 to around 115/75, and she was able to discontinue taking Lipitor and her blood pressure medication.

And these are just a few examples of the great responses Dr. Hall saw in his patients. Since then, the formula has racked up an impressive 82 percent success rate. Most people would look at those results and be satisfied. But Barron wasn't. So he decided to reformulate Glucotor.

The result is a new and improved version of Glucotor (Glucotor v.2), which includes an all-natural ingredient that has been proven to boost the body's insulin response 20-fold. This one addition to the original formula has made the already miraculous Glucotor up to 300 percent more effective than similar products without the potential of toxic side effects.

Make your insulin receptors more receptive

But why reformulate at all when you've already got something with such a high success rate you literally can't keep it on the shelves? Simply put, Barron says the success rate just wasn't high enough considering it's a human statistic. He couldn't see past the 18 percent of people that he wasn't helping.

That led him on a search for other ingredients he could add to boost Glucotor's effectiveness. And once again, he arrived back at cinnamon. But this time he found a specific cinnamon extract, called Cinnulin PF, which eliminated the roadblocks he'd encountered before.

So just what is Cinnulin PF? Well, as Barron puts it, "it's pretty amazing. It's a patented cinnamon extract that operates at the cellular and molecular levels. It actually works to make the insulin receptor sites on your individual body cells more receptive. If you have enough cinnamon every day, you can actually increase your body's insulin response threefold. That's 300 percent—and that's a big deal."

I wanted to find out more about Cinnulin PF so I went straight to the source: Integrity Nutraceuticals Inter-national (INI). INI is a raw material supplier of bulk nutraceuticals including amino acids, herbs, and specialty compounds like Cinnulin PF.

All the benefit, none of the risks

Until recently methylhydroxy-chalcone polymer (or MHCP) was thought to be the active compound in cinnamon responsible for the beneficial effect on blood glucose. It turns out that early research mis-identified the substances responsible for these actions as cinnamon's MHCP fractions. The substances actually providing the blood-sugar-lowering benefits are water-soluble polyphenol polymers called Type-A polymers.[15]

INI created an aqueous cinnamon extract product using a process that removes the potentially harmful compounds from whole cinnamon while leaving the Type-A polymers intact (using no chemical solvents). Extracts made with solvents other than water will actually extract the lipid-soluble portion of cinnamon, which contains the potentially harmful fractions.

Actually, this process makes Cinnulin PF even stronger than it would be without it: The lipid soluble portion of cinnamon has been shown to have no effect on glucose metabolism. But in contrast, the water-soluble portion has been proven to increase glucose uptake by 20-fold.[16]

Early research looks promising

In diabetes,either the body doesn't produce enough insulin or the cells resist it, so the sugar remains in the blood, builds up to higher and higher levels, and ultimately starts damaging protein-based tissue and organs. Cinnulin PF triggers receptor sensitivity to insulin and primes the receptor for glucose uptake.

In one study, researchers tested cinnamon's effects by using a water-based cinnamon extract similar to Cinnulin PF on 28 people with Type II diabetes. Patients received 500 mg of a formula containing water extracts of cinnamon, heshouwu, and mushroom three times per day. Another 29 patients were given a placebo. After two months, researchers found that subjects in the treatment group had a 15 percent reduction in fasting glucose.

In another study, 60 Type 2 diabetics were divided into six groups: three placebo groups and three experimental groups. Participants took 1, 3, or 6 grams of cinnamon daily or the placebo. After 40 days, participants in the cinnamon groups had 18 to 29 percent drops in their fasting glucose. They also experienced 20 to 30 percent lower triglycerides, 7 to 27 percent reductions in LDL cholesterol, and 12 to 26 percent lower total cholesterol levels.[17] There were no significant changes in any of the placebo groups. However, all of the patients in the study were also taking oral hypoglycemic (blood sugar-lowering) medications, so it's hard to say for sure in this case if cinnamon was the sole factor in the improvements.

Recently a placebo-controlled, double blind trial specific to Cinnulin PF was just completed. The study was designed to determine the effect of supplementation with Cinnulin PF on changes in glucose regulation, lipid profiles (cholesterol, triglycerides, etc.), and overall body composition. Final results showed subjects were able to lower their fasting blood glucose by an average of 8.4 percent. Furthermore, participants showed small but significant decreases in body fat (with increases in lean muscle mass!).

New ingredient fares well on its own

If Cinnulin PF is independently getting good results, and so is

Glucotor, imagine the combined effect. Here are a couple encouraging reports INI has gotten over the past few months from people using Cinnulin PF:

G.P. from Springfield, OH wrote to INI saying "My wife saw an article in Parade magazine and suggested I try Cinnulin PF. I have been taking two capsules daily; the results are in the numbers. The VA Center where I go for treatment asked for a brochure on Cinnulin PF to post on their bulletin board. My doctor is not normally in favor of homeopathic medicine, but she was ecstatic with my results. She had read about cinnamon studies and believes it is a good approach."

And another letter, this one from R.J. in Sanford, FL, said: "I use Cinnulin PF to maintain a healthy blood sugar level. It works! I have used it for a month and I take two tablets before lunch and two before dinner. I also recommend Cinnulin PF to all of my friends who have diabetes."

Same size, same price, better results

Barron did note that some people have a problem digesting the capsules quickly enough to get the blood-sugar lowering effects. The problem, as Barron explains, is that many people, particularly as they get older, have burned out their ability to produce stomach acid. Once you get to that point, you no longer have enough stomach acid to easily break down capsules: It takes so long that the Glucotor can't get in place soon enough to block the receptor sites. But taking the formula out of the capsules lets you bypass that problem. So if you don't get the results you expect, try taking the Glucotor v.2 powder out of the capsules and mixing it with a little applesauce or a small glass of water.

And speaking of capsules, the addition of Cinnulin PF hasn't affected the size or swallow-ability of Glucotor v.2. Barron actually had to create a special encapsulation technique in order to contain the desired dosage of Cinnulin PF along with the other proven ingredients. "After a lot of trial and error and changing how we ground and blended the formula, we found we could get the equipment to fill the standard capsules with the desired dose of the new formula. In other words, we were able to add the Cinnulin PF without having to change anything else."

And that's not the only puzzle they had to solve to get this improved formula to you. Adding Cinnulin PF looked as if it would increase the retail price of the new formula 30 percent. So Barron and Baseline Nutritionals thought they would have to choose whether to raise prices or decrease the number of capsules in each bottle. But they found another alternative—one just about unheard of in the supplement industry: They decided not to do either. So you're getting all the existing benefits of the original Glucotor formula plus the added benefit of Cinnulin PF at no additional cost. This is just another indication of the confidence that Barron and the manufacturers have in this formula.

The recommended dosage for Glucotor v.2 with Cinnulin PF is to one or two capsules five to 10 minutes before eating. If you're currently taking medications for blood sugar, cholesterol, or heart disease, talk to your doctor before trying this formula.

CHAPTER SIX

Herbal-tea extract lowers blood sugar and helps patients lose weight—without changes in diet or exercise

Diabetes afflicts over 16 million Americans. The American diet—processed foods high in sugar, low in fiber, and virtually devoid of nutrients—combined with a sedentary lifestyle, has caused the disease to spread rapidly. But Type II diabetes (noninsulin dependent) doesn't happen overnight. It usually takes five to 10 years before a recurring set of circumstances repeats itself enough times and causes enough damage to result in diabetes.

Gerald M. Reaven, M.D., of Stanford University Medical Center, coined the term "Syndrome X" to describe the blood sugar disorder that leads to Type II diabetes. If you have Syndrome X, you're insulin resistant—a dangerous situation since insulin processes the sugar in your blood and converts it to glycogen, which is stored in your liver and muscles for later use.

In the case of insulin resistance, your cells don't respond quickly enough to insulin production and you have high blood sugar levels for longer periods of time. Your body senses that there's too much blood sugar and produces even more insulin.

Instead of being processed by the extra insulin, your body responds negatively and keeps your blood sugar levels high. This is a self-perpetuating cycle that leads to increased resistance to insulin and even higher levels of blood sugar. As a result, your cells don't get the energy they need—leaving you tired and groggy. Your body responds to this condition by craving more sugar for fuel. So you eat again, flooding your system with even more glucose, and heading down the road to Type II diabetes.

Although Type II diabetics usually produce insulin, their bodies are unable to process insulin efficiently and would benefit from a supplement to help transport glucose out of the blood and convert it to glycogen for storage. In some cases, Type II diabetics don't produce sufficient amounts of insulin and may require oral medication or insulin injections.

If you have Syndrome X, it's very likely that you also have elevated triglyceride levels, low HDL ("good" cholesterol), high LDL or VLDL ("bad" cholesterol), high blood pressure, and the slow clearing of fat from the blood.

Factors that increase your risk of contracting Syndrome X include stress, obesity, lack of physical activity, high-carbohydrate intake, a low-fiber diet, excessive alcohol consumption, polycystic ovaries, and smoking. If you're in the high-risk group for Syndrome X and don't do anything to improve your situation, you'll most likely end up with Type II diabetes. While many of the risk factors can be addressed through changes in your lifestyle, reducing blood sugar levels hasn't been very easy if you're insulin resistant. Until now.

Banaba plant lowers blood sugar by 32 percent— in just three weeks

The banaba is a medicinal plant commonly found in the Philippines and Southeast Asia. Its leaves were traditionally brewed to make a tea used to counteract diabetes and high blood sugar. Researchers found that corosolic acid was the active ingredient in the leaves, so they standardized the extract and created a product called Glucosol.™

William V. Judy, Ph.D., of the Southeastern Institute of Biomedical Research in Bradenton, Florida, used Glucosol in animal and human clinical trials to determine if its effects could help mild-to-moderate Type II diabetics reduce their blood-sugar levels. Last year, Dr. Judy conducted five human clinical trials (unpublished) that attempted to reduce diabetics' elevated fasting glucose levels, which averaged 150 mg/dL (normal levels are 70 to 110 mg/dL).

In the first study, 22 Type II diabetics were given 16, 32, or 48 mg of Glucosol per day. The resulting decrease in diabetic symptoms was nothing short of astounding. Patients receiving 48 mg per day had the most pronounced decrease in their blood sugar levels. After just 20 days, they reduced those levels by an average of 32 percent and lost an average of two pounds without making any changes in their diet or exercise regimen. Three other studies using 48 mg of Glucosol per day duplicated those significant blood sugar reductions. The herb appears to work by improving the rate at which sugar is transported out of your blood but doesn't reduce your blood sugar excessively.

Glucosol helps you lose weight without disrupting normal blood sugar levels

To determine if weight loss could be experienced by nondiabetics who take the herbal extract, Glucosol was given to 10 test subjects who did not have a history of blood sugar disorders. The patients were supplemented with 48 mg of Glucosol every day for 30 days. By the end of the test period, the average weight loss experienced by the normal subjects was 2.4 pounds. Two weeks after the end of the test period, the patients had not only maintained their weight loss, they had lost even more weight! Their average weight loss increased slightly to 2.6 pounds. None of the subjects experienced any difficulty with hypoglycemia (low blood sugar), which indicates that Glucosol doesn't transport more sugar out of your blood than is required.

With Glucosol, diabetes doesn't have to be the road to serious health problems

Glucosol and insulin supplements work in different ways. The risks you experience with insulin supplements—either too-low or too-high blood sugar levels—don't happen with Glucosol. Available without a prescription, this herbal extract can help you get control of your blood sugar levels and avoid the serious consequences of diabetes.

Glucosol is available as Sugarsolve.™ For ordering information, see the Member Source Directory.

Part VIII

Memory

CHAPTER ONE

Focus your mind, sharpen your memory with Ayurvedic medicine

Year after year, the car keys seem to go missing more often. Names of distant relatives and household gadgets don't jump to mind the instant you need them. Memories of family events grow hazy. Tasks like balancing the checkbook or preparing a holiday meal become more challenging and more prone to errors. And one day you start wondering if you're edging down that path toward dementia.

Practitioners of Ayurvedic (traditional Indian) medicine, however, have identified several herbs capable of preserving memory and mental acuity and even reversing some age-related cognitive deficits. Practitioners say these herbs, which have been used for centuries, can offset the prime causes of memory loss, namely disease, nerve cell decay, nutritional deficiencies, and stress.

It's a nasty biological fact that our capacity to maintain a sharp memory diminishes as we age. On average, individuals lose nerve cells at a rate of 1 percent a year after age 25. Consequently by age 70, we've lost more than one-third of the cells critical to memory functions. Memory loss can be exacerbated by other factors: stress, depression, disease (including diabetes and hypothyroidism), nutritional deficiencies (especially of vitamins B1 and B12), and certain prescription medications. Trauma, strokes, and heart attacks can reduce oxygen flow to the brain, killing cells and causing memory loss. Sadly, Alzheimer's disease also causes extreme memory loss in one in 10 Americans over the age of 65.

Several Ayurvedic herbs, however, support the brain directly. Bacopa, for example, affects higher-order cognitive processes by rejuvenating nerves and brain cells.[1] Gotu kola helps maintain microvessels in the brain, improving memory and attention span.[2] Mucuna is a natural source of levodopa which optimizes performance of the nervous system, including the brain.[3]

Others bolster cognitive function by strengthening the nervous system. Ashwaganda (or Indian ginseng) fights stress, improves memory, and helps rejuvenate people suffering from general debility, ex-

The right diet may preserve your memory

There are a number of things you can do to regain some lost mental function and improve your concentration. Daily exercise is an excellent way to increase circulation, which helps relieve mind-numbing stress and increase oxygen flow to the brain. Herbs like ginseng and Ginkgo biloba have been used for centuries in many cultures and appear to increase the amount of oxygen-rich blood to the brain. Supplements like phospha-tidylserine and NADH are more recent discoveries that have been found to keep the brain sharp and functioning at its peak. Finally, a diet that includes ample raw fruit and vegetables (the best sources of antioxidants), sufficient protein (which helps maintain nerve cells and healthy blood sugar levels), and cold-water fish (which contain Omega-3 fatty acids and reduce the risk of strokes, blood clots, and heart attacks) protects against many diseases that impair cognitive function. Adding 500-1,000 mg of l-carnitine greatly helps transport these essential fatty acids into cells.

haustion, or stress-induced fatigue.[4-5] Salep orchid is a nerve stimulant. And Morning Glory is an anti-aging remedy that improves memory and intellect by easing nervous debility.

A few herbs also help individuals suffering from memory loss or concentration problems brought on by stress. Muskroot, for example, is a nerve tonic known for its calming effect on the mind.[6]

Now studies indicate that certain Ayurvedic herbs might even offer positive results for severe conditions like Alzheimer's disease and amnesia.

Laboratory tests reveal potential to treat amnesia and Alzheimer's

Scientists at the National Institute of Mental Health and Neuroscience in Bangalore, India, investigated the ability of one formula to treat amnesia. MindCare, a formulation by Himalaya Herbal Healthcare, contains all of the herbs mentioned above as well as Indian valerian (a calming agent) and two herbs that protect against memory-damaging diseases: Guduchi (a tonic that bolsters natural immunity) and Triphala (a combination of three Ayurvedic herbs high in vitamins B and C, which can be depleted by stress). The scientists administered MindCare to laboratory rats suffering from amnesia induced by electroshock therapy.[7] In the medical journal *Probe*, the researchers reported that MindCare "enhances cognition against... amnesia."[8]

Researchers at the Institute of Medical Sciences at Banaras Hindu University in India found that lab rats suffering from cognitive decline due to Alzheimer's disease also responded positively to MindCare supplementation. After two weeks of supplementation, the rats experienced a reversal of cognitive deficits.[9] The researchers discovered heightened concentrations of acetylcholine in the rats' brains—a condition that improves cognitive processes and memory.

Ease the anxiety that can cloud memories
and impair concentration

In other studies, MindCare has demonstrated abilities to ease the stress and anxiety that can exacerbate memory and concentration problems. At the Baranas Hindu University in Varanasi, India, researchers gave rats MindCare for seven days. Afterward, the rats received a drug that increases tribulin—a marker in the brain that indicates the subject is suffering from anxiety. The researchers found that pretreatment with MindCare attenuated the effects of the anxiety-causing drug.[10]

Doctors at Varanasi's Institute of Medical Sciences in India conducted a memory and anxiety test on 20 individuals age 15 to 65. In their study, which was published in the medical journal *Probe*, test subjects received either two placebos or two MindCare tablets twice a day for 12 weeks. The subjects then took a word test to determine the supplement's effect on short-term memory. The individuals taking MindCare showed a 10-point improvement over pre-treatment memory tests. The placebo group improved by approximately two points. The MindCare group registered a similar improvement in anxiety testing. Researchers found "there was a statistically significant decrease" in anxiety after taking MindCare, but the group taking placebos showed no improvement in their anxiety levels.[11]

MindCare is available through Himalaya Herbal Healthcare. Ordering information is in the Member Source Directory on page 529.

CHAPTER TWO

Memory-boosting breakthrough proves "science" wrong by regrowing dead brain cells

First, it's forgetting where you put your glasses… and then finding them sitting on your head.

Then it's missing an appointment because you forgot it was today… or being unable to come up with the name of that acquaintance you ran into at the grocery store.

For years, mainstream medicine has been telling us these frustrating and sometimes embarrassing "senior moments" are an unavoidable part of getting older. Just accept it, they tell us, because there's nothing you can do about them.

They are wrong.

It turns out a single breakthrough—a unique combination of five natural brain-boosters—can have you remembering more tomorrow than you do today… thinking faster today than you did yesterday… delaying and possibly even entirely preventing the frustrations of senility. There's more—this special supplement may even be a knockout blow in the fight against Alzheimer's disease.

It's called NGF and its ability to stop and even reverse cognitive decline is due to one amazing quality. You see, NGF does the impossible.

NGF accomplishes science's 'impossible' dream by regrowing brain cells

I think it was in Mr. Wilson's sixth grade class that I heard it for the first time: Brain cells don't regenerate—if you lose them, they're just gone forever. For as long as I can remember, scientists believed whichever brain cells you were born with, well, those were the only ones you'd ever have. Turns out all of those scientists are being made to eat some crow these days.

You see, we all naturally lose brain cells as we age. Along with the cells go the neurites (the long root-like branches that extend from your brain cells). Neurites make up the network that lets your brain cells communicate with each other.

Losing the neurites disrupts your brain's communication system and your brain cells just can't communicate as efficiently or rapidly anymore. This causes all kinds of central nervous system troubles, including cognitive, memory, and behavioral issues. In short, those unwelcome senior moments.

But groundbreaking research shows that your brain cells can regenerate, and you can regrow your neural connections... as long as the conditions are right. All it really takes is a specific set of premium nutrients and phytochemicals, and your neurites can be replenished. That's a crucial new understanding, because more neurites means stronger brain function.

NGF uses a unique blend of five potent brain-building ingredients to actually regrow your neurites, keeping your neural connections intact and functioning optimally.

Five natural brain nutrients working together to keep your mind crystal clear

NGF impacts brain function so strongly because it approaches the problem of decreased brain cell communication in four unique ways: renovating vital brain cell structures, producing and preserving critical neurotransmitters, supporting the delivery of vital nutrients and oxygen to your brain, and shutting down beta amyloid plaque before it can destroy your brain cells. NGF combines these five important brain ingredients in a single powerful supplement:

- **Acetyl carnitine** increases the effects of nerve growth factor 100 times, allowing your body to regrow brain cells at any age.

- **Acetyl carnitine arginate** neutralizes the brain protein believed responsible for Alzheimer's disease, and acts synergistically with acetyl carnitine.

- **Uridine** supports the regrowth of neurites, which prevents memory loss while improving memory retention.

- **Gotu kola** improves mental abilities by stimulating neurite growth in key areas of the brain.

- **Gingko biloba** extract has strong antioxidant qualities that protect brain cells from free radical damage, and improves blood flow and oxygen supply to the brain.

Combining these five brain-boosting ingredients has a dramatic effect on improving your brain power. That's exactly the purpose of NGF—improved brain-cell health and neurite regrowth can increase your thinking power, restore memory, improve concentration, inspire creativity, boost your mood, even improve your hearing and vision.

Each of the five active ingredients plays a unique role in how NGF works, as you're about to see.

Nerve growth factor is 100 times more effective with acetyl carnitine

Nerve growth factor is a protein produced in your brain—and it has a huge impact on overall brain cell health and vitality. But until relatively recently, no one really knew how to stimulate or regulate its production.

Then in 1991, some scientists discovered that a nutrient called *acetyl carnitine* increased the effects of nerve growth factor by 100 times… making this naturally produced protein 100 times more effective. At the time, this was considered merely an interesting observation, with no real-life applications.[1]

Then, a few years later, scientists discovered that another form of acetyl carnitine, acetyl carnitine arginate, mimicked the effect of nerve growth factor, and could actually cause neurites to grow.[2] Basically, the acetyl carnitine arginate did the same thing as the body's own nerve growth factor! This simple nutrient actually stimulates brain cell regeneration all on its own.

Here's the bonus: When acetyl carnitine arginate and acetyl carnitine were tested together on brain cells, they boosted each other's performance.[3]

Turns out the first one stimulates the production receptors for nerve growth factor and the second one takes advantage of that to produce more brain cells.

This duo has some serious potency. While acetyl carnitine alone boosted neurite growth by 5.6 percent in brain cell cultures, the combination increased neurite growth by 19.5 percent. That's over three times more brain power for you![4]

Preventing Alzheimer's disease and brain aging

The benefits of acetyl carnitine arginate don't stop at its amazing ability to restore brain cells. It turns out it may be your greatest weapon in the fight against Alzheimer's disease (AD). As you know, scientists believe the main culprit behind this debilitating condition is beta amyloid plaque. This plaque is often found in huge quantities in brains afflicted with AD. But instead of expensive drugs that may come with their own side effects, the answer to protecting yourself from this plaque may be as simple as ACA... acetyl carnitine arginate.

Acetyl carnitine arginate literally protects your neurons against the brain cell damage caused by beta amyloid plaque.[5] In fact, one study found that simply adding this nutrient into the mix could wipe out the effects of the plaque all together. When scientists added beta amyloid to healthy human brain cell cultures in the lab, cell death occurred within eight days. But when they added acetyl carnitine arginate at the same time, the cells didn't die, not at all. The nutrient completely protected against beta amyloid toxicity by interrupting its negative impact on healthy brain cells.[5]

But the success doesn't end in a lab sample. Human trials testing acetyl carnitine have also shown very promising results, like

- less pain and improved nerve regeneration in patients with diabetic neuropathy.[6]
- noticeable improvements in patients with mild cognitive impairment and early symptoms of Alzheimer's disease.[7]
- reduced fatigue caused by chronic fatigue syndrome and multiple sclerosis.[8]

Uridine increases memory retention

Uridine is a natural substance found in foods. Scientists used to believe only infants needed it, but new research is showing that it's critical for optimal brain health. More and more research is demonstrating that we need uridine for growth and development throughout our lives.[9]

It turns out that that uridine (which we get mainly from milk)

is our main source of cytidine. Cytidine, in turn, creates phosphati-
cylcholine, a precursor for the neurotransmitter required for proper
memory function and muscle coordination.[10] Phosphatidylcholine
levels naturally decline with age, and that decline seems to play a key
role in memory loss.

I know there are a bunch of ten-cent words up there, so let me cut
to the chase: By simply adding more uridine to your diet, memory loss
can be transformed into memory retention.

Studies into the uridine-human brain cell connection began in
earnest in 2000. One study found that uridine was directly responsible
for brain cell regeneration in the lab.[11] And in 2005, another study confirmed that uridine increased the number of new neurites per cell and
stimulated neurite branching—two events critical for memory retention. Simply by enhancing phosphatidylcholine production, uridine
was able to foster brain cell growth.[12]

Gotu kola, the "brain herb" from India, repairs damaged cells

Gotu kola, a plant native to India, has been used in Ayurvedic traditional medicine for thousands of years. Traditionally, this healing
herb has been used for nervous disorders such as senility and epilepsy,
and as a brain tonic to improve memory. But its brain benefits don't
end there. New research indicates Gotu kola...

- May increase alertness
- May improve cognitive function in Alzheimer's patients.
- May ease anxiety.
- Has been found to increase attention span
- Appears to improve concentration
- May alleviate depression, stress, and insomnia
- Appears to boost learning ability and memory

• May boost the power of nerve growth factor to stimulate the out-growth of axons (key structural components of neurons)

Scientific research into Gotu kola extracts and their impact on the brain only began in earnest in the past few years. The studies have focused particularly on how Gotu kola extracts impacted brain function and structural changes in brain cells.

One of the most important of these studies demonstrated clearly that Gotu kola promoted higher brain function in mice. In that study, Gotu kola extract was given to baby mice, and it stimulated physiological actions that resulted in higher brain functioning... essentially, smarter mice.[13,14]

Another landmark study showed that Gotu kola alcohol extract added to human brain cells (in the lab) caused a striking increase in neurite growth. And when the extract was added to the drinking water of old rats, they demonstrated more functional recovery and increased neurite regeneration. The study authors concluded that Gotu kola extract could be useful for speeding up repair of damaged brain cells.[15]

Ancient herb may reverse the onset of Alzheimer's disease

Ginkgo biloba has been used for many centuries to enhance memory and cognitive function, but modern research on the value of GBE (gingko biloba extract) didn't begin until the late 1950s. In 1965 ginkgo biloba as we know it today was introduced to the European market where it has been widely used for more than 30 years to treat circulation problems and cerebral disorders, including Alzheimer's disease.

Over the past 40 years there have been more than 300 clinical trials of ginkgo biloba, and the evidence from those trials is overwhelming: GBE's excellent antioxidant qualities protect cells from free radical damage, and GBE improves blood flow and oxygen supply to the brain and throughout the body. For most people this results in improved cognitive abilities.

And the results get even better: In October of 1997 the *Journal of the American Medical Association* reported on a study that tested ginkgo biloba against Alzheimer's disease and dementia. That study lasted 52 weeks and included 309 patients. The conclusion: ginkgo biloba is capable of stabilizing and in many cases improving the cognitive performance of demented patients. In the study, this herb was shown to actually stop and even reverse the onset of Alzheimer's disease.

Though there's a large body of research on the individual ingredients in NGF, there haven't yet been any trials performed on this particular combination or using this supplement. But based on the research that is out there, you may notice results in as few as three weeks. And you can boost the power of this already powerful brain-boosting supplement by eating a healthy, antioxidant-rich diet and reducing your stress levels as much as possible.

NGF is available from Vitamin Research Products—you'll find the ordering information for NGF in the Member Source Directory.

CHAPTER THREE

Ancient herb can make your mind young again

New research has led to a breakthrough in the treatment and prevention of brain aging. It's a compound called *huperzine A*, extracted from the Chinese club moss, or *Huperzia serrata*. Used in traditional Chinese medicine for centuries to treat fever and inflammation, this compound has now been shown to bring about significant improvements in cognitive and intellectual performance in patients with Alzheimer's disease and age-related cognitive decline, and it may improve memory and learning in healthy patients as well.

Alan P. Kozikowski, Ph.D., a professor of pharmacology at Georgetown University's Institute of Cognitive and Computational Sciences in Washington, D.C., stated that "according to animal research, it [huperzine A] can actually slow the progression of Alzheimer's disease. In other words, huperzine A has neuro-protective activity, which is really exciting. It makes this supplement really stand out from other treatment modalities."

Researchers at Beijing's Institute of Mental Health conducted a four-week study on huperzine A, administering it to 101 patients with age-associated memory impairment. At the beginning of the four-week study, none of the patients was within the normal range for memory. At the end of the four weeks, however, over 70 percent of those in the huperzine-treated group had improved to within normal memory limits.

How does huperzine A work?

Huperzine A is similar in action to the drugs currently used to treat Alzheimer's disease in that it is a powerful acetylcholine esterase (AchE) inhibitor. AchE is an enzyme that destroys the neurotransmitter acetylcholine and terminates the nerve signal after it has been transmitted. Acetylcholine, which is released at the synapse between two nerve cells, facilitates memory and learning. In some memory disorders, such as Alzheimer's disease, the memory nerve impulse is destroyed before it has been received by the adjacent nerve cell. Thus, by inhibiting AchE, the memory nerve impulse is lengthened in duration, resulting in improved memory and cognitive function.

According to researchers at the Weizmann Institute of Sciences in Rehovot, Israel, and at Georgetown University in Washington, D.C., huperzine A is superior in the following ways to the leading drugs licensed for the treatment of Alzheimer's:

- Huperzine A improves learning and memory in mice better than does tacrine.

- Huperzine A acts specifically on AchE in the brain rather than on the AchE found elsewhere in the body.

- Huperzine A does not appear to bind to receptors in the central nervous system, which can cause negative side effects.

- Its effects last 10 to 12 times longer than those of physostigmine and tacrine.

- Huperzine A is less toxic than the leading drugs, even when administered at 50 to 100 times the therapeutic dose.

A marriage of ancient wisdom and leading-edge science

Huperzine A has been used as a prescription drug for treating dementia in China for years. But we've found an innovative formula that augments huperzine with other brain-specific nutrients.

Brain Protex, created by Nature's Sunshine, combines three powerful antioxidants which cross the blood-brain barrier to protect the brain cells. It also contains two nutrients that act as "brain food," namely Ginkgo biloba and phosphatidyl serine. Together, the antioxidants and the nutrients protect the brain from damaging free radicals and boost mental capacity.

Nutrients found in Brain Protex

Phosphatidylserine (PS) is an essential fatty acid that is necessary for optimal brain functioning. It keeps the membranes of the brain cells fluid and pliant, allowing the cells to absorb nutrients more efficiently. It also stimulates the activity of neurotransmitters, the "messenger" chemicals that relay nerve signals from cell to cell, literally helping you think. More than two dozen controlled clinical trials have demonstrated that supplementation with PS greatly improves learning and memory.

In a recent study of 149 people, age 50 or older, who had "normal" age-related memory loss, some study participants took 100 mg of PS three times a day for 12 weeks while the others took placebos. By the end of the experiment, the people taking PS benefited from a 15 percent improvement in learning and other memory tasks, with the greatest benefit coming to those with the greatest impairment. Furthermore, these significant benefits continued for up to four weeks after the patients stopped taking PS. Clinical psychologist Thomas Crook, one of the study's authors, said the study suggests that PS "may reverse approximately 12 years of decline."

In another 12-week study, 51 people (average age: 71) took PS supplements and improved their short-term memory. They could better recall names and the locations of misplaced objects. They remembered more details of recent events and could concentrate more intently.

Ginkgo biloba is a well-known botanical remedy used in the treatment of circulatory diseases, with particular value in the treatment of brain aging. Ginkgo increases circulation to the brain and is a potent antioxidant, helping to prevent free-radical oxidation in the brain.

Rhododendron caucasicum, also known as the "snow rose," grows at altitudes ranging from 10,000 to 30,000 feet in the Caucasus Mountains of the Republic of Georgia (formerly part of the Soviet Union). Many scientists believe Rhododendron caucasicum, which is regularly consumed in the form of Alpine Tea, is a primary cause of Georgians' remarkable longevity. (One census of the Republic's 3.2 million people, identified nearly 23,000 citizens over the age of 100.) Foreign hospitals have used this plant to treat heart disease, arthritis, gout, high cholesterol, blood pressure problems, depression, neuroses, pychoses, and concentration problems.

In the 1950s, Soviet scientists began vigorously researching Rhododendron caucasicum. Over the next four decades, numerous clinical trials explored the therapeutic values of the extract. It proved to be an excellent free radical scavanger (an "ultra-antioxidant" according to some researchers), capable of protecting the body from cell mutations that can weaken the immune system and cause heart disease, cancer, strokes, kidney failure, and emphysema. It exhibited a tremendous ability (stronger than grape seed extract or pine bark extract) to purge harmful bacteria from the body, while allowing good bacteria (probiotics) to remain.

Rhododendron caucasicum, however, demonstrated special abilities to protect and treat the brain. Researchers discovered that its extract bolsters the cardiovascular system, increasing blood supply to the muscles and especially the brain. Studies also demonstrated that Rhododendron caucasicum increases the brain's resistance to unfavorable chemical, physical, and biological imbalances. At the First Lenin Medicinal Institute in Moscow, researchers treated 530 patients with various forms of neuroses and pychoses with Rhodendron caucasicum. Within 11 weeks of treatment, the majority of the patients regained normal conscious thought and demonstrated heightened mental abilities.

Lycopene is a powerful antioxidant found in tomatoes, pink grape-fruit, apricots, and watermelon. Observational studies have produced evidence that diets high in lycopene may reduce the risk of cancer, especially tumors in the prostate, colon, stomach, lung, or mouth. Re-searchers also believe lycopene may help prevent cataracts and macu-lar degeneration (a gradual loss of vision which is the leading cause of blindness among older Americans).

Alpha-lipoic acid is a sulfur-containing fatty acid found in every cell of the body. It is a key component of our metabolic system, helping to convert glucose (blood sugar) into energy to serve the body's needs. It is also a universal antioxidant, capable of eliminating free radicals in water and in fatty tissue.

Lipoic acid has been most commonly used (particularly in Ger-many) to treat nerve damage caused by diabetes. One randomized, double-blind, placebo-controlled study of 503 individuals concluded that intravenous lipoic acid helped relieve symptoms (pain, numbness, extreme constipation, and irregular heart rhythms) for three weeks.

Researchers now believe lipoic acid may also help retard cataracts and neuro-degenerative diseases, including Parkinson's and Alzheimer's.

Brain Protex can be ordered through The Herbs Place. The recom-mended dose is two capsules at mealtime twice a day. (See the Member Source Directory at the back of this book for ordering information.)

CHAPTER FOUR

Flower power keeps your brain alive

In Alzheimer's patients, chemicals in the brain, called neurotransmitters, go haywire. Neurotransmitters aid communication among brain cells and help electrical impulses jump the tiny gaps (called synapses) between nerves.

In the 1970s, researchers discovered that people with Alzheimer's disease (AD) have low levels of a key neurotransmitter called acetylcholine (a-see-tull-KOH-leen). Not only does acetylcholine help brain cells communicate, but it also plays a vital role in memory, learning, and other cognitive functions. In advanced AD patients, acetylcholine levels plunge by 90 percent. At that point, even the personality is affected.

Acetylcholine is produced in an area of the brain called the basal forebrain. Unfortunately, these cells naturally deteriorate with age and are among the first damaged in the early stages of Alzheimer's disease. When these brain cells die, acetylcholine levels drop dramatically—affecting a patient's memory and capacity for learning.

The problem is compounded in AD patients when an enzyme called cholinesterase is introduced. Cholinesterase cleans up unused acetylcholine in the brain by breaking it down into its component parts. In a healthy person, this is a natural process. But in AD patients, it can add insult to injury and cripple an already impaired memory by further reducing already low levels of acetylcholine.

The current medications for AD, known as "cholinesterase inhibitors," work primarily by stopping the damage of cholinesterase to optimize the levels of acetylcholine. Aside from harsh side effects, such as liver damage, seizures, and depression, their biggest downfall is that they lose their effectiveness within one year.

Does the snowdrop plant hold the key beyond the temporary relief of drugs?

Working with researchers at Life Enhancement Products, a pioneering nutritional development and research company, we've uncovered dozens of recent clinical trials on a natural flower extract that surpasses the effectiveness of prescription drugs.

Galantamine, an extract from the snowdrop flower, daffodil, spider lily, and other plants, has been traditionally used in Eastern Europe to treat a variety of minor ailments. Current research shows its greatest promise is its ability to bring the progress of AD to a virtual standstill and rejuvenate cognitive function.

Like prescription drugs, galantamine blocks the action of cholinesterase—allowing for greater levels of acetylcholine—and *boosts the production of new acetylcholine* neurotransmitters in the brain.[1]

Furthermore, animal studies have found that galantamine does something else no other drug currently being prescribed can do: It stimulates acetylcholine *receptors*, called *nicotinic receptors*, in the brain—over an extended period of time. In AD patients, these receptors wear out and the brain isn't able to transport acetylcholine from one cell to another. In addition, when nicotinic receptors are healthy and active, they're thought to inhibit the formation of beta-amyloid plaque deposits, a hard, waxy substance that results from tissue degeneration and is often found in the brains of AD patients.[2] While the current AD drugs initially help stimulate the nicotinic receptors as well, the effect isn't long-lasting. Nicotinic receptors appear to become desensitized to most drugs over time—often within a year—thus making them ineffective in this respect. Unlike AD drugs, galantamine stimulates nicotinic receptors without appearing to cause desensitization when used for an extended period of time.[3]

Increase memory and cognitive function—and keep it

Scientists in Auckland, New Zealand, found that AD patients in several studies (with 285 to 978 patients taking 24 mg of galantamine per day for three to six months) achieved significant improvements in cognitive symptoms and daily living activities as compared to a placebo-treated control group. They also found that galantamine delayed the development of behavioral disturbances and psychiatric symptoms. After 12 months of treatment, patients using galantamine maintained their cognitive and functional abilities.[4]

Researchers in Belgium conducted a study with 3,000 AD patients enrolled in one of five randomized, controlled, double-blind groups. Various levels of galantamine were tested (16, 24, and 32 mg per day) against placebos, and in every study the galantamine-treated patients maintained their cognitive abilities while the placebo-treated subjects experienced significant deterioration.

Prior to entering each of the five studies, patients were evaluated according to the cognition portion of the Alzheimer Disease Assessment Scale. Each subject's performance was assessed in 11 areas measuring memory and orientation. A score of zero meant the patient made no errors, while a top score of 70 meant he suffered from profound dementia. Results from the patient evaluations showed that moderately severe AD patients treated with galantamine had a seven-point advantage over similarly afflicted subjects in the placebo groups. Researchers found that the optimum dosage of galantamine was 24 mg per day. Groups treated with 32 mg demonstrated no additional improvement in their cognitive abilities.[5]

In another multicenter, double-blind trial, galantamine delayed the progress of the disease throughout a full-year study. Conducted at the University of Rochester Medical Center, 636 patients with mild to moderate AD were given galantamine or a placebo for six months. At the end of the period, patients taking galantamine experienced improved cognitive function in relation to the placebo group. Patients taking 24 mg of galantamine improved by 3.8 points. Additionally, based on clinician and caregiver interviews, the galantamine group performed significantly better in the completion of daily activities and exhibited fewer behavioral disturbances. Moreover, the benefits of galantamine are long-lasting. Baseline cognitive scores and daily function continued to be high when retested at 12 months for patients taking 24 mg of galantamine.[6]

Not only that, but researchers have also determined that galantamine regulates the release of the neurotransmitters glutamate, gamma-aminbutyric acid, and serotonin—all of which play a vital part in proper memory function.[7]

Galantamine fights mental deterioration and increases memory and cognitive abilities— even in Alzheimer's victims

A recent series of comprehensive clinical trials unveiled some exciting new potential for galantamine, not only for treatment but also for prevention and overall cognitive function.

Researchers once thought AD patients who inherited two copies of the apolipoprotein E gene (APOE genotype) believed to cause AD wouldn't benefit as much from cholinesterase inhibitors as other AD sufferers. In four international placebo-controlled clinical trials lasting from three to 12 months, researchers at the Janssen Research Foundation in Belgium studied 1,528 AD subjects with two copies of the APOE genotype and tested the efficacy of galantamine. While those with two copies of the specific gene had an earlier onset of AD symptoms, they received equal benefit from galantamine supplementation as compared with those who had AD from other gene types. So regardless of the genetic origin of AD, galantamine improved cognitive abilities and capacity to handle normal day-to-day activities.[8]

In addition to forgetting things and not being able to draw on previous learning experiences, AD patients have an impaired ability to learn new tasks. In recent animal tests, researchers found that galantamine modifies the nicotinic receptors so there's an increased release in the amount of acetylcholine in addition to acting as an acetylcholinesterase inhibitor. Scientists concluded that daily administration of galantamine over a period of 10 days results in an increase of conditions that are known to augment learning opportunities in AD patients.[9]

Put all these characteristics together, and the overall result for AD patients—as dozens of clinical trials prove—is that the disease slows dramatically and the victim's memory can stabilize and even improve. The latest studies add to the growing body of evidence on the preventative potential of galantamine and its ability to rejuvenate your overall learning and performance.

Rescue your brain—cell by cell—starting today

The proof of galantamine's effectiveness in treating AD is so impressive that it's already being put to use around the world. Under the market name Reminyl,® it has been used widely in 15 European countries. In 1999, Janssen Pharmaceutica submitted Reminyl to the FDA for approval; the FDA sanctioned it for use in AD patients the beginning of March 2001.

But approval by the FDA is only the first step on a long path to getting help for the patient. According to the National Academy of Sciences' Institute of Medicine, important research discoveries can take as long as 17 years before information about them filters down to doctors and hospitals. And even if your doctor knows about a supplement or drug, your HMO or insurance company might not approve it because of the expense. Or they may feel you don't have sufficient need for a particular drug. Regardless of the potential benefits, mountains of red tape and bureaucratic nonsense might prevent you from getting the products you need.

The good news is you don't have to wait. While the pharmaceutical giants, insurance companies, and HMOs fight to get their extracts packaged, marketed, and distributed, you can protect your memory and intellect and put a stop to the advance of AD with the natural form of galantamine.

It's currently available from Life Enhancement Products in a formula called GalantaMind®, which combines galantamine with vitamin B_5 and choline. Refer to page 529 for purchasing information.

Galantamine does have a few minor side effects: nausea, vomiting, and diarrhea. However, they can be significantly reduced and even eliminated by taking smaller initial dosages and working up to the full dosage over a week's time.

The mountain of evidence on the benefits of galantamine for Alzheimer's patients is undeniable. Anyone battling this difficult disease should consider asking his/her doctor about it.

CHAPTER FIVE

Regrow brain cells, fight off toxic proteins, and reverse the signs of Alzheimer's and dementia

By the time symptoms start to appear, it's too late. The damage is done. Alzheimer's disease is insidious, sneaking up on you with stealth, then taking away everything you hold dear.

But this cruel disease can be held off, and some function can be restored. More importantly, you can keep it from ever taking hold in the first place.

With a single safe, natural substance, you can protect the brain cells you have, and maybe even replace some of those that have been lost. What's more, this remarkable brain saver has been helping people suffering from the worst neurological diseases, both preventing and treating Alzheimer's disease and dementia.

Memory of a lion, nerves of steel

With its cascading snowy white tendrils, this mushroom literally looks like a lion's mane—and that's where its name comes from. An ancient staple of Chinese medicine, Lion's Mane (Hericium erinaceus) is relied on for its brain enhancing powers.

In fact, traditionally, Lion's Mane is believed to bestow the memory of a lion and nerves of steel.

Scientifically, Lion's Mane has been found to contain unique active compounds that combat memory loss and decreasing cognitive powers often associated with aging. Specifically, this medicinal mushroom may:

• Improve memory function

• Enhance mental clarity

• Stimulate coordination

• Boost the immune system

• Promote production of NGF (more on this in a moment)

• Regenerate brain cells

That's right—that last point says that Lion's Mane, and particularly a specific patented extract of the mushroom, can help regenerate brain cells, which may be the key to its success in treating Alzheimer's and dementia patients.

100 percent of dementia patients had improvement in daily functioning

Let's start right in with the meat and potatoes here. A small Japanese study[1] looked at the benefits of Lion's Mane in fifty elderly disabled patients (with an additional fifty patients as controls). Of those fifty, seven suffered from dementia.

After consuming 5g daily of Lion's Mane for six months, all seven dementia patients—100 percent!—showed improvement in basic functions based on an objective assessment called FIM (Functional Independence Measure), which measures everyday activities like eating, getting dressed, and walking around.

On top of that 100 percent success rate, six out of the seven also showed improvement in some pretty important ways: They recovered some crucial cognitive powers, like better memory, understanding, and communication.

Those results are nothing short of incredible. And we're just getting started.

Substantial improvement in cognitive function with Lion's Mane

A small 2009 study[2] saw noticeable improvement for patients with mild cognitive impairment (MCI). The patients were split into two groups: One group took yamabushitake (the Japanese word for Lion's Mane mushroom) three times daily, while the other group took placebos. That part of the study lasted for sixteen weeks, and the patients had their cognitive function tested several times during that period.

By week sixteen, 71 percent of the Lion's Mane group had improved by at least three full points on the thirty point scale (that's considered a huge jump). And another 21 percent of that group had seen a two-point increase. In fact, only one of the subjects in the mushroom group was considered 'unchanged,' compared to nearly 87 percent in the placebo group.

But the study didn't end there. Four weeks after the study was completed, the patients were tested again. And this time, the scores in the mushroom group dropped substantially. That lead the researchers to conclude that patients would need to take the Lion's Mane continuously to keep its effects going.

So we know that Lion's Mane can reverse some cognitive decline—even help people regain some independence in their lives. That alone would make it worth trying, but some very dedicated scientists focused on harnessing the mushroom's capability in an even more powerful form.

Powerful extract sparks brain power by growing new brain cells and stopping lethal toxins

Back in 1991, a dedicated scientist named Dr. Hiokazu Kawagishi was hunting for compounds that could get brain cells growing again. But he hit a barrier—the blood brain barrier (or BBB), that is. You see, your brain is highly protected, and very few things can get past the BBB. That makes it very difficult to boost brain power.

Then Dr. Kawagishi stumbled across compounds called hericenones, and found that (at least in the lab), they could stimulate a very special protein called NGF—the very protein that's responsible for growing brain cells. Even better, those compounds, which come from Lion's Mane, were able to cross the BBB.[3]

As he kept working with Lion's Mane, Dr. Kawagishi discovered

---

Aricept: Are the risks worth it?

Aricept (according to the Aricept website) is considered successful if the Alzheimer's patient doesn't get worse, or if his decline slows down—meaning he's still getting worse, but more slowly. And a very lucky few may actually see slight improvement in symptoms.

But that minimal improvement comes with a very disturbing downside in the form of pretty scary adverse reactions. Common adverse reactions (taken straight from Aricept's prescribing information) include things like extremely slow heartbeat and fainting, gastrointestinal bleeding, bladder obstructions, and convulsions.

It gets even scarier when you look at the less common reactions: congestive heart failure, bone fractures, intracranial hemorrhage (that's bleeding in the brain!), strokes (a form called TIA), collapsed lungs, and kidney failure…just to name a few.

When you consider the benefits you might see compared to the risks, is it really worth it?

yet another brain-protecting agent, this one called amyloban. And this fraction does something truly amazing: It protects your brain cells from the toxic damage brought on by beta amyloid peptide—the main component of the brain-destroying plaque that develops in patients with Alzheimer's disease.

Scientists also isolated another active compound from amyloban, known as DLPE (dilinoleoyl-phosphatidylethanolamine). DLPE has shown some very powerful brain cell protection *in vitro* by inhibiting something called ER stress, which is known to destroy brain cells.[4]

With these three active substances—one that protects against toxic plaque, one that protects against deadly ER stress, and one that promotes new brain cell growth—Alzheimer's disease and dementia can be fought on three critical fronts.

So Dr. Kawagishi joined forces with Dr. Cun Zhuang, and together they developed a standardized extract (called Amycenone) that contains both hericenones and amyloban (which, by the way, is patented as an anti-dementia agent in Japan). And that proprietary extract is the key component of a supplement called Amyloban 3399.

One woman's journey from dementia to healthy with Amyloban 3399—a case study

Lin S. was an 81-year-old woman who'd struggled with depression and declining cognitive function for years. After several hospitalizations over several years, she made her way to the clinic of Dr. Inanaga... and her life was immeasurably improved.[5]

He started her on Amyloban 3399 (added to other medications and herbs she was taking). And after just two months, he saw 'notable clinical improvement.' On a clinical scale, her dementia rating went from a score between 20 and 22 (borderline dementia) to 29—a normal score. And the changes in her everyday life are even more compelling:

• Four years earlier, she struggled to name even four vegetables, but after Amyloban 3399 treatment she can name as many as she's asked to without hesitation.

- She couldn't cook before, and now she can.

- She can now solve double-digit subtraction problems, which she couldn't before Amyloban 3399.

- Scary dreams have vanished.

- And she handles separation from her husband much more easily, whereas before treatment she became anxious if he spent more than ten minutes bathing.

While increased scores on scales are impressive, what really matters is every day life. And that's what Dr. Inanaga saw improved for his patient: A true change for the better in her quality of life.

Amycenone takes on Aricept…and wins

Though individual results with Amyloban 3399 are quite remarkable, research on the extract is just getting started, with extremely promising results. Like in this animal study[6], where the Lion's Mane extract was pitted against one of the world's most popular Alzheimer's drugs—donepezil, better known by its brand name, Aricept.

Scientists started with Alzheimer Type Dementia model rats, and gave them either donezepil, a medium dose of Amycenone (the 'equivalent' to how much amyloban extract a person would take), a high dose of Amycenone, or nothing. Then the rats had to fend for themselves in something called the Morris Water Maze Test.

The rats taking either dose of amyloban extract performed much better than the untreated rats, showing huge improvements in learning memory and recognition. Plus, the rats in the high dose Amycenone group did at least as well—and sometimes better—than the rats taking donepezil.

And when it came to increasing NGF levels in their brains, the rats in the high dose Amycenone group beat the pants off all the donepezil group in every test. The medium dose amyloban group did very well, too. In all of the tests, NGF levels were significantly higher in the high-dose extract group than in the drug group. In fact, even the medium-dose extract group had higher NGF levels in half the tests.

Treating dementia and Alzheimer's disease with Amyloban 3399

Amyloban 3399 can protect your brain from cognitive decline and even help turn things around if a slide has already begun.

The recommended therapeutic dose of Amyloban 3399 is three tablets, two times daily. For maintenance or prevention purposes, the suggested dose is lower: two tablets taken twice a day.

You can find ordering information for Amyloban 3399 in the Member Source Directory on page 529.

Part IX

Immune System

CHAPTER ONE

The Scandinavian secret
to cutting colds by 50 percent

I t's that sniffling, sneezing, coughing, headachy, "just go lie on the couch and feel crummy" time of the year again. And that creates a treatment dilemma for a lot of people. You can take popular cold medications, but they don't always provide adequate relief. You can take antibiotics, but ultimately that helps breed drug-resistant bacteria. So the Health Sciences Institute has researched a natural cold remedy/ preventive that promises to be an effective alternative.

Andrographis paniculata, a shrub extract commonly referred to as Indian Echinacea, has been used for centuries in Ayurvedic (traditional Indian) therapies and Traditional Chinese Medicine to treat everything from isolated cases of the sniffles to full-blown outbreaks of influenza. It was credited with halting the spread of disease during the 1919 Indian flu epidemic. More recently, andrographis (under the brand name Kold Kare®) has outsold all other cold medications in Scandinavia for 12 years running. It was named Product of the Year by the Swedish Association of Health Food Producers. And researchers have accumulated considerable data documenting its effectiveness.

Asian herbal extract strengthens your immune system

Andrographis is not an antimicrobial agent. It does not kill the organisms that make you sick—at least not directly. Instead, it boosts your immune system and stimulates your natural antibodies.[1]

Your body makes some very powerful disease-fighting enzymes. If you become ill easily or don't recover quickly from colds and the flu, it's possible that your production of these antioxidant enzymes has been compromised. Andrographis protects those enzymes[2] and consequently enhances your natural disease-fighting ability.

Recover faster and reduce your colds by 50 percent

Chilean doctors tested the effectiveness of andrographis in a three-month, randomized, double-blind, placebo-controlled study in a rural school. Fifty-four students received either two placebo pills or two andrographis tablets every day for three months. A clinician evaluated the students each week to determine if they had symptoms of the common cold. Over the course of the three-month study, 62 percent of the placebo group got colds, while only 30 percent of the andrographis group got sick. Researchers concluded, "andrographis tablets have a preventive effect against common colds."[3]

Scientists at the University of Chile in Santiago conducted a larger study involving 158 adults. It was also a placebo-controlled, double-blind, randomized clinical trial, but it was administered for just five days to determine if andrographis could help patients recover more quickly from colds. Patients suffering from cold symptoms took either four placebo pills or four andrographis tablets a day (a total of 1,200 mg daily), and did a self-evaluation of their symptoms at the beginning of the study, after day two, and again after day four. Researchers reported the andrographis group experienced a significant decrease in intensity of symptoms (especially fatigue, sleeplessness, sore throat, and nasal secretion) by day two. By day four, they experienced a significant decrease in all symptoms. The researchers concluded that andrographis supplements "had a high degree of effectiveness."[4] They also noted that no participants experienced adverse effects from taking four tablets a day.

Meanwhile, doctors in the Hallehalsan Clinic in Sweden conducted two trials of andrographis. They found that cold sufferers experienced significant relief from "throat symptoms" after taking the herbal medication. Even though one of the studies treated patients for only three days, doctors saw "highly significant improvement."[5]

Andrographis reaches maximum potency within two hours

One criticism of herbal treatments is that it often takes a long period of supplementation to generate a benefit. Antibiotics and other prescription drugs work much faster. But, of course, they can also generate some unwanted effects, such as killing beneficial bacteria and creating stronger, disease-causing organisms.

Andrographis is different from most herbal supplements. It reaches maximum levels in the bloodstream 1.5 to 2 hours after it is ingested. Andrographolide, which is the active constituent of andrographis, is "quickly and almost completely absorbed into the blood," according to researchers conducting animal tests at the Guelbenkian Research and Drug Quality Control Laboratory of ADMTA in Yerevan, Armenia.[6] Andrographolide doesn't remain in the body for extended periods of time, which may account for its lack of harmful side effects. According to some researchers, 80 percent of andrographolides are removed via the kidneys and gastrointestinal tract within eight hours, and approximately 90 percent is eliminated within 48 hours.[7]

Andrographis shows other medicinal properties

Andrographis appears to do more than bolster your disease-fighting enzymes. Researchers at the Tongi Medical University in China found the herb can prevent *myocardial ischemia* (inadequate blood circulation in the heart usually due to coronary artery disease) in dogs,[8] while scientists at the National University in Singapore discovered that diabetic lab animals treated with andrographis developed *lower blood sugar levels.*[9] Research has also shown that andrographis can *lower systolic blood pressure* in lab rats bred to be spontaneously hypertensive.[10] Further research has demonstrated that andrographolide treatment *can prevent decreased liver function* in laboratory rodents which were given drugs that would ordinarily impair liver function.[11] Researchers at Yerevan State Medical University in Armenia also found that andrographis could *inhibit the formation of blood clots.*[12]

Such research is very preliminary and limited to animal experiments at present, so the herb's potential to influence these conditions in humans isn't yet known. Extensive human trials of andrographis have only measured the product's impact on cold symptoms and occurrences. Those trials have never identified any adverse side effects. However, you should consult with your health care practitioner before supplementing with andrographis, especially if you suffer from high or low blood pressure, a blood-sugar disorder, or vascular problems.

This andrographis supplement is available under the brand name Kold Kare. Kare N Herbs, the formulator of Kold Kare, recommends that you take one tablet four times daily to fight colds or the flu. If you're suffering from allergy symptoms or have sinus problems, you can also use Kold Kare for relief, but at a reduced dosage of two tablets daily. For ordering information, refer to the Member Source Directory on page 529.

CHAPTER TWO

An immune revolution begins: The miraculous protective yeast culture that's been one company's secret weapon for decades

It was a little over two years ago now when executives at a small, family-owned animal feed ingredient supplier in Cedar Rapids, Iowa put two and two together and came up with an answer that's poised to take the supplement industry by storm. And believe it or not, it all started with an outcry from the company's manufacturing plant workers—disgruntled, because they hadn't gotten sick. At least, not nearly as often as they deserved.

A workweek's worth of perfectly good days off had gone to waste, year after year—and, they insisted, it just wasn't fair.

If you thought this was going to be a losing battle—and, like me, I'm sure you did—you'd be mistaken. In response to what might be the oddest personnel protest in history, the plant workers finally got their way. They'd be able to use those five complimentary days at their own discretion—because, as it turns out, they had a very good point.

As years passed, many administrative and sales employees of the company submitted your typical deluge of medical bills, easily piled up from a bad case of the flu or one of those nasty seasonal sinus infections that it seems like just about everyone gets. But the plant workers? Well, they didn't register so much as a blip on the radar. And because of it, Diamond V's insurance premiums hadn't budged—even while national rates skyrocketed up a colossal 11.2 percent.

Mysterious? Maybe to some. But to Paul Faganel, the unfolding of events was a little less unlikely than anyone might have thought.

Insurance premiums—and debilitating diseases—stopped in their tracks

Faganel, now the president of Embria Health Sciences, was among the first to pick up on the baffling trend. In 2004, he was working on the operations side of Diamond V Mills, with access to the health insurance records, as well as the payroll, which reflected the surplus of unused sick time in question. But it didn't stop with paperwork and insurance premiums—the stories floating around the plant bordered on the unbelievable, too.

Take the plant's manager, for one. Half of a pair of fraternal twins, both he and his sister had been diagnosed with macular degeneration. After 30 years at Diamond V his own vision is still amazingly intact, while his sister's vision has suffered substantially, registering in at only 20 percent—leaving her practically blind. Another long-time employee was diagnosed with multiple sclerosis before she joined Diamond V—and in her 14 years at the plant, the disease has not progressed at all.

The company was riding a stroke of luck that looked nothing short of heaven sent. But as it turns out, this was a different kind of guardian angel at work: the company's flagship fermented yeast culture. The idea seemed odd, but not unthinkable—after all, the super substance had been keeping farm animals healthy since the family business started in 1943.

Yeast: the secret weapon of farmers everywhere

You probably already know a little something about yeasts. They're single-celled, microscopic fungi, best known for their crucial role in making bread and beer. But you may not have known that farmers have been feeding yeast to animals for years—initially in the form of farm-produced "mash" (maybe the term "slop" sounds more familiar)—only to discover that this unusual food was actually keeping their livestock healthy.

We see it all the time—fermented grapes create wine, for example, which has benefits that compound and surpass those of the grapes alone. Over the course of the fermentation process, mediums such as grains or grapes will take on a whole new nutritional value—becoming enriched with B-vitamins, minerals, amino acids, and other metabolites that are necessary to a sturdy constitution.

But to really get to the bottom of yeast's benefit to Old MacDonald, let's review a few highlights from Farm Feed 101. (Warning—if you already aced this course, you might find these next few paragraphs a little tedious.) Cattle, among the most common of the barnyard animals, are known as ruminants, and their digestive systems are far different from other animals. They have an additional organ, called a rumen, where most of their digestion takes place. Unlike humans, who naturally produce digestive enzymes in their small intestines, a cow's rumen acts as a fermentation vat. The naturally occurring beneficial bacteria living in the rumen produce the necessary enzymes to break down food—especially cellulose, the primary cell wall of green plants (a big part of the cow's diet, for which no mammal innately has a digestive enzyme).

Up to 80 percent of the cow's daily requirement for energy results from this fermentation process. That's why including yeast culture in its diet helps encourage the naturally occurring rumen bacteria to do a better job of digesting the cow's food. For this reason, yeast culture supplementation helps cows absorb more nutrition from the food they eat and produce the maximum amount of high quality milk.

The product that sets Diamond V apart from the pack

Diamond V was founded by a former farmer who saw a market for producing and selling this type of product on a large scale. But more than that, he had a very different method for manufacturing his products—one that, in his experience, was a lot more effective than your run-of-the-mill slop.

According to Faganel, most animal nutrition companies simply mix dry active yeast (similar to what you would buy at a grocery store) into cereal grains as feed. In this case, the yeast cells are young, and though they are still a good source of nutrition (rich in beta glucans, a polysaccharide known to stimulate immune function), they only just begin to ferment by feeding off of the nutrients and oxygen available in the grains. While the fermentation process has started to occur, boosting the nutrient content to a degree, there really aren't any substantial biochemical changes in the feed.

Diamond V, however, was the first to bring the yeast culture to the market, an aromatic granulated substance that contains both the metabolites that result from the fermentation process and the nutrients inside the yeast cells themselves. In their product, the yeast cells achieve full fermentation with a proprietary nutritional medium—the specifics of which are a well-guarded business secret—before they're ever added to the feed.

Mother Nature might be smarter than you think

If it's been a while since you broke out the chemistry books (I know it had for me), the differences here might be looking a little murky. So, I'll do my best to explain the process to you simply. Anaerobic fermentation begins when yeast cells have run out of oxygen and nutrients. When the yeast cells are added directly to a medium, they continue to feed on that—growing and reproducing exponentially—for some time. But as their oxygen and nutrient sources begin to wane, they sense their impending death and begin to secrete a variety of byproducts under the stress of survival—all of which are imparted to the medium, accounting for its fermentation.

In manufacturing their yeast culture, Diamond V lets the yeast cells reach full fermentation in their secret medium first, allowing all of the nutrients to develop completely. Both the cells and the medium are then dried. The result is a complex substance that goes way beyond the typical nutritional profile of regular yeast and contains loads of undefined nutrients.

Those undefined nutrients—birthed by the secret proprietary fermenting medium and preserved by a patented drying process—make this particular yeast culture downright impossible to imitate, as one of literally thousands of unique combinations. As it turns out, Diamond V's products not only work to aid digestion in ruminants like cattle, but they also support the health of other animals—like chickens, pigs, or even fish. And of course, as company executives ultimately discovered, humans are no exception. As consulting director Dr. Stuart Reeves so bluntly put it: "Mother Nature is not stupid." And it appears that some of her gifts truly are universal.

The ultimate immune modulator that's better than berries at fighting free radicals

Shortly after Diamond V dodged the bullet of mounting insurance premiums, company executives knew it was time to investigate future possibilities. Based on the anecdotal accounts he'd heard, Faganel had been pressing for this all along.

Once the paperwork was in place to back up the stories, he knew that they had the makings of a revolutionary product. The first order of business was to conduct a preliminary study to find out what—if any—benefits were actually brewing in the bodies of Diamond V's plant workers.

Ten employees of the manufacturing plant participated in the study, along with a control group of 10 other gender and age-matched subjects that had not been exposed to the company's immune-boosting yeast culture. The study, which included blood and saliva samples from each of the 20 participants, yielded astonishing—though not altogether surprising—results

The samples of the 10 plant employees exhibited a number of significant differences. Blood tests revealed higher-activity natural killer (NK) cells, despite being lower in their actual numbers. The number of CD-8 (immune suppressor) cells was lower, accompanied by a higher ratio of CD-4 (immune helper) cells. There were also notably lower levels of the immune complexes that are common culprits behind inflammation and tissue damage. A closer look at saliva samples—to measure salivary IgA, the immunoglobulin that builds a barrier in your body's mucosal tissue—spawned comparable observations. The plant employees had a salivary IgA level that was 68 percent higher than the unexposed study participants.

When researchers looked at the yeast culture itself, it also showed some impressive characteristics. Most notable was its score on the oxygen radical absorbance capacity (ORAC) test, which measures the antioxidant power of any given substance. The yeast culture had a value of 613. That's a formidable number, making such antioxidant powerhouses like blueberries and raspberries pale in comparison—it's a value nearly 300 percent higher than either of those fruits.

Subsequent in-vitro studies and a brief 30-day single-dose study reinforced all of the above findings—and the connection between the yeast culture and a quantifiably heartier immune system moved well beyond the status of mere suspicion. But I wondered: Diamond V's plant workers weren't actually eating the stuff. How, then, did they arrive at a recommended human dosage?

Faganel explained that the 500 mg dosage decided upon for each capsule was a pound-per-pound estimate based on the typical effective dosage for other, larger animals. And what was deemed effective for animals was based on over 60 years of research within the feed industry. While tests measuring the particulate matter in the air of the manufacturing plant showed that employees would have ingested only around 10 mg of the yeast per day, Faganel suspects that its positive effects were cumulative—based on daily exposure over the course of at least a decade.

Exhaustive safety studies on the yeast culture also demonstrated that the product is completely non-toxic, won't interfere with drug metabolism, and doesn't cause gene mutation or cell proliferation.

With more concrete proof to support a foray into the nutritional supplement world, Faganel launched Embria Health Sciences. This spin-off is devoted to exploring the vast potential of their parent company's yeast culture on the human health market. Embria's main task—and arguably the most important one—was to hone in on and maximize the antioxidant and metabolite profile of Diamond V's original yeast culture to maximize its benefit to humans. EpiCor® is the fruit of that labor.

And according to Reeves, now a consulting director at Embria, even more studies are underway to solidify the company's body of evidence, "including a slightly longer term clinical study," he told me, "and an in-house human study."

A preventive approach that upholds lifelong health

This extensive research is one of the many qualities that make Embria's yeast culture unique in its niche of preventive health. But as Faganel points out, the niche itself is enough to set EpiCor apart from the pack. "A lot of the supplements out there are indication-specific," he notes. "But if you take EpiCor when a cold is coming on," he emphasizes, "it's just too late—it won't help."

"It will be about three to four weeks before you'll see any improvements," he told me. "And then you'll notice that if you do get sick, you recover much quicker."

According to Faganel, after enough time taking EpiCor, a good night's sleep is usually all it takes to knock out a cold or the flu. And Faganel can vouch for that personally, having benefited from the initial sample capsules that the company has been using in its research. Since his college days, not a year has passed without a sinus infection cropping up like clockwork. But, he tells me, the two years that he's been taking EpiCor have been absolutely free of sinusitis—a shocking feat as, he admits, his overall habits are far from the healthiest.

But there are lots of stories within the company to match his—even from the die-hard skeptics. Faganel told me that the Vice President of Technology Research, a tough-to-convince scientist with a penchant for marathon running, noticed that he stopped getting cold sores after his grueling training sessions—a common occurrence when your body's under unusual amounts of physical stress. When he stopped taking EpiCor, they immediately came back—and, Faganel tells me, the runner was first in line for a refill of his samples.

Another Embria employee broke his arm while waterskiing, severing enough nerves to lose use of his right hand—doctors said there was a chance that he would never regain function. But, to their surprise, he recovered—and fast. When he returned for his six-week follow up, his bone had healed and he had already regained half of the function in his injured hand. His doctor told him that, within six weeks, his body had accomplished six months' worth of healing—and then invited him to participate in a study that he was planning to conduct on a collection of extraordinarily resilient patients.

It's hard not to wonder what kind of impact a product like this will have in an age where antibiotics are handed out like candy and irrational fears of pandemic flu outbreaks abound. One thing's for sure: If EpiCor is even half as effective as all of the stories (and studies) around it suggest, these signs of the times aren't likely to last long.

CHAPTER THREE

Protect yourself from a flesh-eating hospital horror with this natural life-saver

Imagine this: You go into the hospital for routine surgery, expecting to be home in just a couple of days, no problem. Next thing you know, one nurse is too busy to wash her hands between patients, and you're staring down the superbug of the century: MRSA.

You've seen it in the news, but new studies are revealing it's becoming more common than ever. Antibiotics don't kill it, and MRSA infection can result in some really horrifying stuff—like flesh-eating pneumonia. It's enough to give you nightmares and make you swear off hospitals forever.

Nancy Rattigan's story starts normally enough. In February 2007, she had hip-replacement surgery. Not a big deal, she thought. She'd had her other hip done in 2000. A self-described "can-do girl," she knew she would recover in time to take her granddaughter to Disney World in June.

But two weeks after her surgery, Nancy started feeling like she had the flu and what felt like an arthritis flare up. She chalked it up to the pain medication. And the fact it had been 7 years since the first operation—she wasn't getting any younger. Nothing to worry about. After all, her recovery seemed to be going well.

A week later, she was shocked to find she couldn't get out of bed. Nancy was weak and disoriented. Something wasn't right. The incision from her surgery wasn't looking so good—certainly not like it was healing.

At the hospital, her doctor found that Nancy's white blood cell count was over 100,000 (normal is 5,000-10,000). The surgical site was looking worse and worse. Her doctor ran some tests. And that's when the nightmare began—one that would last for more than a year.

The hospital won't protect you— your health is in your hands

Methicillin-resistant Staphylococcus aureus (MRSA). If you've been following the news, those words are enough to stop your breath. But you might not know that MRSA's actually quite common—the bacteria can lurk on the skin and in the nose and throat of a healthy person without ever causing an infection.

There are actually two kinds of MRSA: hospital-acquired (HA) and community-acquired (CA). CA-MRSA is easy to pick up in places like schools and gyms—combining shared gym equipment and unwashed hands, for example. It most often shows up as a swollen, painful skin infection. Since it usually amounts to a surface infection, it's more easily treated than HA-MRSA.

HA-MRSA, on the other hand, preys on those with weakened immune systems, which is why it can spread like wildfire through hospitals and long-term care facilities. Sure, hospitals have sanitary procedures, but overworked and tired staff don't always follow them. If HA-MRSA gets into the body through a wound or through the site of an invasive medical device like an IV or catheter, it can attack internal organs. Or worse—MRSA-related necrotic ("flesh-eating") pneumonia and blood poisoning are associated with high death rates.

If that's not scary enough, it's becoming increasingly difficult to treat. Because they're on an evolutionary "fast track," bacteria that survive antibiotic treatment quickly pass on their resistant traits, at the same time learning to resist other antibiotics. Now think about the antibiotics that find their way into our food and water, and about doctors' eagerness to whip out the prescription pad—we've basically been breeding these superbugs.

This antibiotic-resistance is what turned Nancy's infection into a major ordeal. When she tested positive, it was assumed that surgeons would clean out the surgical site and that would be that. On the morning of the cleanup surgery, she felt optimistic.

Until she felt that the hospital bed was wet—her incision, which had taken 66 stitches to close, had opened. Imagine Nancy's horror at finding a large abscess going all the way down to the joint! She was rushed into surgery, and part of the implant was removed.

An ominous yellow isolation notice was taped on the door of her room. The same notice appeared on four of the 20 doors in the joint-replacement recovery area. As the nurses came in and out with their disposable instruments and gloves, Nancy wondered how many of the 16 others would be back to have yellow cards slapped on their doors.

But she didn't have much time to think about it, being awake only about six hours of the day. The antibiotic Nancy was given was so caustic it could actually burn her veins. The drug had to be pumped directly into her arteries.

For all the danger to her body, it didn't even work. Nancy could feel the fluid building up at the surgical site again. There was talk of amputation. Nancy's doctor could only insert implants, so she was sent to specialists who gave her a difficult decision to make. The replaced joint had to come out. Otherwise, she could lose her leg. But the surgery itself could kill her.

Nancy spent her birthday in surgery. And then 10 weeks without a hip, artificial or otherwise—she had to wait until the MRSA infection was cleared before a new implant could go in.

Ten weeks after her surgery, Nancy had that new hip. But her fight wasn't over yet—it would take a blown knee, 10 weeks in a special brace, months of physical therapy, and a mix of conventional and alternative medicine before Nancy considered herself well again. And she'll *never* be declared fully MRSA-free.

Even now, she has good and bad days. The pain in her joints sometimes gets so bad she can't carry a load of laundry up the stairs. And there's her immune system—ravaged by MRSA, it is weakened for good.

Still, she considers herself a survivor. Over the past year, Nancy corresponded with others in similar situations. About half the people are still alive. The odds aren't good when it comes to MRSA. But despite the threat of a medical meltdown, not much is being done to protect hospital patients. As usual, it's all left up to you.

A common leaf succeeds where conventional medicine fails

If this doesn't sound like an impending epidemic, I'm stumped. A 2007 report shows that the number of MRSA cases nationwide had more than doubled since 1999. Then, there were 127,000 reported cases of MRSA infection. In 2005, there were 278,000. Deaths rose from 11,000 to 17,000. And the numbers are only going up. It's estimated that in the United States alone 95 million people carry Staphylococcus aureus, with 2.5 million carrying MRSA.[1]

Not scary enough for you? Well, a study reported by the Mayo Clinic estimated that 46 out of every 1,000 hospital patients are infected or colonized with MRSA.[2] While hospitals in some countries have minimized the spread of MRSA by screening incoming patients, the CDC has not followed suit in the United States.

It's getting so bad that hospitals are turning to some very dangerous drugs. The primary type of antibiotic used to treat MRSA, called glyco-peptides, can cause kidney damage. And no matter how powerful the drugs, it's a losing battle. The new MRSA strains are almost four times more deadly and are resistant to more anti-biotics than past strains.

So what is one to do? If you're planning a hospital stay, or if some-one you love lives in a nursing home, you need to build up protection *now*. And there's one particular weapon you'll want to arm yourself with.

Grown as far back as 3000 B.C., the olive tree is called the "tree of life"—and for good reason. It's been used for thousands of years as a treatment for colds and flu.

Olive leaf's active components were isolated in 1969, and when researchers for the American Society for Microbiology tested those components, they inhibited or killed off the more than 50 viruses, bac-teria, fungi, and protozoa thrown at them.[3]

Those powerful components, phytochemicals including oleuro-pein and hydroxytyrosol, keep pathogens from replicating. They also disable infections long enough for the immune system to find and kill them. By supporting the immune system instead of trying to replace it, olive leaf succeeds where conventional antibiotics fail.[4]

So how does it work? It is thought that oleuropein inactivates mi-croorganisms by dissolving the outer lining of the cell. Once they get their "in," the other components of olive leaf work together to weaken the unwelcome guest. Olive leaf also helps to build the immune system by stimulating phagocyte (cells that ingest and destroy foreign matter) production.[5]

A 1999 study demonstrated the "broad antimicrobial activity" of the polyphenols in olive leaf, leading researchers to conclude that it could be a potential source of antimicrobial agents.[6]

It's shown promise against chronic fatigue syndrome, breast and prostate cancer, HIV, and arthritis. And then there's MRSA. Olive leaf has worked so well against MRSA that it is used in hospitals in Hungary as an official infectious-disease remedy.[5]

One brand retains the power of the whole olive leaf

Search "olive leaf" on any popular online pharmacy and about 200 items pop up. Most of these products have one thing in common—the original leaf has been altered to pump up the oleuropein, only one of the phytochemicals in the olive leaf.

But, as I described, oleuropein doesn't work alone to wipe out invaders. And there's one company, working under the motto "Nature made it right," that preserves all of the disease-fighting components of the olive leaf in a 100 percent pure organic extract.

Seagate is an unusual company. Instead of developing a formula and then outsourcing production to the cheapest bidder, they do everything themselves—from the production of the raw materials to the final bottling.

In the case of the olive leaf extract, the leaves are harvested by hand from local olive trees, and the extract is produced by cold-press extraction. This freshwater method uses absolutely no chemicals. The goal? To preserve the delicate structure and balance of the olive leaf.

In independent testing, Seagate's olive leaf products killed off all introduced MRSA colonies within the first hour. The nasal spray gave particularly impressive results, killing off all colonies in 15 seconds. Other nasties were also wiped out—Strep, Candida albicans (which causes dangerous fungal infections in chemotherapy and transplant patients), and E. coli—among others.

Before putting the olive leaf extract on the market, Seagate performed a "challenge" test required by the FDA. At an independent lab, very high concentrations of bacteria, fungi, and mold were injected into the Seagate Olive Leaf Nasal Spray (simply the liquid form of the powdered leaf extract) and tested over the course of one month.

99.9 percent of all bacteria colonies were killed within 60 seconds, with all of the bacteria dead by the time a second sample was taken six hours later. It was the same story with fungi and mold. Every time more bugs were introduced, the olive leaf killed them. These results exceeded FDA standards.

Unlike antibiotics, there are no toxic effects associated with olive leaf extract, even when taken in large amounts.

When I asked Richard Lentz, the founder of Seagate, what he would recommend for someone planning a hospital stay, he suggested taking Seagate's olive leaf extract caplets ahead of time, generally two to four capsules per day. He suggests doubling up with the nasal spray, which kills pathogens in the sinuses.

Richard also recommends olive leaf extract for use before traveling on an airplane or going into other crowded environments. It is effective against colds and the flu when taken at the first sign of illness, and his daughter got rid of a bad case of food poisoning in about a day by taking 10 olive leaf extract capsules every two hours.

Ordering information for Seagate's olive leaf products can be found in the Member Source Directory on page 529.

CHAPTER FOUR

Scientists rediscover 3,000-year-old wound-healing marvel

Until just a couple of weeks ago, my experience with honey was strictly culinary. A spoonful in my evening cup of tea, or drizzled over English muffins in the morning. Then I came across a small yellow tube of Wound Honey. What I learned after that has made me look at my favorite sweet treat in a new light.

Conventional wound treatments leave a lot to be desired. Who hasn't winced as a bandage has torn away delicate new skin around a wound? And, even worse, most of the antiseptics used in modern medicine actually cause tissue damage, leaving behind ugly scars or even preventing wounds from healing properly.

You need something better to heal your wounds—quickly and safely. While modern medicine tries to convince us that the secret is in a lab, it actually rests in a remedy that's been around for thousands of years.

Revered across many cultures for centuries as a medicine and salve, honey shows up in the most ancient of writings. Around 350 B.C., Aristotle wrote that honey is "good as a salve for sore eyes and wounds." Dioscorides (ca. 40-90), an ancient Greek pharmacologist, declared a local honey to be "good for all rotten and hollow ulcers."

The Koran describes bees being taught to build hives to produce "a drink of varying colors, wherein is healing for mankind," and the prophet Mohammed strongly recommended honey for healing. For over 3,000 years, there's been a lot of respect for honey in traditional medicine.

Of course, once modern medicine started taking over, "old" came to mean "bad," and honey's medicinal use faded away. Still, some research popped up here and there. In 1892, researchers isolated honey's antibacterial properties. The fact that those properties are increased when honey is diluted, as when applied to a wound, was reported in 1919.

But it wasn't until about 70 years later that honey really started getting the recognition it deserves. In 1989, an editorial writer for New Zealand's *Journal of the Royal Society of Medicine* argued that the "therapeutic potential of uncontaminated, pure honey is grossly underutilized." The article goes on to urge conventional medicine to "lift the blinds off this 'traditional remedy' and give it its due recognition."[1]

Researchers at the University of Waikato in New Zealand heard this call to action and formed the Honey Research Unit in 1991. Their research focused on the natural healing properties of honey, especially those of one very special variety.

Honey beats conventional treatment in fighting all kinds of wounds

Manuka honey has been used for generations as natural medicine by the Maori of New Zealand. It's produced when honeybees gather nectar from the flowers of the manuka (*Leptospermum scoparium*) shrub, which is native to New Zealand and southeast Australia. The honey is darker and richer than most of the honey you'll find on the shelf at the grocery store. And it just happens to have extraordinary antibacterial, antiseptic, and antifungal properties.

Before I tell you about what makes manuka honey special, let's back up for a moment. *All* kinds of honey actually demonstrate antiseptic ability. Though people didn't know it when they were slathering honey on wounds a couple thousand years ago (they just knew it worked—and that's what matters, right?), there are several factors that go into the healing power of honey.

Honey's viscosity provides a protective barrier that prevents new infection. It also draws fluids from tissues, lifting bacteria, dirt, and debris away from the healing tissues. This osmotic effect also helps to create a moist healing environment, which helps new tissue grow and prevents scabbing. With conventional wound treatment, a moist environment can invite bacteria. But because of its other healing properties, this is not a danger with using honey.[2]

Many strains of bacteria need water in order to multiply. But the sugar molecules in honey interact strongly with water molecules, leaving very few H20 molecules free for bacteria to use. The sugar content of honey has another benefit. Bacteria will feed on glucose in preference to amino acids. This produces lactic acid instead of the foul-smelling byproducts of the use of amino acids. The bad odor associated with some wounds just fades away.

In most honey, the most effective healing property is the production of hydrogen peroxide. When honey is made, bees secrete an enzyme called glucose oxidase into the nectar. When honey is diluted (as in a wound), this enzyme reacts with water and oxygen, releasing hydrogen peroxide.

Hydrogen peroxide is a well-known and effective antiseptic, but in recent years there's been a backlash against its use. You see, it has a tendency to cause inflammation and tissue damage. The concentration of hydrogen peroxide produced by honey is about 1,000 times less than that in the 3 percent solution found in drugstores. It's still strong enough to heal, but doesn't cause the same problems as bottled hydrogen peroxide.

When it's diluted in a wound, honey produces a "slow release" of hydrogen peroxide, meaning the antiseptic power lasts longer. The hydrogen peroxide released by honey also promotes anabolic metabolism, prompting cell growth.[3]

Honey also speeds up the healing process by encouraging granulation in wounds. Granulation tissue is the connective tissue that replaces the fibrin clot in healing wounds. It aids the healing process and protects against pathogens. A doctor in one study observed that granulation occurred at a remarkable rate in wounds treated with honey.

All of this makes for a pretty impressive natural healing agent. Clinical studies have shown that honey can be diluted up to 10 times its original strength and still kill the seven species of bacteria most commonly involved in wound infection.[2]

I can't help but wonder why honey still isn't accepted by conventional modern medicine. Take the study of 59 cases of wounds and ulcers. Despite various conventional treatments, these wounds had gone unhealed from one to 24 months. When treated with honey, all of the wounds were sterile in one week. New tissue developed rapidly, and there were no adverse effects.[3]

In one particular case study, a patient was suffering from a deep pressure sore that was not responding to conventional treatment. When dressed with honey, the wound healed completely in six weeks.[4]

The "wow" moments kept coming as I read through more and more reports of successful trials. In one, honey went up against silver sulfadiazine, the most widely used agent to clear infections in burns. After seven days, 91 percent of the burns treated with honey were completely sterile. In the same amount of time, infection was merely controlled in 71 percent of the burns treated with silver sulfadiazine. The patients treated with honey had better pain relief and less scarring.[3]

In another study, nine infants with large, infected post-surgical wounds that weren't responding to intravenous antibiotics were treated with honey. After 21 days, all of the wounds were closed, clear, and free of infection.[4]

One unique variety packs a double dose of potent antibacterial action

When the Honey Research Unit started testing honey, they quickly discovered something special about manuka. When the enzyme catalase was added to destroy the hydrogen peroxide in honey, only manuka showed any significant antibacterial activity. Because catalase is present in the tissues and serum of the human body, the bacteria-fighting power of hydrogen peroxide can only last so long. Manuka honey, on the other hand, can keep fighting infection even when it can't produce hydrogen peroxide.

Manuka honey doesn't require oxygen to activate the full scope of its antibacterial properties. So it can wipe out infection in deeper tissue of the body. It can also be used with all kinds of wound dressings without fear of weakening its power.[5]

Unlike other varieties, manuka demonstrates strong antifungal action. Antibiotics are ineffective against fungal infections, making them difficult to treat. In studies treating fungal infections, manuka honey did the job when other varieties could not. Less dilution was needed to fight fungal infection than bacterial infection, making manuka honey ideal for treating drier surface infections.[2]

Of course, as with any natural food product, there is variation from crop to crop. Once the news of manuka honey broke, many companies started selling inferior varieties, some with undetectably low levels of antibacterial activity.

So how can you tell if the manuka honey you're buying really works? To determine the non-hydrogen peroxide antibacterial levels of manuka honey, the team at the Honey Research Unit came up with a grading system called "unique manuka factor" (UMF). The UMF number corresponds to the concentration of phenol (a common conventional antiseptic) that has the same antibacterial activity. So a manuka honey product labeled "UMF 15" has the same power as a 15 percent concentration of phenol.

Most professionals use honey designated as UMF 10 or above, as this is the only kind to yield consistent results in clinical studies. In studies using UMF 12 honey, widespread serious skin ulcers have healed rapidly. And we're talking ulcers that simply hadn't responded to modern conventional treatment. Some people in one study had been in intensive care for nine months. Treated with honey, their wounds healed at an astounding rate. Three separate studies have proven UMF 12 honey's ability to heal MRSA-infected wounds. Many wound types are counted among the success stories: venous leg ulcers, diabetic foot ulcers, pressure ulcers, unhealed graft sites, boils, and surgical wounds.[3]

Heal ulcers and sores in days with Wound Honey

With memberships in the American Podiatric Medical Association and the American Sports Medicine Association, Dr. Randolph Nordyke is no stranger to treating pain. He's spent the past few years perfecting a wound-healing formula that combines UMF 12+ manuka honey with aloe vera and vitamin B to soothe wounds as they heal. Dr. Nordyke has used Wound Honey on more than 100 patients, with some incredible results.

When I visited the Wound Honey website, I found images of a foot with a very large and painful-looking diabetic ulcer. This foot belongs to Adrien Goldbaum, who applied Wound Honey to the ulcer after having no luck with other treatments. It healed completely in only a few days. Other images show similar results with a large wound on the bottom of another patient's foot.

Another user of Wound Honey, N.W. of California, wrote to Dr. Nordyke about a post-surgical ulcer with a "horrible odor." After N.W. used Wound Honey for about eight days, the ulcer was completely healed. N.W. says Wound Honey is "nothing short of amazing."

Doctors using Wound Honey on their patients echo that amazement. Dr. Scott Roberg, DPM, notes that he would not have believed the effectiveness of Wound Honey had he not seen it himself. He uses it on all of his wound-care patients, and calls it an "incredible success."

Wound Honey can be used on all kinds of wounds, large and small, for rapid healing. Unpasteurized organic manuka honey makes up 98 percent of the formula. The rest? Aloe vera soothes the wound and decreases inflammation. Panthenol, a nonirritating form of vitamin B, moisturizes the area of the wound.

When I got my hands on a tube of Wound Honey, I didn't have any reason to try it. One of my cats, Bartleby, decided to help me out in that department. Agitated by a stray cat hanging out on the deck, he turned and sank his claws and teeth into my leg. After cleaning the cuts (including one where he really dug in), I smoothed on some Wound Honey.

I didn't have a bandage wide enough to cover all of the damage, so I put a Band-Aid over the deepest scratch. Of course, Wound Honey is very sticky. Soon, my other leg was smeared with honey. You'll need some kind of dressing with Wound Honey.

Because the scratches were so spread out, I continued putting Wound Honey only on the deepest one. Now, about five days after the "attack," there's hardly a trace of that wound, while the smaller ones are red and scabbed.

Granted, the wounds I'm treating are nothing compared with the serious ones Dr. Nordyke's patients are healing with Wound Honey. But it just goes to show that Wound Honey could be a practical addition to any household. If you'd like to try it for yourself, ordering information is in the Member Source Directory on page 529.

CHAPTER FIVE

Peruvian herb completely eliminates Lyme disease—no matter how long you've had it

It sounds like a bioterrorist attack: A hard-to-detect microbe that embeds itself in your heart and brain, potentially causing dozens of easily misdiagnosable symptoms. A microbe that can change shape, so your immune system can't identify and kill it. And it's believed to already infect as many as one in six people on the planet.

The bacteria that causes Lyme disease (which is called *Borrelia burgdorferi*, or Bb) may sound like a science fiction villain—but it's all too real, very easily spread, and nearly impossible to diagnose and cure.

With mainstream methods, that is…

Because there is a natural cure for Lyme disease, one that comes from the depths of the Peruvian rainforest—a vine called *uncaria tomentosa*, more commonly known as cat's claw. And a special and very rare type of this Amazon plant may be the only way to knock out Lyme disease once and for all… once it's been correctly diagnosed, that is.

The 'Great Imitator' hides behind misdiagnosis

When you think Lyme disease, you probably imagine its hallmark sign: the bullseye rash. But what you probably don't know is that many people (and some researchers believe up to 90 percent of people) infected with Lyme don't get that rash at all... and that's the first step toward misdiagnosis.

Step two: misdirection. Instead of claiming symptoms that could define the disease, it mimics other ailments to throw off accurate diagnosis. The attack starts with fever, weakness, and lack of energy, which most doctors write off as a simple case of the flu. And because the flu is a virus, they don't prescribe the antibiotics that could actually get this bacterial infection under control before it gets out of hand.

And while *B. burgdorferi* causes symptoms very much like other ailments, it acts very differently than other bacteria. It's not like your garden variety salmonella or E. coli. In fact, it's a spirochete (meaning it has long, heavily coiled cells that look like spirals) in the same family as the bacteria that causes syphilis.

Spirochetes aggressively embed themselves in tissue—muscle, tendons, even heart and brain. In fact, these spirochetes can penetrate into your brain in as few as three weeks after you've been infected with the Lyme disease.

And Lyme disease, like syphilis, gets harder and harder to wipe out as the infection progresses.

Ticks get all the blame

It's common knowledge that Lyme disease is caused by deer ticks. But, unfortunately, they are not the only ones spreading it. Other ticks, mosquitoes, fleas, and bot-flies can all also carry Lyme disease. And the disease is now known to spread by human-to-human contact as well.

Three stages of Lyme disease triple your risk of serious symptoms

Lyme disease isn't just a one-shot illness. Rather, it has three distinct stages, each with its own set of debilitating symptoms. And since these stages can occur months—even years—after the initial bite, they're often diagnosed as something else entirely, and treated incorrectly.

Stage I starts with the infection itself (whether by bug bite or through human-to-human contact), and develops symptoms within two or three weeks. If you're "lucky" enough to get the telltale symptom, the bullseye rash, you may be among those diagnosed and treated correctly and quickly.

But the other Stage I symptoms—the ones that are much more common than the hallmark rash—are very easily written off as other things (like the flu, or normal signs of aging). These symptoms include:

- Fatigue
- Joint pain (especially in your knees)
- Muscle pain
- Headache
- Fever
- Lymph node ailments (like swollen glands)

Stage II symptoms can show up weeks, even months, after the initial bite. Again, these symptoms are usually misdiagnosed, as they seem to have no clear cause. But the joint pain (officially known as arthralgia) and muscle pain that show up at this stage can become debilitating—and they may persist until the Lyme is cured.

And then there's Stage III, which appear years after the original infection. So even if you think your Lyme disease is gone, its symptoms can still affect you years later. The most common Stage III symptom is severe, erosive arthritis of your large joints, particularly your knees.

But Lyme disease doesn't stop there.

You may be struck with occasional vomiting, back pain, muscle weakness, nerve pain, and sudden chills. Or perhaps you'll end up with a stiff neck, insomnia, night sweats, or heart problems. Some people even get symptoms that look just like Parkinson's disease or ALS (amyotrophic lateral sclerosis, better known as Lou Gehrig disease).

And because these symptoms come so long after the initial infection, and seem completely unrelated, there's a strong probability that you'll remain misdiagnosed, mistreated, and very ill—all because of one very tough bacteria that has quite a few tricks to play.

Bb hides in plain sight, evading antibiotics, and biding its time

B. burgdorferi is different than most bacteria—and not just because of its spiral shape. This bug follows a very unusual (and dastardly) life cycle. Bb actually goes dormant and hides inside other cells, sometimes in a cyst-like form where it's protected against antimicrobial agents.

For one thing, standard treatment is a two-to three-week course of oral antibiotics, which may kill off some of the bacteria but can't even come close to the hidden Bb cells.

Those Bb bugs can hide out anywhere from two weeks to eight months, just biding their time until they can strike again.

And when your body is under stress, those cysts burst out of their hiding places, and storm back into your bloodstream where they once again take their spirochete form.

That's when they resume their damaging ways… but it's also when they're once again vulnerable to attack.

Finally, a proven cure for Lyme disease

Believe it or not, there is a complete cure for Lyme disease—it just takes time, patience, and stealth to eradicate every single spirochete. And one remarkable rainforest herb can do the trick, without causing undue harm to your body (unlike some powerful antibiotics).

In a moment, we'll talk about just how this miraculous extract works to wipe out Lyme disease once and for all. But first, let's take a look at some real results that prove just how completely effective this herbal medicine—called Samento—can be.

Because when doctors put Samento to the test, their patients saw dramatic improvement... and many of them were completely cured.

Back in March 2002, Dr. John Kule started using Samento in his practice—and wrote about the results in a report for the *British Naturopathic Journal*. He treated sixty patients (some of whom were diagnosed with Lyme disease) with the cat's claw extract... and 59 of them showed 'distinct clinical improvement.'

Many patients reported increased energy and reduced inflammation, two hallmark symptoms of Lyme disease, among other things. Only very few mild and transient side effects were reported, though some patients experienced what's known as the Herxheimer reaction (see sidebar).

Then in 2003, renowned cardiologist Dr.William Lee Cowden

Beware the Herxheimer reaction

When your body is riddled with bacteria, killing off that multitude of microbes can occasionally cause something known as a Herxheimer reaction.

Basically, when medication kills off bacteria, those bacteria may release toxins, which can send your immune system into overdrive and may cause some unpleasant side effects. So, you may feel worse before you feel better—but that just means the treatment is really working.

pitted Samento against antibiotics in a small pilot study of documented Lyme disease patients. Thirteen of those patients were treated with Samento, plus a regimented diet and detoxification program. The fourteen in the control group were put on standard antibiotic treatment. Of the fourteen in the control group, three saw slight improvement, three got worse, and eight saw no change.

But *everyone* in the Samento group improved dramatically—and 85 percent of the group (eleven patients) tested negative for the Bb bacteria at the end of the six-month study.

Samento's unique makeup makes it the best solution to Lyme disease

Samento is a potent and unique extract of cat's claw, a Peruvian vine scientifically known as *uncaria tomentosa* (and called *una de gato* by local healers).

Now you've probably heard of cat's claw before, but you've never seen this specific form. Samento is made from a rare type of *u. tomentosa* that's rich in POA—pentacyclic oxindole alkaloids—and FREE of tetracyclic oxindole alkaloids (TOA).

That rare mix gives Samento its unique effectiveness against the Bb bacteria. Because while POAs increase germ-killing, TOAs can cancel out the POAs work. Most varieties of cat's claw (and most cat's claw products that you'll find at the health food store) contain a mix of POAs and TOAs—and it's anyone's guess as to how much of each you'd be getting.

With Samento, there's no question: You're getting straight, healing POAs without any potentially blocking TOAs.

POAs help your immune system gear up to fight Lyme disease

The key component of Samento—POAs—impact your immune

system on the cellular level, in several ways, all of which help knock out the insidious Bb bug.

First, POAs increase your body's germ-killing power by special white blood cells called granulocytes. They got their name because they contain minute granules that hold very powerful chemicals and enzymes that your body uses to destroy foreign invaders.

Next, cat's claw seems to help cells called lymphocytes survive longer.[3] Their key responsibility is specific resistance to disease, attacking invaders in just the right way to kill them. The POAs also seem to manage lymphocyte production by setting off a special compound—something that those TOAs (which Samento does not contain) can inhibit.

Another benefit of POAs: they boost *phagocyte* function. Phagocytes, also known as scavenger cells, work by engulfing bacteria and then destroying them through a digestion-type process.

Finally, POAs act as modulators for the immune system, stimulating it when necessary, then reining it back in when the job is done.

Samento contains more than just POAs

Though potent POAs (and zero TOAs) make this cat's claw extract special, Samento also contains plenty of other healing agents.

- Organic compounds (called multiple quinovic glycosides) that unleash antimicrobial powers against Lyme disease
- Ursolic acid, which offers liver protection, antiviral activity, and antioxidant powers
- Special polyphenols, called OPCs (oligomeric proanthocyanidins), which offer a whole host of health benefits including preventing DNA damage to cells, keeping inflammation in check, and boosting the powers of natural killer cells.

The combination of natural compounds in cat's claw work together to empower your immune system and destroy the Bb bacteria.

Cat's claw tackles inflammation, easing Lyme symptoms while it knocks out the disease

And on top of its Lyme disease-curing properties, cat's claw is known to be a powerful anti-inflammatory agent. That's particularly important here because the Bb virus can set off very powerful inflammatory reactions.

This added benefit is partly due to the herb's antioxidant powers, and partly because cat's claw can inhibit TNF-alpha (tumor necrosis factor-alpha). TNF-alpha is a major cause of inflammation, especially when your immune system is fighting toxins.

And one study found that a mere nanogram (a miniscule 1/1000 of a microgram) of cat's claw could curb TNF-alpha expression, reining it in by 65 percent to 85 percent. And that translates to a much milder inflammatory reaction—a true blessing for Lyme sufferers.

Antibiotics can't stand up to Lyme disease

For a few people who are diagnosed correctly and quickly, and immediately placed on a two-week course of the right antibiotics, these drugs may knock out the Bb bacteria. But we know that some of the bacteria hide, and the drugs can't touch them—so a two-week course may not wipe out the bug completely. In fact, a short course of even the most potent IV antibiotics can't get to the dormant bacteria, which may just build up resistance to the drugs.

To really knock out this insidious threat, you need long-term treatment, long enough to wipe out those initially dormant Bb when they wake up and rear their ugly heads again. And therein lies the problem: Long-term treatment with pharmaceutical antibiotics can be extremely dangerous, causing many severe side effects… some that are even worse than Lyme disease itself.

Samento goes the distance to knock out Lyme disease once and for all

Unlike pharmaceutical solutions (meaning megadoses of antibiotics), Samento can be used safely for as long as it takes to wipe out all the spirochetes, no matter how long that is.

In fact, some researchers believe that TOA-free cat's claw formulations are the "best alternative treatment for Lyme disease," even going as far as possibly fixing damage to the immune system caused by the Bb bacteria. And scientists studying the TOA-free form of the herb (like you'll find in Samento) suggest that cat's claw treatment last from eight to twelve months in order to eliminate all spirochetes from the body.

The manufacturer recommends putting one to fifteen drops into a glass, then adding four ounces of water. Then wait one minute before drinking the solution. In order to avoid a potential Herxheimer reaction, they suggest you start at the lowest dose, and slowly work your way up to the maximum dose. Start with one drop (in four ounces of water) two times daily, and slowly increase that dose up to fifteen drops (in four ounces of water) two times per day. It's also recommended that you work closely a medical practitioner as you fight Lyme disease.

You can find purchasing information for Samento in the Member Source Directory on page 529.

CHAPTER SIX

Secret germ antidote knocks out Flu in 8 hours

I n 2002, National Geographic published an article that related the details of how the Chernobyl nuclear accident destroyed a nearby anthrax research lab, releasing live anthrax into the wind and affecting villages for more than 60 miles.

What National Geographic didn't cover is what happened in response to this disaster. The Russian military directed classified researchers at the State Scientific Center Research Institute of Highly Pure Biopreparations, located in Saint Petersburg, Russia, to develop protection against such biological warfare agents.

Starting in 1980, the team studied more than 600 products. Only one exhibited effectiveness, low cost, and high safety. The Russian microbiologists discovered a special strain of lactobacillus bacteria with powerful immune-protecting properties. Lactobacillus occurs naturally in your nose, mouth, throat, and intestines.

With all the recent hype about probiotics, you've probably heard about the benefits of lactobacillus. Well, take that concept and put it through special training and you get the powerful immune-boosting formula developed by the Russian scientists—a formula that helped one pharmacist give his daughter back a normal life.

Knock out flu in less than a weekend

I recently spoke with that pharmacist, John Sichel. He told me that, in his profession, he comes into contact with quite a few product manufacturers—and all sorts of product samples. Most of the time, this is just a run-of-the mill part of his job. But in 1999 he received a sample of this supercharged lactobacillus formula. When Sichel's daughter, Pamela, came down with the flu that winter, he gave her the sample. It completely knocked out her flu symptoms in just eight hours. Sichel was impressed, but he didn't think much more about the supplement again until several months later, when he received a heart-wrenching call from Pamela.

For several years she had been experiencing symptoms of hepatitis C—brain fog, fatigue, depression, and flu-like symptoms that would not go away. Now, though, her doctor told her she had a viral load of about 250,000 (a healthy person would typically have a viral load of 0), and her immune system just wasn't handling the attack.

Sichel remembered giving her the Russian immune-boosting product to beat the flu and how well it had worked. So he suggested she try the same formula again, although he had no idea if it could pack the same punch against the more serious, aggressive illness his daughter was facing this time. But to his astonishment, once again, the virus was no match for the product. Within just a few months, all of Pamela's hepatitis symptoms were completely gone. She began taking the formula daily—her viral load quickly normalized, and she remains in good health today.

This time, he was so impressed that what had been "just another product sample" quickly became the new focus of his career.

After 50 years working in the pharmaceutical industry, Sichel understood that unless the product became mainstream—accepted under the watchful eye of U.S. agencies—there was a good chance that his daughter's deliverance would not be available to her, or anyone else, in years to come.

To ensure that this didn't happen, he went to pretty extreme measures. He learned enough Russian to be able to effectively communicate with the product's developers and actually traveled from his home in Boulder, Colorado to Russia. Sichel spent the next three years working with the original formulators to devise a plan of action to manufacture this extraordinary product in the USA.

Now, this product, known by many aliases—Lactoflor, Matrix E., Preparate, Extrabiolate, and its current moniker Del-Immune™—is not only available in this country, but it's also 10 times more powerful than the original formulation.

Breaking down walls to build stronger immunity

When he arrived in Russia, Sichel's first priority was to learn as much about the product as possible. The Russian microbiologists explained to him that they'd worked with scientists in Bulgaria to supercharge the lactobacillus agent. The Bulgarians showed the Russians how to break the cell walls of this potent lactobacillus, because their research proved that the immune-protecting properties in lactobacillus exist as proteins inside the cell.

Unless the cell wall is broken, our immune systems are unable to "see" these proteins, which are necessary for a dramatic immune response. Once the cell wall is successfully broken, the resulting cell pieces are called "cell wall fragments." Cell wall fragments have been found to contain highly active proteins, amino acids, and complex sugars that account for the effect upon the immune system. So the researchers used these fragments to create a supplement by freeze-drying them, crushing them into a fine powder, and encapsulating them.

Small quantities of this product were brought to the United States, and Sichel was one of the few people who received samples. Subsequently, nothing came of this technology until Sichel formed a partnership with the Russian researchers.

Fans of the original have even higher praise for U.S. version

Since the manufacturing technology was transferred to the U.S., further refinements, involving innovative culture nutrition and precisely controlled manufacturing procedures, have produced significant improvements in potency over the original Russian product.

The U.S.-made product is estimated to be 10 to 30 times more potent than the Russian counterpart—with three times more proteins within the cell walls. This is due to over a year of diligence by the U.S. team, using the lab's experience in culture nutrition and modern technology to produce and test the product. They paid special attention to laboratory analysis, DNA formatting, and the development of good manufacturing practice (GMP) standards. Currently, quality control using DNA and other contemporary analysis methods ensures that every batch of Del-Immune is pure and identical.

Sichel told me that many of the original product users were asked to try the new U.S.-made version and report their impressions. More than 50,000 doses of the new Del-Immune product were evaluated in human subjects for comparison, and the results were great news for all of us. Since each capsule is equal to more than two capsules of its predecessor, many users who were taking two or more capsules a day were able to cut their dose in half, saving money in the process. The higher potency also appeared to decrease the amount of time it takes for the product to "kick in" and start working.

He explained that typical use for Del-Immune is to provide effective, reliable, safe, and immediate immune system support. Users have provided anecdotal reports with its application in flu, West Nile virus, colds, coughs, bronchitis, fatigue, hepatitis C, certain skin infections, yeast, non-healing fractures, constipation, and side effects of chemo and radiation therapies. Essentially, Del-Immune acts like your body's specially-trained secret virus-fighting agent.

You can't get this immune boost
from yogurt alone

To understand how Del-Immune works, you need to understand some basics of your immune system. According to James L. Wilson, N.D., Ph.D., "The immune system comprises an innate immune system and an acquired immune system. A portion of this elaborate network of immune defense is functional at birth; this is the innate immune system. When called upon, it moves with great speed. A second immune system develops as the body interacts with the environment (and reacts to such influences as vaccination); it is the acquired immune system and works slowly. The host is protected by both the innate and the acquired immune systems, working together."

White blood cells, called T-cells, are a part of the innate immune system. The T-cells first act as a command center that issues combat orders. Then, this part of the immune system fights viral and bacterial invaders directly—think of it like hand-to-hand combat.

Meanwhile, the B-cells of the acquired immune system act as the artillery. Keeping a safe distance from the invader, B-cells deliberately fire round after round of antibodies toward the perceived enemy without having direct contact with it.

Del-Immune helps the two systems work together more effectively in viral combat situations.

Wilson explained that he was so impressed by this idea and his own clinical experiences, he started investigating the scientific basis for immune enhancement with lactobacilli cell walls and cell wall fractions. Of the various combinations commercially available, the cell wall fractions of specific strains of Lactobacillus bulgaricus (L. bulgaricus) appear to be the most potent. One of the significant discoveries the U.S. team made was to identify this strain using modern technological advances—technology not available to the Russian lab at the time of original strain identification.

Wilson explains that the difference in performance between "these immune enhancing strains of L. bulgaricus and yogurt cultures or the common lactobacilli preparations sold for intestinal bacteria replacement is…vast."

Your secret agent in the fight against colds and flu

I told you about Pamela Sichel's fast relief from the flu and from hepatitis C after taking Del-Immune, but she isn't alone. I spoke to several people who swear by its protective effects.

After taking Del-Immune at her daughter's recommendation as a quick fix for her flu symptoms, one woman began taking it as a daily immune-support supplement. As a fifth-grade teacher, she was constantly battling whatever bug her students were passing around. But since she started taking Del-Immune daily, she told me, she has yet to bring home any illnesses from school.

Perhaps even more striking is 56-year-old Matthew R.'s story. He told me that Del-Immune sent the reinforcements his system badly needed to heal after major surgery and cancer treatment: "Two years ago I had two major surgeries. One was to remove a tumor, and, unfortunately, a type of lymphoma cancer was found. Lymphoma affects the immune system and I caught a very bad cold after leaving the hospital. I got down to 112 pounds from 140 pounds and was very weak. John Sichel heard about my illness and offered me some packets of Del-Immune powder. I have taken one dose every day since. Only once in two years did I get sick. That was when I ran out of it… As soon as I started Del-Immune again, things got better. No more colds or flu. I have made sure I don't run out again, as I am convinced the Del-Immune is keeping my immune system working."

Primetime cover-up?

In the course of my research, I had a chance to watch a never-aired documentary from a major network news program on Del-Immune. According to the tape, it appears that Del-Immune is not just for colds, flus, and biological pathogens; if your body's immune system needs support, it seems to benefit from this product.

In 1992, after the Cold War, the product—no longer classified—was used clinically in the treatment of breast, lung, and liver cancers, serious hospital-type infections, and contagious disease at the State Cancer Hospital in St. Petersburg, Russia. The product was also used to boost the immune systems of patients undergoing chemo and radiation therapies, allowing the patients to complete their therapies without the usual debilitating effects. Numerous Russian studies document the remarkable cancer-related uses of this secret agent. The doctors reported that the patients on Del-Immune looked and felt better and had more energy.

With such promising reports and potential benefits, it's tough to fathom why the piece never aired, but if I had to guess, I'd say it probably had something to do with the all-too-familiar red tape so many effective natural treatments encounter when they're brought to the public. But despite the suppressed news coverage, Del-Immune is now available in this country, and, as you've read, it's already becoming the answer to many people's immune concerns.

Fast relief without the side effects

Del-Immune offers both consistent long-term support and immediate support. The recommended daily dose as a dietary supplement is one to three capsules daily, or as directed by a healthcare provider. The fast-acting remedy dose—two capsules immediately, followed by an additional two capsules 12 hours later—should be taken at the first sign of cold or flu.

After taking Del-Immune, you can expect the boost of immune support to begin in approximately six to eight hours. Relief is often as fast as 24 hours but varies for each person.

There are virtually no reported side effects and it is shown to be very safe—even at high doses of up to 15 g per day. According to the manufacturer, during testing, massive dosages—50 to 100 times the suggested dose—caused gastric upset in some subjects. Dr. Elin Ritchie, a medical doctor with a practice in Taos, New Mexico, remarks that, "I have used Del-Immune in more than 20 patients in the last few months, since it became available to me. None of the patients have experienced any side effects."

Many of the testimonials in the never-aired documentary mentioned that they were especially confident in the safety of the product. And because it is grown in a special media, not cultured in milk, some lactose intolerant users have reported they experience no problems taking it.

See the Member Source Directory on page 529 for complete ordering information.

HSI's immune-boosting all-stars

All too often these days, just as you find a natural alternative that works—poof! It's no longer available, but there are three others I wanted to mention.

These few products aren't necessarily "late breaking news," but they are effective in helping boost your immune system. And in a time where our effective natural options are dwindling fast, it's more important than ever to be aware of what we still do have access to.

N-acetylcysteine (NAC) is a naturally occurring derivative of the amino acid cysteine. Your body uses NAC to manufacture another compound called glutathione, which acts as a master antioxidant and liver detoxifier. As such, glutathione plays a critical role in supporting the immune system—fighting disease and protecting the vital systems of our bodies.

Glutathione stores can be depleted by injury, strenuous activity, chronic disease, or radiation exposure. Supplementing with NAC will help restore and maintain optimum intracellular (inside the cell) glutathione levels.

According to one human trial, NAC significantly increased immunity to flu infection. Over a six-month period, only 29 percent of those people taking NAC developed symptoms of the flu, vs. 51 percent of those taking a placebo.[1]

NAC is widely available in health-food stores and through mail-order companies.

The second featured product is ImmPower (AHCC). AHCC is an extract of a unique hybridization of several kinds of medicinal mushrooms known for their immune-enhancing abilities. On their own, each mushroom has a long medical history in Japan, where their extracts are widely prescribed by physicians. But when combined into a single hybrid mushroom, the resulting active ingredient is so potent that dozens of rigorous scientific studies have now established AHCC to be one of the world's most powerful—and safe—immune stimulators.

Since 1987, various clinical trials conducted in Japan have demonstrated that AHCC has the ability to support normal immune function. More than 700 hospitals and medical clinics in Japan recommend AHCC as part of a regular immune maintenance program. It's available in America as ImmPower™ AHCC®.

Typically, each soft-gel capsule contains 300 mg of AHCC. Dosage recommendations range as follows: For maintenance of general health and prevention of disease, 1 to 3 grams per day; for treatment or prevention of cancer drugs' side effects, 3 to 6 grams per day.

Our third standout—lactoferrin—has literally been around forever. In fact, lactoferrin, an iron-binding protein in breast milk, was the very first immune booster. It has two specific functions: First, it binds to iron in your blood, keeping it away from cancer cells, bacteria, viruses, and other pathogens that require iron to grow. And it also activates very specific strands of DNA that turn on the genes that launch your immune response.

Numerous studies on rats as well as patient case histories have documented the benefits of lactoferrin in helping to combat many types of viral and bacterial illnesses, as well as malignancies.

The general recommended dose is 100 mg each day, taken at bedtime.

For product information and how to order, see the Member Source Directory on page 529.

Part X

Vital Health Secrets

CHAPTER ONE

Nature's perfect food: Discover the amazing health benefits of the fruit from the Amazon's "tree of life"

If you get your health guidance from the mainstream media, you'd think the healthiest way to live is to guzzle red wine and drown everything in olive oil.

That's basically what they've told us in recent years. First, it was the "French paradox"—the fact that the French, who generally eat lots of cheese, cream, and butter; drink lots of wine; and smoke like chimneys, are healthier than Americans. Scientists told us it was all in the wine—specifically, in the *anthocyanins*—the antioxidant flavonoid that gives red grapes their deep color.

Then it was the "Mediterranean diet," the traditional way of eating in regions of Italy and Spain, where olive oil is a staple. We learned that olive oil is a good source of essential fatty acids that are processed right out of many Americanized foods.

I'm not discounting the benefits of either of these phytochemicals. In fact, in a minute I'll explain exactly why both are so important to good health. I just question the *sources* recommended in the headlines.

There's got to be a better way to get these valuable nutrients than guzzling wine and drowning in oil.

As it turns out, there is. I learned about it from HSI panelist Jon Barron. He told me about a single superfood from the Amazon that, fresh from the tree, can provide over 30 times the amount of anthocyanins as red wine *and* all the beneficial fatty acids of olive oil in one delicious, all-natural package. And this is just the beginning of this food's health benefits. It's virtually impossible to over-do this food—which is certainly not the case with red wine or olive oil.

Get the healing power of many phytonutrients in one delicious package

There's no disputing the health benefits of anthocyanins and essential fatty acids. Both have proven to be powerful nutritional tools in the quest for good health.

Research has shown that plant pigments like anthocyanins are potent antioxidants. The cardiovascular benefits are the most well known; studies show that anthocyanins can help prevent blood clots, improve blood circulation, relax blood vessels, and prevent atherosclerosis.[1,2] But scientists have also uncovered a whole host of other powerful effects from anthocyanins, including antiviral and antiallergenic properties.[3] Some research even suggests that anthocyanins can prevent cancer, by blocking carcinogenesis on a molecular level and encouraging tumor cell death.[4]

Essential fatty acids have proven just as powerful. Oleic acid, a monounsaturated omega-9 acid, and linoleic acid, a polyunsaturated omega-6 acid, help lower LDL and maintain healthy HDL levels. They also increase the absorption of fat-soluble vitamins like vitamins A, E, D, and K, which are essential to good health. Research has even suggested that oleic acid may prevent against cancer and hypertension.[5]

Olive oil may be the best known sources of these nutrients, but it is certainly not the only one. It's the pigment in red grapes that gives wine its anthocyanins—and that same pigment can also be found in other red and purple fruits and vegetables, such as blueberries, red cabbage, and purple sweet potatoes. Oleic acid is also present in pecans and seed oils, and linoleic acid is found in peanuts.

But there is one food that delivers it all—plus other healthy nutrients like fiber, phytosterols, and vitamins C and E. For centuries, it's been a staple for people in Brazil, yet virtually unknown to anyone outside the region—until now.

Discover the health secret of generations of Amazonian Indians

It's called *açaí* (pronounced ah-sigh-ee), and it's the fruit of a palm tree that grows in the rainforests of the Amazon—a tree Brazilians call the "The Tree of Life." About 90 percent of the small, round fruit is its hard, inedible pit—but that's OK, because it's the outside skin that holds the treasure. That dark purple skin is what contains the anthocyanins.

The natives puree the skins, creating a treat that can be served warm as a sauce over fruit or grains or frozen like a sorbet. They've been eating it for centuries, passing down recipes from generation to generation. (The native people have also passed down the story of how açaí was discovered; see the sidebar on the following page for the Legend of Açaí.) Because fruit itself is perishable, its popularity never spread beyond the region.

Then, a few years ago, two friends from California went to Brazil on a surfing expedition and tasted açaí for the first time. Before they even knew the health benefits, they were hooked on the taste. But once they learned that the tasty treat was also a nutritional powerhouse, they knew they had to find a way to bring açaí to the rest of the world.

Superfood fights heart disease, cancer, prostate enlargement, and more

Since then, the news about açaí has been steadily spreading—and the evidence of nutritional and health benefits just keep piling up. Consider this: a 100-gram serving of açaí contains only 90 calories, just 2 grams of fat and no cholesterol. Plus, it delivers 3.5 grams of dietary fiber, something we could all use more of in our diets. Improved processing of the fresh fruit is making it possible to preserve more of the fruit's healthful attributes. Currently, the puree provides more anthocyanins than red wine and has antioxidant concentrations that well outweigh blueberries.

Subsequent research has shown that in addition to anthocyanins and essential fatty acids, açaí also contains a healthy dose of plant sterols, another class of phytochemicals that have been shown to reduce

---

The Legend of Açaí

For centuries, açaí has been a traditional food of the native people of the Amazon—and part of its folklore, finding its way into legend as well as onto the table.

Once upon a time, there was an Amazon Indian girl named Iaca, whose father was the tribal chief. His tribe had grown so large that there wasn't enough food to go around. So the chief decreed that all newborn babies must be killed. And when Iaca, his own daughter, bore a child, the chief had his decree carried out.

Iaca mourned her baby's death alone in her hut for days, until she thought she heard a baby crying. When she went outside in search of the baby, she saw a palm tree shooting up from the earth, covered in fruit. Full of despair, she lay down under the tree and died.

The next day, the tribe found Iaca's body under the new tree. The tree's fruit satisfied their hunger and renewed their energy, and the chief lifted his harsh decree, declaring that the fruit would be named for his daughter (açaí is Iaca spelled backwards). With abundant food for all, the tribe grew and flourished.

cholesterol, protect the immune system, and relieve prostate enlargement.[6] In fact, it turns out açaí is in the same family as saw palmetto, a common herbal treatment for prostate enlargement. And researchers at the Federal University of Rio de Janeiro have discovered that açaí extract can be used to fight infection, like the parasitic infection *schistosomosis* which affects 10 million Brazilians each year and the common bacterial infection *staphylococcus aureus*. It seems there's no end to this miracle fruit's health benefits.

Thanks to those Californian surfers, açaí is now available to just about anyone. Their special recipe is based on one created by Brazil's Gracie family, the founders of Brazilian Jui Jitsu, which is the fastest growing martial art in the world. The recipe combines the powerful health benefits and great taste of açaí with the sweet syrup of the guarana fruit, which has long been touted for its beneficial effects on stamina and concentration.

In some parts of the U.S., you can purchase açaí in Whole Food Markets. Or you can order direct over the phone or via the Internet. (See the Member Source Directory on page 529 for complete ordering information.) So instead of trying to emulate the French or the folks in the Mediterranean region, consider taking a cue from the native people of the Amazon.

CHAPTER TWO

Learn what may be causing your bladder control problems— and what you can do about it

Recently I came across some exciting information about an all-natural supplement that is proven to help relieve one of the most common causes of urinary urgency and pain. According to its developers, it's completely safe with no side effects or contraindications. And it's readily available without a doctor's prescription.

Because bladder control problems are so common and because there aren't any safe, natural solutions, we decided to bring this new product to you as quickly as possible. But, before I tell you more, I need to share one concern raised by our Medical Advisor, Martin Milner, ND. When we spoke, Dr. Milner explained to me that there's still a possibility that this compound may reduce the level of hydrochloric acid in your stomach and your ability to digest protein and dietary forms of calcium.

Although the manufacturers acknowledge the importance of stomach acid and suggest they've put this concern to rest, Dr. Milner advises anyone trying this product to do so with discretion—on an "as needed" basis. (If you have bladder control problems, you're probably asking what "as needed" can possibly mean. Be patient. You'll see.)

Here at HSI, we'll follow up on these issues with Dr. Milner's help. Let us hear about your experiences. When we learn more, we'll let you know.

Millions depend on Depends waiting for real help

According to the Internet site urologychannel.com, about 13 million people in the U.S. experience incontinence on some level. Sometimes it's just a sudden and frequent urge to urinate. Sometimes it's difficult or even painful urination. And sometimes that urge is just a little too sudden—and then it's an embarrassment and an impediment to a full, independent life.

Unfortunately, too many people suffer with these problems for years without relief. Many are reluctant to talk to their doctors about them. Even if they did, conventional medicine doesn't offer much in the way of help. (Recently, the pharmaceutical companies have developed drugs to help with combating an overactive bladder. But that's a very specific type of problem, involving involuntary spastic contractions of the muscles surrounding the bladder—and these drugs are far too new to know much about their long term safety and reliability.) If you're among these millions, you may have just given up hope.

Of course, there are many different kinds of bladder control problems with many different root causes. According to urologychannel.com, urinary tract infections, prostate enlargement, bladder stones, urinary cancer, and neurological disorders like multiple sclerosis and Parkinson's disease can all be underlying causes. Even some prescription drugs list incontinence as a side effect.

That's all the more reason to bring this up with your doctor and have a full checkup to rule out any undetected health problems. But many times, the doctor can't find a reason—and that means you can't find relief.

Another possibility is a diagnosis of *interstitial cystitis*. Interstitial cystitis (IC) is defined as chronic inflammation of the bladder, resulting in difficult and/or painful urination, increased urgency, and increased frequency of urination. The diagnosis is fairly new, but already authorities estimate that as many as one million people—about 90 percent of them women—suffer with this problem.

If you've been living with symptoms like these, you may take heart in having a name for your suffering, but unfortunately a diagnosis of IC doesn't do much good. Because according to conventional medicine, the cause of IC is unknown—and so is the cure.

Yet for years, there's been a growing body of anecdotal evidence to suggest that something very basic may be behind many of these unexplainable and incurable bladder problems. Something we all take into our bodies every day: our food and drink.

Your diet may be sending you to the loo

Believe it or not, it may be that simple. Many people report that certain foods and beverages exacerbate their bladder control problems—particularly people with diagnosed IC. And the foods that seem to cause the most problems are those that are highly acidic: cabbage, coffee, tea, soda, tomato-based foods, fruits, fruit juices, beer, and wine.

At first glance, it seems like such a simple solution to such a troublesome problem. But when you think about the reality of eliminating many of your favorite foods from your life forever, you can't help but want a better way.

There is one. It's an all-natural formula that actually reduces the acid in food. And it's been clinically proven to reduce painful and embarrassing symptoms in people diagnosed with IC.

Works on the food, not the person

The active ingredient is *calcium glycerophosphate*, a dietary mineral that combines calcium and phosphorus in a 1:1 ratio. When it is added to acidic foods, the mineral acts as a base agent, actually bringing the pH of the food toward a neutral level. According to the manufacturer, it "works on the food, not on the person." (That's an important distinction, because we know that interfering with the body's natural acids can be disastrous.) In fact, there have been no reported side effects from using this formula—just powerful results.

According to studies conducted by the manufacturer, calcium glycerophosphate significantly reduced the acid level of common foods and beverages—some by as much as 99 percent. With just one tablet, the acid in an eight-ounce glass of iced tea was reduced 99 percent; a six-ounce cup of coffee was reduced 95 percent; and an eight-ounce cola, reduced 98 percent. Three tablets reduced the acid in a four-ounce glass of chardonnay by 80 percent and the acid in a 1/2 cup of bottled pasta sauce by 60 percent.

Research suggests that these results translate into real relief for real people. Urologists at Graduate Hospital in Philadelphia, PA, studied the effects of the mineral-based supplement on more than 200 IC patients. When using it, 61 percent of the participants reported a reduction in urinary urgency, and 70 percent experienced less pain and discomfort when eating acidic foods.[1] Another study presented to the Quebec Urological Association in 1998 tracked the results of the supplement on 200 IC patients. Using visual analog scales to assess pain severity and urge intensity, participants reported significant relief in both areas after using the formula for four weeks.[2] These results led the Interstitial Cystitis Association (icihelp.org) to recommend the supplement to its membership in its quarterly publication, *ICA Update*. In every study, there were no adverse side effects.

Convenient, easy to use—and no change in taste

The product is called Prelief®, and it's available in both tablet and granule form. You can decide which delivery method works best for you: You can either swallow the tablets whole, dissolve them in your acidic beverage, or sprinkle the granules in your acidic food or beverage. (The manufacturer notes that the granules will not dissolve in alcoholic beverages; for these acidic drinks, Prelief tablets are recommended instead.) Users say that it doesn't change the taste of most foods; if anything, you may detect a slight mellowing of the food's "bite" due to the acid reduction. The amount used depends on the food or drink you're using it with; a handy Prelief pocket guide included in the package tells you how much you'll need to reduce the acid in your favorite foods.

Prelief is available at major retail, drug and grocery stores; the website includes a search function to help you find a store near you. You can also order it directly either online or by phone. See the Member Source Directory for complete ordering information on page 529.

CHAPTER THREE

The Polish mothers' secret indigestion remedy

Any country that considers sauerkraut and pierogies fried with onions as dietary mainstays <u>needs</u> a good remedy for indigestion. So for generations, Polish mothers have been mixing shredded black radish with fresh farmer's cheese as a cure for any number of digestive ailments. It works. Believe it or not, there's research to prove it. But I'm certainly not in any hurry to whip up a batch and chow down the next time I have an upset stomach. It fact, the thought of it sort of <u>turns</u> my stomach. But I found a better way—or at least a more appealing one—to get the same benefits in a single supplement..

It's called Raphacholin (or Raphacholin C), and it's been used in Eastern Europe for over 45 years. It contains a blend of five ingredients, each with a long history of traditional use and a bevy of modern research to back it up. But somehow, this trusted Polish remedy has remained a secret outside the region—until now.

I spoke with Peter Karpinski, Ph.D., president of QLife®, the dietary supplement company based in New York that imports Raphacholin from Poland. He told me that growing up in his Polish household, it was an everyday part of life. "My mother used Raphacholin tablets regularly," he says. "In my household, as in many Polish households, Raphacholin tablets are always in the medicine chest in case of indigestion or almost any stomach trouble."

Natural ingredients aid digestion, reduce inflammation and protect liver

The name Raphacholin is a combination of two of the formula's main active ingredients: black radish (*Raphani sat. nigri*) and cholic acid, a bile acid. These two ingredients mimic the old folk remedy recipe I mentioned above (the cholic acid takes the place of farmer's cheese). The other active ingredients are artichoke (*cynara scolymus*), peppermint oil, and a special herbal charcoal preparation derived from linden tree bark.

Turns out each of these old world folk remedies has some real science behind it. In one animal study, Hungarian scientists found that black radish root granules could effectively reverse the changes seen in rats' colons after they ate a high-fat meal. Untreated rats experienced a reduction in the number of enterocytes (intestinal lining cells) and goblet cells (specific enterocytes that secrete mucous) and a proliferation of inflammatory cells after eating a high-fat meal. But treatment with black radish effectively nullified these effects, returning enterocyte and goblet cell counts to normal levels and reducing the inflammation.[1] Black radish has also been shown to have antiviral and antibacterial properties.[2]

Research also supports the traditional folk wisdom that artichoke promotes bile secretion, protects the liver, and relieves dyspepsia.[3,4] According to Karpinski, Polish workers in the viscose fiber plants used to receive artichoke extract tablets each day at work, to protect them from liver damage caused by poisons like carbon disulfide, which were everyday hazards in the factories.

And peppermint oil is known to soothe the stomach and decrease intestinal spasms; in one study, peppermint oil proved to be a more effective anti-spasmodic agent than a prescription drug for patients undergoing gastro-intestinal endoscopy.[5]

Relief from acid reflux, constipation, and more

While Raphacholin has been safely used in Eastern Europe for generations, some people should probably think twice before trying this remedy. First, Raphacholin contains 75 mg of charcoal, which can absorb some medications in the stomach and render them ineffective. If you depend on regular medication, talk to your doctor before trying Raphacholin. Also, because of its bile-inducing effects, Raphacholin is not recommended for people with bile-tract obstructions, gallbladder disease, or those who have had their gallbladders removed.

But if those conditions don't apply to you, Raphacholin may offer effective relief from acid reflux, bloating, flatulence, and constipation. QLife recommends that healthy adults take one or two tablets, one to three times a day as needed with fluids. For laxative effects, take two tablets in the morning and two in the evening 30 minutes before meals.

There are two Raphacholin formulas available today in the U.S. with different names. QLife's product is called Raphacholin-C, and it is imported directly from its Polish manufacturer, Herbapol. But Herbapol also makes a private label Raphacholin formula called Digest RC for a company called CX Research. The names may be different, but both products contain the same ingredients in the same formulation. For complete ordering information for both Raphacholin C and Digest RC, see the Member Source Directory on page 529.

CHAPTER FOUR

The key to good health is hiding in your bone marrow: Wake up your stem cells without stirring up controversy

These unsung heroes of the human body have finally found their place in the sun. Unfortunately, the magnifying glass accompanying the research on stem cells has put them in the hot seat, as well. And this seat's not just hot—it's on fire. These days, even the most casual mention can get you into trouble.

But unless you're living in a plastic bubble, you'd better get used to it. Like it or not, this particular controversy is here to stay.

Perhaps you're wondering why I would even bother to bring up one of the sorest subjects in the U.S. these days. Am I trying to rub salt in the country's collective wounds?

Allow me to assuage your fears. Here at HSI, we're all about healing. So when a bottle of StemEnhance landed on my desk, you'd better believe I took notice. According to the formulators of this unique product-the very first of its kind to debut on the alternative health market, under a new category dubbed "stem cell enhancers"—the key to good health has been hiding in our bone marrow all along.

Packing the punch of a million microscopic healers into one convenient capsule

StemEnhance actually evolved from another supplement. In the August 2005 *Members Alert,* we told our members about Aphanizomenon flos-aquae (AFA)—the aquatic superfood from Klamath Lake that took nutritive healing to another level. It's chock full of vitamins and minerals (nearly 64) and omega-3 fatty acids (excellent aids in reducing inflammation), and it even contains a molecule (called pheny-le-thylamine, or PEA) that's known to elevate the mood, increase alertness, and alleviate depression.

In that article, we also told you about some of the studies suggesting that two of the blue-green algae's active compounds might be responsible for boosting the circulation of your own stem cells. If you ask Christian Drapeau, a scientist with years of AFA research under his belt, he'll tell you that the connection between stem cell circulation and a turn for the better in health is no coincidence. According to Drapeau, AFA's compounds have been tapping into what he believes is the human body's innate ability to heal itself.

So he was hardly shocked by the testimony that continued to pour in—reports ranging anywhere from the recovery of old injuries and the easing of painful inflammation to the reduction of symptoms associated with the most dreaded neurodegenerative diseases. Certain that they had hit something big, Drapeau and his colleague, Dr. Gitte Jensen, were bound and determined to isolate the two compounds credited with this effect, packing the punch of a million regenerative chameleon-like characters—your very own stem cells—into one convenient capsule.

I wondered how a higher circulation of adult stem cells would result in healing of such biblical proportions. It sounded like a serious stretch to me. Sure, adult stem cells from bone marrow are used in therapies today for post-chemotherapy and radiation cancer patients. Stem cells are harvested from the patient's marrow before the damaging high-dose treatments, and re-injected later to repair a ravaged immune system. Stem cell transplants are also used in order to replace the defunct blood cells of patients with leukemia, lymphoma, and various other genetic diseases.

Whatever the example, the current use of adult stem cells is a complicated and invasive process, not accessible to the average Joe, and reserved—so far, at least—for treating only the most serious blood disorders. But are the possibilities really endless?

Drapeau believes that he and his colleague have switched on our own stem cells' superpowers with StemEnhance. And what's more, he claims that it can help everyone with healthy marrow—no matter what his or her condition.

Send your stem cells to work in as little as one hour

According to Drapeau, adult stem cells from bone marrow are much more capable than most scientists would confidently claim today. Embryonic stem cells are widely considered the more useful variety, due to their ability to morph into nearly every type of tissue in the entire body. The National Institutes of Health maintain that, while studies are still underway, adult stem cells able to give rise to all cell and tissue types have not yet been found. But Drapeau insists that they absolutely can serve this purpose, based on tidbits of the latest research that look remarkably promising, if still incomplete. A rebellious stance, for sure—but one worth considering.

Patented in November 2004, StemEnhance is a botanical extract of Aphanizomenon flos-aquae that, as mentioned earlier, isolates two of the algae's most essential compounds—L-Selectin ligand and polysaccharide—to make up a high-molecular-weight fraction of AFA. What that means in lay terms is this: The beneficial effects that AFA consumption has on your stem cell circulation can now be found in the form of a supplement that cuts directly to the chase. Not only does it promote your stem cells' more rapid release from the bone marrow, but it also increases their homing mechanism—that is, their ability to get to the damaged tissues that need them the most.

Isolated from its algae origins in StemEnhance, the L-Selectin ligand blocks the receptors on your stem cells that keep them anchored in your bone marrow, allowing them to enter circulation. While the exact function of the polysaccharide is unknown, it forms what Drapeau refers to as a synergy with the ligand. According to Drapeau's studies, consumption of the two components together results in approximately a 27 percent increase in stem cell circulation within an hour.[1] And that's about as soon as you might start seeing results, because at that point, the stem cells have cleared from the blood and have supposedly made their way to their final destinations, where they take up the task of repairing your body.

While there's no solid evidence to back the conclusion that the stem cells have actually gone to work at damaged tissue sites, Drapeau believes that this is the case, based on the results of his studies on natural killer cells in response to AFA consumption. In one preliminary experiment, he worked with a breast cancer patient who had just had her brachial lymph nodes removed following a mastectomy. In general, he told me, lymphatic fluid (which is composed of red and white blood cells and a fat-and protein-based digestive substance called chyle) is very hard to study. But when there is a drain to collect fluid from swelling in this area, as after an operation, you have access to these fluids that you otherwise wouldn't.

This gave Drapeau something to go on. When natural killer cells have entered your tissues to fight a viral infection, they eventually return to your blood by way of the lymphatic fluid. If, after he fed the patient some AFA, the number of natural killer cells circulating in her blood spiked and quickly cleared, he'd know that they had visited her tissues if they showed up in her drain, into which the lymphatic fluid would empty. The high number of natural killer cells that Drapeau found in the patient's drained fluid—many more than there were before she consumed the algae, he tells me—was in keeping with his theory. Based on this one instance, Drapeau believes that the compounds in StemEnhance send our stem cells-the behavior of which seems to have mimicked natural killer cells so far-to work in the tissues as well.

New answers to an ancient problem

It's hard to say what's really happening here. Maybe Drapeau and Jensen's hunch was correct-if not entirely, at least partially. I'm reminded of a recent article I read in The New York Times' health pages, highlighting the role of stem cell research in regenerative therapy.[2] While many hail this technology as the hope of the future and others revile it as repugnant to the laws of both nature and ethics, there remains a small contingent that transcends the argument in favor of a much more radical theory. And this one's as old as time itself: evolution.

Consider how readily the liver repairs itself. After thousands of years of attack, whether from poisonous plants and rotten berries when we were still a hunting and gathering species or from the airborne toxins, preservatives, and pesticides of the 21st century, this organ has mastered the art of regeneration like no other in our body. We know that it can replace up to 2/3 of its own mass within two weeks, or grow and shrink to any size in order to meet its needs. Why shouldn't every organ follow this one's example? Could it be that the rest of our body has simply lost its touch?

After all, the very animals with which we share at least one identifiably regenerative gene—salamanders and zebra fish, to name a couple—are capable of replacing everything from severed limbs and spinal cords to damaged retinas and hearts. But it's not because a bunch of stem cells rush like an army to the rescue. On the contrary, the cells that are already in place revert back to their most primitive state, forming what is called a blastema, in order to reenact the birth of the missing or damaged piece. In short, the cells aren't taking orders from the surroundings that remain. As if through some bizarre bodily will to power, they create themselves—and the genesis of their new surroundings follows. Could it be that somewhere hidden deep within us remains the memory of this power, begging to be unleashed?

The subject polarizes scientists on every possible level, and until more is known the research will carry on and the conversation—and controversy—will continue. While most doctors and research scientists swear by the limitations of adult stem cells, so much remains in the dark. The only thing we really know is that we don't know. And while the science behind the formulators' claims might raise an eyebrow, who's to say they aren't true? I don't know if StemEnhance operates the way Drapeau says, or in some other, as yet, unknown way. But I'd ask if it really matters. Many of history's greatest breakthroughs had their roots in shockingly radical hypotheses. Besides, at the end of the day, actions always speak louder than words.

So all of this begs one important question: Does StemEnhance actually work? Well, it would appear that the answer to this question largely depends on who's volunteering it.

2 years of excruciating pain erased in 5 days

Doing my best to keep an open mind, I gave Celia Monilaws of Calgary, Alberta a call. And let me tell you, she was more than happy to talk with me.

Her story begins as many do—from the bottom of a steady and heartbreaking decline. At the age of 52, Celia had suffered from fibromyalgia for 15 years and osteoarthritis for eight. A slow surrender of her favorite activities left her 150 pounds overweight. Both of her hips eventually gave out. She had been living in excruciating pain for nearly two years, unable to walk without two (yes, two) canes and otherwise confined to her couch. But she continued to go to work each day, adamantly steering clear of painkillers—except for once, she confessed, when she took some ibuprofen at the end of one of her worst days. She was on the waiting list for a hip replacement, each day inching closer to quitting her job.

After a close friend of hers who also happens to be a naturopath gave her StemEnhance, she told me, her life was completely changed. Within five days, like magic, she rose from bed one morning and stood to her feet—no canes, nothing. She's been walking—without even so much as a limp—ever since. For now, the hip replacement is looking like it won't even be necessary. Her nearest and dearest are in awe, she tells me, at how she's reclaimed her life. I asked her if anyone else she knew had tried it.

According to Celia, everyone—friends and family alike—wanted a bottle. After seeing her results, they expected a miracle too. Did they get one? Well, no. None quite like Celia. They did, however, notice a lot of benefits: Sleep was more sound and energy was less elusive. Blood sugar readings balanced, cholesterol levels lowered, migraine headaches, sinusitis, and nagging aches and pains just about disappeared. Not exactly miracles, but if you take the results for what they are, you've got to admit, it still sounds pretty appealing.

The recommended dosage of StemEnhance is one to two capsules twice a day along with plenty of water. Dark greens and algae can be a significant source of vitamin K, which may not be clearly stated on the label. According to Dr. Martin Milner, HSI's medical advisor, this could be an area of concern in terms of drug interactions (especially ones that thin the blood). If you're currently taking medication to treat a health condition, he recommends that you check with your doctor before using StemEnhance.

As sometimes happens with AFA, StemEnhance can cause a detoxifying reaction (headache, diarrhea, or skin eruptions). If you experience discomfort, you may want to drop your dosage and increase it incrementally, as your body adjusts. Everybody is different, so experiences with StemEnhance will vary. While some notice immediate results, many find that it takes eight to 12 weeks for visible changes to occur.

CHAPTER FIVE

Steam up your sex life with this native secret from south of the equator

Sometimes, a name can speak for itself. Take *huanarpo macho*, for example.

I probably don't have to detail the traits of this potent Peruvian herb for you to have a pretty good idea of what it does. But I will anyway—and I'll start with a few of its unique physical characteristics.

It's a shrubby tree that grows to about 35 feet in height, adorned with blooms of rich, red flowers. You'll find it in the Amazon's Maranon river valley. And the young branch stems are shaped an awful lot like, well… the aroused male anatomy.

In case you haven't guessed yet (though I'm betting you probably *have*) huanarpo macho (known as *Jatropha macrantha* in technical circles) is an Amazonian aphrodisiac—a secret love potion that delivers a serious boost in sexual stamina. And in case you haven't also guessed, HSI panelist (and resident rainforest expert) Dr. Leslie Taylor introduced it to me.

It probably seems fitting that the secret to a better sex life would be hiding in a remote jungle somewhere. And the truth is, quite a few of them are. We've already shared a lot of these with you—like muira puama, maca, and catuaba. But when it comes to increasing your sexual performance, you'll probably agree that less *isn't* more—and every little bit of help you can get counts.

Obviously, I couldn't wait to share huanarpo macho with you—not least of all because I was pretty certain you'd never heard of it before. After all, I hadn't. And as it turns out, there was a very good reason for that.

The most popular libido-booster you've <u>never</u> heard of

Up until recently, indigenous Peruvians were practically the only ones able to benefit from huanarpo macho's power. It's so popular in its native territory, in fact, that the local government has occasionally been forced to restrict its harvest. This—and the almost complete lack of suppliers in the States—means that you aren't likely to hear much about it outside of the jungle it grows in.

"I've known about huanarpo macho for many years now," Taylor told me. "Anytime I asked another herbalist, herbal doctor, or native healer what they used for impotency or male sexual stimulation, huanarpo macho was usually named first, or at least in the top three."

But just as appealing to Taylor as its revered role in native medicinal preparations was that fact that not a single side effect had been reported with the use of this wildly popular herb. In fact, there's been no incidence of negative reactions whatsoever in huanarpo macho's long history of local use.

And as you no doubt already know, that's a *lot* more than can be said for the usual suspects on the erectile dysfunction drug market today. With their notorious lists of side effects (like swelling, shortness of breath, vision changes, headaches—and even worse, *painful* erections) good sex is likely to be the *last* thing on your mind.

Packed with plant chemicals
to help you get up—and stay up

Laboratory analysis has revealed that huanarpo macho is rich in a number of disease-fighting, energy-boosting compounds, including sapogenins, flavonoids, alkaloids—and a particularly large number of a class of polyphenols called proanthocyanidins. These compounds are widely known for their ability to fight inflammation and arthritis, stave off heart disease, and scavenge cancer-causing free radicals from your body.

But it's only been more recently that scientists have started investigating the potential these proanthocyanidins might have to reverse erectile dysfunction in men. The primary target of these studies has been pycnogenol, an extract of pine bark that's another extraordinarily rich source of proanthocyanidins—and which has been shown not only to restore long-lasting erections, but also to enhance fertility in both humans and animals.[1,2]

In 2006, a team of Italian researchers verified that huanarpo macho stems contain a comparably wide range of these fertility-boosting pro-anthocyanidins—concluding that this finding "is in agreement with the traditional use as an aphrodisiac of the plant under investigation." They also confirmed that, among these plentiful compounds, proanthocyanidin B-3 is the most abundant.[3] And although scientists aren't certain yet, this distinguishing factor may hold the key to huanarpo macho's extraordinary abilities.

Studies show that proanthocyanidin B-3 exerts a particularly positive influence on a hormone called bradykinin, a key player in proper physiological and cardiovascular function.[4] And this relationship is very important, because bradykinin has also been revealed as essential to the relaxation of the penile cavernous smooth muscle—a necessary step in the formation of an erection, and one that's often negatively affected by high blood pressure.[5]

Regulating bradykinin could put an end to this kind of erectile dysfunction—and prompt a massive increase in the frequency and duration of your erections. But that's not the only vital sex hormone that research shows huanarpo macho extracts can influence.

In a 2003 study, researchers observed two groups of mice: One that received 5 grams of huanarpo macho in their water each day, and another that received regular water. At the end of the 30-day test period, study authors found that the mice that had consumed the extract experienced significant increases in blood testosterone levels. And as you probably already know, testosterone plays a key role in boosting your libido, increasing the frequency and firmness of your erections, and in giving you the energy you need to get going—and stay going all night.

Early reports reveal greater energy— in more ways than one

With so much research still yet to be done on the exact mechanism of huanarpo macho's performance-enhancing powers, I'm sure you're eager to hear how the herb has fared in real-life cases. But because it's still so new, few have even tried it.

But those that have used the extract report definite changes. Several experienced major boosts in energy and vitality. And the effects seemed to be stronger with regular use. One man reported a surge in his libido with consistent doses—and another claimed: "I don't feel as energetic since I have not been taking it."

Still, the best testimonials remain those of the millions of Peruvians who swear by this herb's extraordinary powers. Ask any of them, and I'm sure you'd get the same answer: Huanarpo macho is one of the strongest natural aphrodisiacs south of the equator.

Huanarpo macho extract is available as a liquid tincture. Taylor recommends using 60 drops, two to three times a day as needed (between meals is best). And you can take it any way you prefer—either straight, or add it to juice, water, or any other beverage. You'll find ordering details in your Member Source Directory.

CHAPTER SIX

Beat depression, migraines— and everything in between—with this single serotonin-boosting breakthrough

*P*sychiatrists Top List in Drug Maker Gifts.

That's the bone-chilling headline that caught my eye from the pages of *The New York Times* just a few short months ago. And while I can't say that it came as a surprise, it did serve to point out how desperately so many patients are seeking help—and how few of them are actually getting it.

I'm acutely aware of some of the more common risks of antidepressant use: Insomnia, weight gain, sexual dysfunction, nausea, constipation, dizziness, memory lapses, agitation, and anxiety.

And if you guessed by now that I'm about to write about a new natural treatment for depression, you'd be right.

But here's the twist: If you guessed that I'd write about migraines, low sex drive, irritable bowel syndrome, tinnitus, or even fibromyalgia, well… you'd be right about those, too. As it turns out, every one of these conditions can be traced back to the same imbalance that causes depression—and a new product called Seratonin can alleviate them all.

The dangerous truth behind low serotonin— and the drugs used to "treat" it

Seratonin is the life's work of Dr. John Allocca, a medical research scientist and pioneer in the field of natural migraine treatment. As was the case with so many breakthroughs we've covered in the past, Dr. Allocca developed his formula in an attempt to combat his own relentless migraines.

Having suffered from these debilitating headaches for 40 years, he devoted his career to finding a cure. The fruit of this research was his invention of the very first migraine brain chemistry model in 1997. What he discovered in the course of making this model is that imbalances of two important neurotransmitters, norepinephrine and serotonin, are responsible for this painful phenomenon—and a whole lot more.

The first of these neurotransmitters, norepinephrine, is a stress hormone released from the adrenal glands and converted into epinephrine (adrenaline) during a typical "flight or fight" reaction. Whether it's the result of daily stress, a traumatic event, or an injury, your body's sympathetic reaction will always be the same, responding with high blood pressure and pulse, insomnia, aggression, glucose release, inhibition of the gastrointestinal tract—and also a depletion of the second important neurotransmitter, serotonin.

Most serotonin is produced in your GI tract and later stored in your platelets—while there, however, it can't be used by your central nervous system, as the molecule is too large to cross the barrier into your brain. Instead, your brain relies on serotonin's precursor, tryptophan, to enter the brain via an albumin carrier, where it is converted into serotonin afterward.

But there's a catch: When faced with outside disturbances (like stress or anxiety), an array of competing enzymes is introduced, leaving tryptophan to be metabolized before it ever has a chance to be transported. The result is low serotonin in your brain—and this state has been linked to all of the conditions I mentioned earlier, including depression, migraines, insomnia, and fibromyalgia.

The complicated tree of neuro-chemical pathways that causes migraines and depression would be impossible to explain to you fully here. But the general rule of thumb is this: Problems typically occur only when reserves of norepinephrine and serotonin are exhausted at a faster rate than they can be replaced. Without enough stores of these neurotransmitters on hand, messages in the central nervous system can't be relayed properly.

That's the conundrum addressed by your typical antidepressant. After serotonin and norepinephrine are shot across your brain's synapses, they are reabsorbed into their original cells—an action called "reuptake." Antidepressants inhibit this process, however, forcing more of one or both neurotransmitters to remain active on the synapse while increasing levels of free serotonin and norepinephrine in the brain.

This interrupts your brain's natural processes, though—and the problems associated with that interruption can be *very* dangerous.

Some of the most sinister tragedies in recent times have been linked to these prescriptions. Consider the shootings at Columbine… or worse, the mass murder of 32 students and faculty members on the campus of Virginia Tech. In both cases, the gunmen were taking popular antidepressants. And—as recent research has shown—in both cases, the deaths of many might have been avoided.[1]

Several studies have now linked depression drugs to major hostility events like these—and all U.S. labels currently list anxiety, agitation, panic attacks, irritability, hostility, aggressiveness, impulsivity, and mania as possible side effects. During the course of his migraine research, however, Dr. Allocca came to realize that risks like these aren't necessary evils at all—not if you provide your brain with the appropriate blend of nutrients.

He discovered that it is possible to enhance the natural function of your brain's neurotransmitters without a single dangerous side effect. And his new formula Seratonin does just that.

Your ultimate defense against serotonin depletion

I've already mentioned stress as a potential cause of neurotransmitter imbalance. But really, there are a number of causes (some of which you might have already guessed) that can contribute to this problem. These include inflammation, allergic reactions, hormonal changes, systemic candidiasis, unstable blood sugar, and dehydration.

Balancing all of these factors obviously requires a comprehensive

---

Beware the hidden dangers on your dinner plate

Tyramine content isn't something that you'll find listed on a nutrition label—but if you've had problems with depression, migraines, or mood swings, it's definitely something you want to watch out for. Even some of the healthiest foods could be contributing to your low serotonin levels. Some of these include:

- cheese
- mustard
- berries
- sourdough
- yogurt
- miso
- tofu
- any aged or fermented food
- alcoholic beverages (including beer and red wine)
- chocolate
- onions and garlic
- avocado
- tamari
- soy sauce
- vinegar
- smoked/cured meats
- yeast and brewers extracts

approach—and all 14 of Seratonin's nutrients serve a manifold purpose. First, they help your brain to manufacture and maintain serotonin and norepinephrine. Additionally, they aid in decreasing allergic reactions while controlling glucose levels (these are two of the most common stressors to your body, both of which contribute significantly to serotonin depletion).

5-Hydroxytryptophan is arguably the most important ingredient. With the recent controversy stemming from a supposed contaminated batch of tryptophan, the real thing has become very hard to find (we alerted you to one of the only sources back in November 2004). But while the supply of true tryptophan has dwindled, this form of the molecule—called 5-HTP for short—enjoys a slightly wider availability. It's extracted from the African tree Griffonia simplicia, meaning that it's not a synthetic compound like its predecessor—and it's also one step closer to serotonin in the conversion chain.

More important, though, is that it delivers equally profound benefits. A double-blind clinical trial performed by Swiss researchers in 1991 showed that it's as effective as fluvoxamine (a popular antidepressant) in relieving depression, while being superior in tolerance and safety. And while it has loads of research to support its effectiveness against panic and anxiety disorders, insomnia, and migraines, more recently the spotlight has turned on its clinical effectiveness against fibromyalgia—with clinical studies showing that it significantly improves symptoms with only mild, short-lived side effects.

The one notable drawback of supplementing with 5-HTP is that at higher dosages (like the 200 mg you'll get in Seratonin), you could find that it causes some temporary nausea, especially on an empty stomach—but taking it with food will usually help with this.

In addition to this key ingredient, Seratonin also contains a blend of vitamins and nutrients to block serotonin depletion from every angle:

• B-vitamins (including niacin and folic acid) are vital to the production of neurotransmitters and also inhibits depletion.

- Vitamin C and copper facilitate norepinephrine production.

- Magnesium and calcium boost nerve transmission and vasomotor control.

- Zinc promotes a calm mood (deficiencies of mineral are linked to anxiety).

- Choline increases magnesium uptake.

- Quercetin stabilizes cell walls, reducing allergic reactions and inflammation.

- Trimethylglycine helps convert norepinephrine into epinephrine.

- Alpha lipoic acid is a potent antioxidant.

- Vanadium and chromium increase insulin receptivity and control glucose fluctuations.

By now, you might have already guessed that replenishing your serotonin supply isn't as simple as just adding a daily supplement to your routine. Paying strict attention to your diet is also essential.

That's especially true when it comes to foods containing an amino acid called tyramine. Tyramine displaces norepinephrine from nerve endings, resulting in the sympathetic "fight or flight" reaction I described earlier (high blood pressure, insomnia, aggression, and increased glucose release). And the result of this is a depletion of norepinephrine, epinephrine, and serotonin reserves. (For a list of high-tyramine foods to watch out for, see the sidebar above.)

But it's not just food that's naturally high in tyramine that's a threat. In fact, tyramine can increase exponentially through the process of aging and fermentation—meaning that even a food that's naturally low in tyramine, like a banana, can become a problem when it's overripe.

Other foods that negatively affect your serotonin level are ones with a high glycemic load—in simpler terms, any foods that are high in sugar or other simple carbohydrates. These boost your insulin production, stressing your body and sparking inflammation, which in turn depletes your serotonin reserves. Also, you should avoid any food that might be hiding neurotoxins (which includes just about any processed, preservative-packed product you'll find at the grocery store these days).

The bottom line: Even while you're taking Seratonin, you want to keep your food fresh, and low in tyramine and sugar.

Years of pain and depression reversed in a single month

None of this may appear to be very new or exciting—but the truth of the matter is, Seratonin is one of the only successful treatments (pharmaceutical or natural) that you'll find for migraines or depression on the market today.

Dr. Allocca has received floods of testimonials detailing how Seratonin has changed his clients' lives—many of whom were confined to their beds in excruciating daily pain. But as one woman from Louisiana wrote in: "Within a month I was headache free for the first time that I can remember." She goes on to say: "I feel like a new person, and I would love to share this with as many people as possible." This same experience was shared by countless others, all of whom have stayed permanently migraine-free when nothing else had worked.

But what's even more impressive is that Dr. Allocca is currently in the process of wrapping up a large-scale clinical trial called the American Migraine Prevention Study. And preliminary results show that this approach, unlike many others, actually works—although a complete summary of the study won't be out until next year.

If you suffer from migraines, chances are good that your doctor's orders have never reached beyond the limits of simple (and usually ineffective) pain management. And if you suffer from chronic depression, the outlook for a future of safe and effective solutions has become even bleaker. The same goes for other neurotransmitter-related conditions, like fibromyalgia, tinnitus, or IBS—in fact, you may have been told by more than one doctor already that you'll just have to learn to live with them.

But it's simply not true. And if nothing else, Seratonin's lengthy track record is proof of that.

CHAPTER SEVEN

Forget dangerous HRT... You can balance your hormones safely and naturally—without adding a single hormone to your body

The hot flashes, the night sweats, the low energy and mood...

Think you just have to learn to live with your menopause symptoms? If you've been an HSI Member for a while, you certainly don't want to mess around with hormone replacement therapy (HRT). (For more on the dangers of HRT, search "hormone replacement therapy" at www.hsionline.com.)

So you've decided to tough it out—but how much longer can you really do that?

Well, finally there's an answer. You can balance your hormones *without* the dangers of HRT. In fact, this could beat even bio-identical hormone replacement therapy in terms of safety and effect.

Because this method doesn't involve adding hormones to your body at all. Instead, it relies upon a vegetable, revered for thousands of years in Peru, that helps your body to balance its *own* hormone production.

And it's been rigorously tested in numerous published clinical trials over the past five years. These studies prove that this non-HRT approach to menopause not only relieves the symptoms of post-menopause, but can also go a long way to helping your heart health and bone density.

After all, the transition to menopause should be relatively symptom-free. And it has been for generations of women, thanks to a dietary staple that can only be grown in their native Peru.

The Peruvian vegetable that's been beating menopause for generations of women

Though it's grown all over several South American countries, only maca (*Lepidum peruvianum*) from Peru has been significantly researched and shown to have a therapeutic benefit. In fact, growers who have tried to cultivate this miracle vegetable elsewhere in the world have been largely unsuccessful.

But it's no wonder they keep trying. Maca boasts a long list of benefits. Traditionally (perhaps for thousands of years), it's been used to treat fatigue, anemia, and infertility, as well as to enhance stamina and as an aphrodisiac.

And that's not even getting into what it's been doing specifically for women for just as long. Peruvians used (and still do use) it to treat "female conditions" including menopausal symptoms and decreased libido.

Modern research is backing up the many uses of maca. Studies have shown benefits in production of sex hormones, enhanced sex drive, stimulation of body metabolism, control of body weight, increased energy, stress reduction, antidepressant activity, and memory improvement.

Maca has the power to balance hormones without containing any hormones itself—so it can't be lumped in with other natural menopause remedies like red clover, black cohosh, and soy isoflavones.

Maca may target the same symptoms, but its action is very different.[1]

That's because maca is an adaptogenic plant, meaning it helps regulate and balance the body's systems, particularly hormone production. Adaptogens modulate the body's response by supporting it in dealing with a variety of stressors—physiological, biochemical, and psychological.

They are among the more useful medicinal herbs, helping people cope with fatigue, anxiety, depression, and sleep problems. Other well-known adaptogenic herbs are American ginseng and Siberian ginseng.

However, those other herbs don't seem to have the same effect on menopausal symptoms that maca does. Researchers theorize that maca stimulates hormonal reserves by strengthening the body's ability to regain and maintain hormonal balance in the face of stressors.

Unlike HRT, maca can actually increase the body's own production of estrogen, instead of simply adding estrogen to the body. It stimulates the hypothalamus, pituitary, adrenal, and ovarian glands in order to rebalance the body's production of hormones and treat menopause symptoms as a whole.[1]

One particular formulation of maca, called Maca-GO, has proven itself over five years of clinical trials. Research reveals an 84 percent success rate in the reduction of menopausal symptoms (hot flashes, night sweats, fatigue, mood swings, and so on); increased bone density; enhanced absorption of iron, calcium, and other trace elements; and a better ability to maintain a healthy weight, optimal cholesterol, and triglyceride levels.[2]

Menopause symptoms reduced by 84 percent

When hormone production is regulated and balanced, it's easier for your body to achieve overall harmony. This means fewer menopause symptoms and an overall improvement in general health.

Maca-GO has a leg up on HRT because it works with your own

body to balance the levels of key hormones: FSH, estrogen, LH, and progesterone—and nothing is more natural than your own hormones.

Maca's benefits have been reported in many publications over the past 20 years.

It's been shown to enhance sex hormone production, stimulate body metabolism, increase energy and vitality, reduce excess body weight, relieve stress and depression, improve memory, and enhance a person's sex drive.

But in the past five years, the first standardized maca formulation (Maca-GO) has been studied specifically in menopausal women. And Maca-GO is the only formulation to demonstrate statistically significant improvements in both menopause symptom relief and hormonal balance.

In addition to relieving the symptoms of menopause, use of Maca-GO has been shown to lower total cholesterol in menopausal women, with significant reductions in triglycerides and BMI. It's also led to increases in HDL cholesterol and significant reductions in LDL cholesterol.

One study was carried out in five urban gynecological clinics in two culturally different cities in Poland—researchers wanted to see Maca-GO's effect on a wide variety of women.

Use of Maca-GO led to a highly significant increase in initially low estrogen levels after one month and again after two months. Initially elevated FSH levels dropped significantly as estrogen production normalized. After two months on placebo, two months on Maca-GO brought significant increases in estradiol. And after those two months, patients experienced a highly significant increase in HDL and a decrease in LDL, as well as lowered triglycerides and total cholesterol. When patients were switched back to a placebo, menopause symptoms and hormone levels went back to untreated levels.

Though Maca-GO benefited patients after only two months, researchers noticed trends toward metabolic adjustments that could require about three months to show any difference, such as positive effects on total cholesterol and bone density.[3]

Another study, conducted over the course of three months (one month on placebo, two months of treatment), explored the effects of Maca-GO on women who had ceased menstruation and were not using HRT prior to the study. The formulation alleviated symptoms of menopausal discomfort, and researchers observed an overall balancing effect on sex hormone levels.[4]

A four-month trial on women taking Maca-GO measured several attributes of menopause. The women, who were all in early postmenopause, took Maca-GO twice a day with meals. Each month, hormone levels were measured and a gynecologist conducted interviews. Patients were weighed, blood pressure was registered, and menopause symptoms were analyzed.

Maca-GO was shown to significantly alleviate symptoms of discomfort, with an 84 percent reduction. There were significant increases in estrogen and progesterone levels and reductions in blood pressure, body weight, triglycerides, and cholesterol.

Also, it was shown to significantly stimulate estradiol production, to help regulate the thyroid, and to increase bone density.

Researchers concluded that Maca-GO could be a valuable non-hormonal plant preparation for alleviating symptoms of menopause, including frequency of hot flushes, incidence of night sweating, interrupted sleep patterns, nervousness, depression, and heart palpitations.[5]

Ten years of menopause symptoms reversed in two weeks

Maca-GO is available in a supplement from Natural Health International called Femmenessence, which many women all over the world are describing as a "miracle."

Linda Ackerman, a woman in California, calls Femmenessence a "wonderful nutritional addition to my life." She's been taking it for four months and has found that her hot flashes and insomnia have decreased significantly. Also, without altering her diet or exercise, she's lost about 10 pounds.

Gail Kennedy, a 54-year-old woman in Australia, has been suffering through menopausal symptoms for 10 years. After only two weeks on Femmenessence, her energy picked up, she felt more motivated, and her sex drive started returning.

And when women aren't speaking up about their success with Femmenessence, their doctors are. Naturopath Peter Bablis described a 53-year-old woman who had been dealing with menopausal symptoms for seven years. She was experiencing night sweats, hot flashes, fatigue, poor memory, increased weight, and a decreased libido. She also felt depressed and had no motivation.

Her life was more or less controlled by her symptoms. She'd tried all the usual medications, but absolutely nothing had helped.

Then she started taking Femmenessence. Taking one capsule twice a day, she noticed a slight improvement in her hot flashes in about five days. Once she started taking two capsules twice a day, they stopped altogether.

And after six weeks, her fatigue disappeared, her memory started getting better, and she'd lost 5 pounds without even trying. After 12 weeks, things were even better. She'd lost 12 pounds, again without dieting or exercising, and didn't feel depressed at all. To her surprise, her libido even returned.

Naturopath and professor Tori Hudson, who has been specializing in women's health for 25 years, has also seen much success with Femmenessence. She notes that she's impressed by the level of commitment to research of the product. And in her clinic, she's seen some pretty amazing results.

She usually sees benefits in two to three weeks, though it can take up to three months to see truly significant results. Most frequently, there's a remarkable reduction in the number of hot flashes as well as overall improvement in mood and energy.

There is actually a range of Femmenessence products, for women in each stage of life. There's a variety for young women seeking relief from premenstrual symptoms, one for preparing the body for optimum fertility, and varieties for women dealing with pre- and post-menopausal symptoms.

Natural Health International has naturopathic doctors on staff who can talk through any concerns or questions you may have about Femmenessence.

Ordering information for Femmenessence is in the Member Source Directory on page 529.

CHAPTER EIGHT

Stop sleep apnea in just one night— and throw out that bulky mask

Do you toss and turn all night, never falling deep into sleep? Do you wonder why you even bothered going to bed at all because you wake every morning feeling like you got no rest at all? Do you snore so loudly it wakes you up, or stop breathing for 5 seconds or more as you sleep?

You could go to an expensive sleep clinic, where they'll hook you up to various machines and monitor your sleeping for a few nights. A couple thousand dollars later, they'll probably tell you that you have sleep apnea— a condition in which your breathing stops as you sleep. And then you'll be given a Continuous Positive Airway Pressure (CPAP) machine that delivers compressed air through a bulky mask you have to wear all night. Or you could have surgery to remove the excess tissue blocking your airway.

Or you could start feeling relief now—without uncomfortable contraptions or going under the knife—thanks to one of HSI's most trusted sources.

Breathe easy with a formula that fights apnea at the source

If you've been an HSI Member for a while, you know I'm a big fan of Peaceful Mountain. I don't go on a trip without my Travel Rescue kit ("Quit feeding superbugs—silver knocks out bacteria without conventional dangers," December 2008). And when founder Steven Frank started his new line, Nature's Rite, I jumped right on their Leg Relaxer ("Clam the gnawing of restless legs in minutes with targeted herbal relief," July 2009).

So when he told me that praise was pouring in for their new Sleep Apnea Relief, I knew I had to tell you about it. Especially because of the way Sleep Apnea Relief came to be—out of Steven's own need for it.

You see, Steven had been struggling with sleep apnea for five years. He'd tried everything out there, but nothing worked. Each episode of apnea lasts about a week, during which time he would wake every 60 or 90 seconds throughout the night. Obviously, the man was getting no rest.

So he decided to do something with those sleepless nights. He read all he could about apnea until he fully understood the cause—a problem with the signaling between the brain and diaphragm muscles during the transition to stage 2 sleep (the intermediate stage right before deep sleep).

Once he understood that, the search was on for an herb that would increase the communication between the brain and those muscles. He found that in lobelia, a flowering plant traditionally used by Native Americans to treat respiratory and muscle disorders. It's a relaxant that can soothe the nerves and ease tension.

Steven decided to add thyme, which enhances the activity of lung membranes, to the lobelia in the hopes of getting more use out of each breath. He took it, went to bed... and slept. He tried it the next night, and the next, and it kept working. Amazingly, he'd hit on the right herbs on the first try. As he told me, he was "beyond excited" because it didn't just prove his theory—it ended that five year struggle.

That was about five years ago. In that time, he's been working on tweaking the formula, adding more herbs to increase the effectiveness. He added cramp bark, which relaxes stressed muscles. Chamomile also has relaxing effects, and meadow sweet ensures that the other herbs are fully absorbed.

When he was finally happy with it, he called it, quite simply, Sleep Apnea Relief, and started sharing the blend that had saved his nights.

Steven is quick to say that Sleep Apnea Relief won't necessarily work for everyone (after all, nothing does). Some people have such bad obstructions that they need more direct physical help. But for MOST people suffering from sleep apnea, this formula means not having to sleep with a machine on the floor next to your bed, pumping air through a mask strapped to your face.

Steven calls that freedom, and wants to share that with everyone who needs it.

Even with the worst obstructive sleep apnea— Sleep Apnea Relief can help

If you have obstructive sleep apnea, you might be thinking your condition is just too much for any herbal formula to handle. But don't resign yourself to that bulky oxygen machine yet.

With obstructive sleep apnea, your airway is blocked by either a sagging soft pallet or other tissues. Even though this blockage contributes to your inability to breathe through the night, it's not the real cause of the problem.

When you sleep, your brain reduces the intensity of the signals to your skeletal muscles so you don't act out your dreams. Well, as we age, other signals start getting reduced, too. Including the signals to your diaphragm, which controls your breathing rate.

If the signals going from your brain to your diaphragm are reduced too much, you can stop breathing altogether. This causes your blood oxygen level to decrease—when it drops so low that it's dangerous, your brain sounds the alarm, causing you to take an immediate deep breath. With obstructive sleep apnea, this fast intake of breath sucks the sagging tissue into your airway, causing a loud snort that disrupts your sleep.

So if you take care of the brain-signaling problem that causes your breathing to stop, the obstruction of the airway is no longer an issue. Sleep Apnea Relief increases your respiration intensity so you don't stop breathing.

Start sleeping soundly in just a couple of days

Are you already thinking about how good a full night's sleep is going to feel? If the response Nature's Rite has received from happy customers is any indication, it's going to feel *great*. They've found that many people come back and order another six months' worth of Sleep Apnea Relief at a time—and have some pretty great words for it when they place those orders.

Annette found relief in only two days. She used to fall asleep behind the wheel of her car because she was so tired during the day after so many sleepless nights. But now she feels rested and alert. Her daughter also tried it—and it stopped her snoring.

Stan had to use a CPAP for four years, but is now a firm believer in Sleep Apnea Relief. He says he "won't go back to that machine again!"

Maybe Carol puts it best. She wrote to Steven to say: "Before Sleep Apnea Relief neither one of us were able to sleep because of my husband's severe apnea and snoring, especially the snoring. The first time he tried those natural herbs all that changed! I was so excited the first night that I literally cried. Even our 18-year-old daughter noticed the change in my husband after he had been able to sleep and breathe at night instead of choking and snoring. I think the person who developed this herbal remedy should be awarded a Nobel Prize."

Now, you do have to make sure to take Sleep Apnea Relief every day if you have sleep apnea every night. There is no cumulative effect with the herbs in this formula. Some people have sleep apnea only periodically—you can take Sleep Apnea Relief just during those episodes.

Ordering information for Sleep Apnea Relief is in the Member Source Directory on page 529.

CHAPTER NINE

"Nothing—and I mean nothing— has ever had such a wonderful healing effect on my eczema"

She'd been battling eczema for years with no relief in sight. Sometimes it burned so badly that she burst into tears.

But nothing worked—the medicine cabinet full of lotions and creams might as well have been tubes of water for all the good they did for her burning skin.

So Claire figured she'd just have to live with the pain. But that was before Eczema Rescue (originally Eczederm Rescue).

It's absolutely the only thing that's worked for her. And it works fast—in a matter of *days*, the stinging pain and redness simply started fading away.

Eczema Rescue is an expert blend of herbs famous for their antifungal, antiviral, and antibacterial properties. And it comes from one of HSI's most trusted sources.

Once again, the mainstream offers up nothing but side effects

There still isn't much of an explanation for eczema. Some doctors use the term for any unidentifiable rash. It most commonly causes dry, reddened skin. Intense itching or burning is usually the first symptom. Eczema can lead to blisters and oozing lesions—and a whole lot of embarrassment and discomfort.

The mainstream may not have an answer for it, but that doesn't keep them from trying. The medical standard is to use topical corticosteroids in short bursts to suppress symptoms. Long-term use is avoided because those steroids can cause skin atrophy and lesions.

Even used short-term, they can be of little use, because as soon as you stop using them, the eczema can come right back.

In extreme cases, doctors prescribe systemic corticosteroids to cut down on inflammation. But their use can lead to gastrointestinal intolerance, weakness, muscle problems, and increased infection.

Recently, two new topical treatments for eczema were approved by the FDA—tacrolimus and picrolimus. Their long-term effects are unclear, but several studies have shown an increased prevalence of skin cancer in lab animals treated with the compounds.

The long and short of it is this: No drug deemed effective at suppressing outbreaks has yet been approved for long-term use without the possibility of side effects.

Thanks to Peaceful Mountain, however, there is a powerful herbal answer to eczema—Eczema Rescue.

Stop the symptoms of eczema from interfering with your life

Eczema Rescue is a topical cream that captures the power of herbs with antifungal, antiviral, antibacterial, and tissue-regenerating properties.

No matter the cause, or how long you've been suffering, it works. From the day Eczema Rescue was introduced, success stories like Claire's have been pouring in.

When Deon in Denver, CO, developed eczema, his doctor was completely baffled. Though Deon tried everything, nothing cleared up the rash—and the itching was unbearable. The moment Eczema Rescue touched his skin, he knew it was different from anything else he'd tried. It cooled the burning, and he reported that, in just days, his eczema was well on the way to being completely cleared up.

Holly, who lives in Kansas City, MO, wrote to Peaceful Mountain to "gush over" Eczema Rescue. A massage therapist, Holly relies on her hands for her livelihood. But for the past five years, she's been suffering from eczema so badly on one hand that nothing would help the symptoms.

She was amazed at how quickly Eczema Rescue healed her hand. "It has been years since my hand has looked this good," Holly reported. The symptoms are gone and, perhaps more importantly, Holly's self-esteem is back.

Melissa, of Mustang, OK, has been suffering from eczema for about 20 years. She'd tried prescriptions, natural products, elimination of certain foods, and countless other treatments. At some points, the rash has covered all of one of her hands.

Then, as I'm sure you've already guessed, she found Eczema Rescue. After only a week of using it, she reported that the burning, itchy rash was 70 percent better, and getting better every day.

Stories like these are common at Peaceful Mountain. And they've recently been backed up by a promising clinical trial.

Starts healing eczema in a matter of days

Eczema Rescue was put to the test against a placebo in a four-week clinical trial conducted by an independent lab. Over the course of the trial, participants recorded the daily severity of a number of symptoms—sleep interference, itching, pain, overall discomfort, redness, crusting, and overall appearance. Symptoms were rated on a scale of 1-9 (from nothing at all to as bad as it could be).

Participants using Eczema Rescue reported a significant drop in symptoms as compared with participants using the placebo. The most notable differences were in discomfort, crusting, and appearance.

At follow-up visits after the study period, continued improvement was observed. Researchers concluded that there was a clear benefit over placebo after only two weeks.[1]

A separate report on side effects concluded that Eczema Rescue causes minimal side effects. The most commonly reported ones were dry skin, temporary staining of skin, and stinging upon application.

The stinging may have been due to applying the gel to open sores, and only occurred when it was first applied. The same side effects were reported by people who used a placebo in the trial.

The report pointed out that the benign nature of Eczema Rescue means it can be used as a maintenance treatment without the risks of skin atrophy and lesions that come with corticosteroids.[2]

Soothe and heal your skin with an arsenal of herbs

All of the herbs in Eczema Rescue have traditionally been used for relief from the itching and pain of eczema, dermatitis, and rashes.

Bloodroot has been shown in several studies to have antimicrobial and anti-inflammatory properties. Its high concentration of the compound sanguinarine reduces inflammation when used topically. The antibacterial action of bloodroot has actually won it FDA approval for inclusion in toothpaste. In Eczema Rescue, it helps to prevent infection in the affected area.

Bacterial infection is a concern if you have eczema, as it can be introduced through broken skin after you scratch the itch. This secondary bacterial infection can feed the inflammation cycle in eczema—bloodroot prevents the infection and quells that inflammation.

Used for a host of skin conditions, pokeroot has immune-stimulating properties. It contains tannins, which protect tissues.

Neem is an herb derived from a tree in the mahogany family. In India, the tree is known as "Nature's Drugstore" for its many properties—it's antifungal, antibacterial, antiviral, and anti-inflammatory.

Neem is considered a major component in Ayurvedic medicine and is often prescribed for skin disease. There have been many reports of success using neem for eczema—the leaves are commonly used as a bath for eczema sufferers.

St. John's Wort adds to the antimicrobial properties of Eczema Rescue. It's been used with great success to treat first-degree burns. Traditionally, St. John's Wort is used for inflammation and pain. Hyperforin, a major constituent of the herb, has been found to have antibacterial properties strong enough to kill MRSA.

Chapparal, calendula flowers, and arnica contribute further to the anti-inflammatory effects of Eczema Rescue. These herbs also have analgesic properties when applied topically—helping to soothe the pain of eczema.

Arnica in particular has been the subject of various studies that have demonstrated its usefulness in treating pain. When used topically as a gel (as it is in Eczema Rescue), it's been found to have the same effect as NSAIDs like ibuprofen in treating the painful symptoms of hand osteoarthritis.[3]

White willow bark shares arnica's pain-killing properties. In fact, it's a precursor to aspirin. Studies have shown that it's useful against pain caused by inflammation.

While comfrey leaf shares the anti-inflammatory properties of other herbs in Eczema Rescue, it really shines as a healing agent—it increases the rate at which new skin can be formed, maintaining the integrity of skin. This is because it contains allantoin, a cell proliferant that speeds up the natural replacement of body cells.

The herbal extracts in Eczema Rescue are combined with several oils (olive, avocado, macadamia nut, and kukui nut) that provide essential fatty acids as well as vitamins A and E. Additionally, vitamin C has been added to adjust the pH and to assist healing.

Rounding out the formula is aloe vera, known for its antibacterial and analgesic effects. Altogether, Eczema Rescue is a product that's brought relief to many people, including a few of us here at HSI.

Several days ago, one of my colleagues described an itchy red rash she had developed on one arm. She showed it to me, and I immediately handed her the tube of Eczema Rescue that was on my desk. The next day, I asked her if it was working. "It smells a little funny," she said, "but it works!" The rash had faded considerably, and she didn't find herself scratching at it nearly as much.

Ordering information for Eczema Rescue is in the Member Source Directory on page 529.

CHAPTER TEN

Astonishing nutrient turns the tide on Alzheimer's disease, dementia, even strokes!

"It's Alzheimer's disease." That may be the scariest sentence you'll ever hear... and it's usually said without any hope. No chance of a cure, but the very real possibility that your loved one will disappear right before your eyes, every day sliding further and further away from you.

The doctor may tell you about medications that might possibly slow the disease down—but not so much that you'd notice, and not enough to stop the damage. And he'll probably tell you to start thinking about long-term care, while his eyes carefully avoid the tears streaming down your cheeks.

But it doesn't have to be that way. Because there is real hope— a chance to substantially slow down the disease, even noticeably improve quality of life and keep memories alive.

Why your doctor can't help... and HSI can

As usual, mainstream medicine takes a short-sighted, profit-driven approach to treating Alzheimer's disease. They focus on a single facet of the problem, and hit it with a sledge hammer. They claim their drugs offer 'statistically significant' changes for Alzheimer's patients—but that doesn't really translate into noticeable improvement.

And, like the vast majority of pharmaceutical drugs, these medications come with some highly damaging side effects and very high price tags, while delivering nothing of value. Actually, that's not true, they do worse than nothing. Because they offer the promise of possibility that they simply do not deliver.

Your doctor may hold them out as the only choice... but he's wrong.

We here at HSI have uncovered an astonishingly effective natural medicine that does more than impact some numbers on a made-up scale. It can make a difference in people's lives—whether they're stricken with Alzheimer's disease (AD) or watching someone they love suffer through it. And if you're looking to prevent that horrible fate, this alternative cure can help you do it.

So while mainstream medicine has nothing much to offer here—except dangerous, expensive medications that do, well, nothing—natural medicine, once again, holds the key.

The nutrient your brain can't live without can turn AD around

Not surprisingly, this natural brain protector targets some of the same issues as pharmaceutical drugs—but in a gentler and much safer way.

The natural medicine you'll learn about here is the real deal. In fact, some doctors have already been using this complex nutrient as medicine in Japan to treat strokes and brain injuries. And researchers are just beginning to understand how it can improve brain function... even for Alzheimer's and dementia patients.

This miracle nutrient is called citicoline (or CDP coline, which stands for cytidine diphosphate choline), and it's crucial for healthy brain function. In fact, your brain literally can't function without it.

So far, citicoline's success has been pretty amazing. And it makes me wonder why more mainstream doctors don't know about it.

- It halts progression of Alzheimer's disease, and even improves quality of life for Alzheimer's patients (helping them maintain independence, for example)[1]

- Improves brain function of stroke patients (when taken within 24 hours of the stroke)[2]

- Citicoline improves mental function in some dementia patients

- Citicoline helps both prevent and treat age-associated memory impairment

- Can improve memory, especially in people who suffer from memory impairment

- It may even help coma patients recover more quickly

Actually, it's really American mainstream doctors who aren't working with citicoline. Japanese and European doctors have been using it successfully for years.

Scientists finally see (literally!) how citicoline boosts your brain power

In November 2008, researchers published the first study that clearly showed just how citicoline impacts the brain. Using special imaging technology, these scientists were able to see exactly how citicoline changes brain activity, specifically in the frontal lobe.[3]

Citicoline keeps your eyes in tip-top shape, too

What's brain power without eyesight? Luckily, with citicoline, you may never need to worry about that. One 12-month study found that the nutrient improved retinal and visual function in glaucoma patients. And an 8-year study showed that citicoline substantially improved vision.

Citicoline actually increases brain function in the frontal lobe, which handles things like attention span, learning, memory, and creativity. In fact, your front lobe is considered the management center of your brain, and when that center gets damaged—as can happen with Alzheimer's disease—all of those functions will suffer.

Some of these scientists most important discoveries explain citicoline's success in boosting brain power. For one thing, it substantially increases a critical brain chemical called phosphocreatine, which provides extra energy and helps reduce fatigue.

The researchers also learned how essential citicoline is for brain cell protection—it increases specific lipids (phospholipids) that help maintain cell integrity and turnover, and your brain simply can't work without this.

Another surprising discovery: citicoline seems to increase alpha brain waves, the ones associated with relaxation. In fact, these brain waves are the ones responsible for getting your brain into the much-desired awake relaxed state. And since one of the defining symptoms of AD is extreme agitation, boosting alpha waves can make life for the patient and his caregiver much less stressful.

And that's not all they found out—they uncovered exactly how citicoline powers your brain, and helps keep your memory and cognition intact.

- Increases blood circulation to your brain
- Boosts your brain's energy reserves
- Increases efficient oxygen use
- Enhances production of acetylcholine
- Maintains optimal dopamine levels

By making sure your brain has all the blood, oxygen, and energy it needs, citicoline can turn memory problems around. And by boosting production and maintenance of key brain chemicals, it can do so much more than that.

Acetylcholine—the super brain chemical that powers your mind

One of the key benefits of citicoline is that it increases production of acetylcholine, the most plentiful neurotransmitter in your brain, and one that's responsible for a lot of key functions. In fact, acetylcholine deficiency is a key player in Alzheimer's disease (and a big focus of pharmaceutical drugs that try to manipulate the chemical artificially, with little success but plenty of dangerous side effects).

What can boosted acetylcholine levels do for you?

• Help increase attention span

• Improve your ability to concentrate

• Increase coordination

• Ease depression

• Slow down memory loss

• Maintain better sleep

In fact, you can read this article because your brain has a healthy amount of acetylcholine. But when someone develops AD, his acetylcholine declines and is more quickly broken down by an enzyme called acetylcholinesterase (AChE). And when acetylcholine levels drop so dramatically, they can cause memory loss and decreased learning capacity, among other things. Taking citicoline can help make sure that your brain has more acetylcholine—and that means better memory, concentration, mood, and sleep for you.

Citicoline boosts many more critical brain chemicals to keep your mind sharp

Citicoline affects a lot more than acetylcholine, though. It also plays an important role in other brain-critical compounds like dopamine, norepinephrine, uridine, and phosphatidylcholine (PS).

Let's start with dopamine, a crucial brain chemical that citicoline helps your body manage and maintain more efficiently. Dopamine is especially important because deficiency of this chemical has been implicated in Alzheimer's—and correcting that problem could help treat the disease.

Norepinephrine is another crucial brain chemical, and citicoline seems to increase its levels. Many AD patients have been found to lack norepinephrine, so restoring higher levels could help turn the disease around. And this neurotransmitter is well known for increasing alertness and attention span, and enhancing memory and learning.

Then there's uridine, which has been found to be directly responsible for brain cell regeneration in lab studies. It's also been found to clearly support memory retention. It also plays a key role in the generation of phosphatidylcholine (you'll see how important that is in a second). Most important, uridine is being looked at as a possible treatment for Alzheimer's disease because of its ability to improve brain function.

Phosphatidylcholine (PS) is an essential fatty acid that your brain needs to function at its best—and citicoline increases the total amount of PS in the brain. In fact, it can even restore deficient levels to normal, and that can make a huge difference in brain power. It helps keep your brain cells in peak condition, and boosts neurotransmitter activity so that cell messages get where they need to go. And dozens of studies show that adding PS to the mix greatly improves learning and memory.

Real people are seeing real results

Citicoline—sold under the brand name Cognizin®—can do wonders for people suffering from Alzheimer's disease and dementia, but

---

The top three prescription medications for AD—Aricept, Exelon, and Razadyne—are cholinesterase inhibitors. They work by stopping cholinesterase, with the hope of leaving more acetylcholine for the brain to use. But they cause some pretty harsh gastrointestinal side effects, and in rare cases, seizures and liver damage. Plus, they also tend to lose any effectiveness within a year.

it can also improve everyone's memory, mood, and cognition. Here are just a few examples of the kind of difference citicoline can make.

Gina is a 55-year-old retired housewife. She said, "My husband has been ill for several months and since I have been taking Cognizin it's helped me keep my husband's medications straight and deal with his problems and his doctors, because of this Cognizin has reduced my level of stress. I'm a little more focused and don't seem as stressed. Plus, every once in a while I can answer a question or two on Jeopardy—it seems that something has come back!"

Walter, a 52-year-old corporate executive also saw his daily life improve. "When I started taking Cognizin several months ago I almost immediately found myself more focused more relaxed. I was able to look at budgets and figure out percents very quickly, everything seemed to work better. I'm more relaxed, I have more energy, and I seem less stressed about things."

And then there's Patty, a 65-year-old realtor whose husband *really* noticed the Cognizin difference. "My husband asked me the other day, 'What's going on? You are not as emotional as usual and you have not lost your car keys in over a month?' I told him that I have been taking Cognizin… and you have pretty much made me believe that it is working if you see the differences. The mood swings that I was having have reduced 95 percent and things just seem to be very clear, the fog of trying to remember names or places has been lifted."

Cognizin® is the only reliable source of citicoline

Cognizin® is the brand-name of the best source for citicoline. In fact, Cognizin® is identical to the citicoline used in the studies that show just how effective it is for improving brain power.

The manufacturer's recommended dose of Cognizin® is one or two 250 mg tablets each day, taken with meals. You'll find ordering information for Cognizin® Citicoline in the Member Source Directory on page 529.

CHAPTER ELEVEN

The government tried to keep this life-changing supplement from you... but HSI is giving you direct access

Government persecution almost kept you from access to one of the world's most progressive healing supplements. Almost.

But a group of dedicated professionals and researchers, and one highly committed Japanese scientist worked tirelessly to make sure that you would not have to suffer any more. That you would not be denied access to this unique natural substance.

And this single supplement may be the answer to just about everything that's ailing you: osteoporosis, arthritis, atherosclerosis, kidney stones, Alzheimer's disease, insulin resistance, and much more.

Calcium—every cell in your body counts on it

If there's one thing our bodies can't do without, it's calcium. We need this essential mineral for dozens of functions, not the least of which are cellular-energy production and nerve, brain, and heart functions. And when we don't get enough calcium, every system in the body suffers.

Most of your body's calcium supply is stored in your bones, where it also provides strength and rigidity to the skeleton. If there isn't enough calcium circulating in the blood to supply the body's cellular needs, your body will steal calcium from its "reserves" in the bone. And if your calcium intake is chronically low, your bones will eventually become porous, weak, and prone to fracture.

But even a sufficient calcium intake may not be enough—if you aren't getting the right kind of calcium, a form your body can easily work with, it's almost the same as not taking it at all.

The Calcium Paradox

Weakened bones is just the tip of the calcium deficiency iceberg, though. And while that is a severe health problem, things can get a whole lot worse, thanks to what Dr. Fujita calls the "Calcium Paradox."

When you aren't getting enough calcium, your body reacts in a very predictable—but dangerous—way. Calcium deficiency triggers your body to produce more parathyroid hormone (PTH). Excess PTH stimulates a process called bone resorption, which literally leaches the calcium out of your bone and into your bloodstream, causing decreased bone mass (and potentially osteoporosis) along with calcium abundance in your blood.

But since that calcium hasn't gone through the normal digestive process, it doesn't go just where it's supposed to... and that's when serious risk sets in.

That calcium enters your soft tissues—like your blood vessels and your brain—and wreaks havoc. It can actually cause these organs to deteriorate, and cause many health problems. Arthritis, for example, can result from excess calcium deposits in the joints. Atherosclerosis can be brought on by calcium deposits in your blood vessels. And excess calcium in your brain could lead to senile dementia.

And while it might seem counterintuitive, the solution to the calcium paradox is to give your body more calcium. As long as you take a highly absorbable supplement, that is. Then your body gets the right kind of calcium, and sends it to the right places, reducing or even fully stopping that excess PTH activity and preventing the mineral from invading your soft tissues.

This almost-banned supplement may be the true key to preventing calcium paradox diseases entirely. In fact, one study[1] found that it reduced red blood cell calcium levels substantially better than calcium carbonate (the most commonly taken calcium supplement—but far from the best choice). The reason? This supplement does something the others can't: It sends more of the mineral directly where it needs to go, because your body can absorb it better than any other form.

If you can't absorb it, your body can't use it

As nutrients go, calcium is very poorly absorbed—only a small percentage of the calcium we take actually makes it into the bloodstream.

Experts estimate that in order to supply the body's cellular needs and build and maintain bone stores, we need to consume 1,000 to 2,000 mg of elemental calcium every day, starting in adolescence.

Unfortunately, the average American diet only provides about 500 mg of calcium daily. And to make matters worse, our ability to absorb calcium declines as we get older. When we're babies, we absorb about 70 percent of the calcium we take in. By the time we're adults, that drops off to about 50 percent... and when we hit the senior years, we only absorb about 30 percent of the calcium we ingest.

But Dr. Takuo Fujita found a way around that problem, and brought us a real solution to the calcium paradox.

Scientific breakthrough breaks through absorption obstacles

Dr. Fujita has dedicated a considerable part of his life to searching for a form of calcium that could be more efficiently absorbed and used by the body. Driven by his firm belief that reversing calcium

LaneLabs Trounces FTC in Stunning Victory

When HSI first broke the AdvaCal story back in July 1999, we had no idea of the drama, intrigue, and suspense that would follow.

Soon after we wrote about AdvaCal, LaneLabs (the product manufacturer) got scolded by the FTC. The company responded to an FTC consent order by agreeing to refrain from making any claims about their health products unless they could support the claims with scientific evidence.

Fast forward to 2006, when the FTC started picking on LaneLabs about AdvaCal, and the (solidly backed) claims the company was making about their one-of-a-kind supplement. Then in 2007, the agency filed a motion against LaneLabs holding them in contempt of the consent order—and asking for a $24 million fine to boot.

Now with all the proof behind their products, you've got to wonder why the government would pick on LaneLabs. It really makes no sense. There were NO customer complaints about the products—NONE. The FTC couldn't show that the products caused anyone any harm. And even the FTC's own witnesses wouldn't say the products were risky or ineffective. Add to that numerous published studies that stand behind every word LaneLabs says about their products—a wealth of solid science.

If this seems like a slam dunk for LaneLabs—it was, though it took a long time to get to the basket. But in July 2009, a full ten years after HSI first told you about AdvaCal, Judge Dennis Cavanaugh of the U.S. District Court of New Jersey found in favor of LaneLabs... and sent the FTC packing.

deficiency is the solution to osteoporosis, the calcium paradox, and many other age-related health conditions, Dr. Fujita was determined to find the solution.

The first breakthrough came in the discovery of a compound called AAACa, a unique form of calcium derived from oyster shell—but it didn't come without two major drawbacks. First, the oyster shell often contains other heavy metals (including lead) which can remain in the finished product. Second, oyster shell contains the poorly absorbed calcium-carbonate form of the mineral.

But Dr. Fujita sidestepped both of these problems with a unique processing technique.

Instead of just being ground into powder, the oyster shells are heated to extremely high temperatures (800° C!), which creates a fine ash. This process burns off any heavy metals that might have been present in the natural shell... and it also breaks down calcium into a much more digestible form. In fact, studies show that AAACa is absorbed more than twice as well as calcium carbonate.

AAACa plus special algae quadruples the effectiveness

The next breakthrough took AAACa to a whole new level. Dr. Fujita discovered that AAACa's absorbability could be boosted even more by adding a certain specially processed algae. This algae preparation (which has been translated from the Japanese as "Heated Algae Ingredient," or HAI) doesn't actually contain any calcium, but it is a highly rich source of amino acids.

Studies conducted by Dr. Fujita show that HAI substantially increases the intestinal absorption of calcium, possibly because of its amino-acid content. And when HAI is added to AAACa (a combination sold as AdvaCal), the result is an extremely high-potency calcium supplement that is absorbed four times better than typical calcium-carbonate supplements.

Dr. Fujita's research leaves no question that AdvaCal is far more bioavailable than typical calcium supplements. But even more important: Can it effectively prevent and treat osteoporosis, a test that all other calcium supplements to date have failed? To answer that question, Dr. Fujita embarked on a number of long-term, double-blind, placebo-controlled trials… with groundbreaking results.

AdvaCal vanquishes osteoporosis… and more

AdvaCal has been proven effective over and over again—even against osteoporosis. This miracle mineral also reduces fracture risk, may decrease kidney stone formation, could take on Alzheimer's disease, and seems to be the solution to the deadly calcium paradox.

Let's start with osteoporosis, where AdvaCal is affecting some substantial changes. In fact, every study that's ever been done on this calcium supplement has shown that it significantly boosts bone mineral density—in premenopausal women, postmenopausal women, men, and elderly women. Every single study! We'll look at just a few…

- One study of 58 elderly women (with an average age of 82) showed that AdvaCal increased bone mineral density (BMD) of the spine by over 3 percent after two years![2] That's an astonishing result, especially when you consider the age of the women in the study. And by comparison, the women taking standard calcium-carbonate supplements saw only a slight (0.6 percent) increase of spinal BMD, while women taking a placebo *lost* almost 2 percent.

- A larger study conducted by Dr. Fujita showed that AdvaCal can not only prevent osteoporosis, but can actually reverse bone loss caused by the disease. In a trial of 136 patients (ages 51 to 83) already suffering from osteoporosis, those taking AdvaCal had an increase in spinal BMD of 8.0 percent after three years.[3] By comparison, the subjects taking a placebo lost about 3.5 percent.

- Another small study found that AdvaCal increased trabecular (that's spongy bone) forearm bone density in women by more than 6 percent in just four months, while the women in the placebo group saw no increase. And what's alarming is that while women in the calcium carbonate group saw only a negligible increase in trabecular bone, they suffered a significant *decrease* in cortical bone (the hard outer layer of bone).[4]

AdvaCal is a formidable ally when it comes boosting your bone density. But it can do so much more.

Turn back the clock—and turn on good health—with AdvaCal

Not only does AdvaCal dramatically increase bone mineral density, it can knock down PTH levels… reduce fracture risk… inhibit kidney

---

How do popular calcium supplements compare?

Calcium carbonate (Caltrate, Tums) is one of the more concentrated forms of calcium (it contains about 40 percent elemental calcium). It's also relatively in-expensive, making it very popular with supplement manufacturers.

The problem with calcium carbonate, though, is that this form of calcium is very hard for your body to break down and use—and that means only about 22 percent of the mineral actually gets absorbed by your body. It's even worse for people with low levels of stomach acid (which naturally decreases as we age), and absorption can be as low as 4 percent.

Other calcium supplements (Citracal, for example) use a slightly more expensive compound called calcium citrate. This form is easier for your body to break down and absorb… but it comes with its own drawback. Calcium citrate contains only about 20 percent elemental calcium, so you would need to take a lot more of it to get enough calcium—and that translates to an awful lot of pills to swallow every day.

stones… and maybe even protect you from Alzheimer's disease.

Let's start with how dramatically AdvaCal can impact your health by reducing your PTH levels. We already know that calcium deficiency sets off PTH, and that PTH kicks off bone-calcium theft, wreaking havoc on your bones and virtually every other cell in your body. That's because too much calcium in any cell leads to decreased cell function… and eventually cell death.

Decreased cell function is associated with many (if not most) signs of aging: changes in your hair and skin, hearing loss, cataracts, irritability, forgetfulness—the list goes on. We saw earlier how AdvaCal actually reduces red blood cell calcium levels, and that can make a noticeable impact.

Studies also show that AdvaCal can significantly reduce circulating PTH levels in both men and women—knocking them down by almost 30 percent after just 5 days in one study[5]! But the unlucky participants getting placebo saw a 5 percent increase in their PTH levels.

Then there's the reduced fracture risk: A 2004 study[6] found that elderly women who got AdvaCal for two years suffered fewer fractures (thanks to an increase in their lumbar BMD). Unfortunately, the women in the calcium carbonate group fared no better than the placebo group and saw no decrease in fracture risk.

And how about kidney stones? While the Women's Health Initiative found that supplementing with calcium carbonate actually increased the risk of kidney stones, a study run by Dr. Fujita found that AdvaCal seemed to inhibit the formation of kidney stones.[7]

And, finally, research seems to point toward a the role of AdvaCal in possibly warding off Alzheimer's disease. It appears that calcium overload in brain cells which prompts cell death may lead to neuronal dysfunction—like memory loss, cognitive problems, and the dreaded 'sundown syndrome' suffered by many AD patients. In a groundbreaking study, researchers found that AdvaCal helped correct the evening calcium decline, while the placebo did not. And that correction may just help turn the tide when it comes to sundown syndrome.[8]

Easy to swallow, easy to absorb

On top of its superior absorbability and its widely documented health benefits, AdvaCal comes with yet another distinct advantage over typical calcium supplements: it's very easy to swallow.

While most calcium supplements come as hard-pressed tablets (a.k.a. horse pills) which can be extremely difficult to take and digest, AdvaCaL comes in small capsules, assuring that 100 percent of the active ingredients are released for absorption.

Six capsules a day provides 900 mg of highly absorbable elemental calcium, the amount proven effective in multiple scientific trials. According to Dr. Fujita's research, you can boost the effectiveness of calcium therapy by taking three capsules, half of the daily dosage, at bedtime.

You'll find ordering information for AdvaCal in the Member Source Directory on page 529.

CHAPTER TWELVE

The single herb that combats cancer, Alzheimer's, heart disease, and more...exclusive access for HSI Members

"It sounds like science fiction. A simple natural substance that can take on cancer... and so much more. This unique herb can stand up to Alzheimer's disease, hyperthyroidism, and many other diseases.

It sounds too far-fetched to be real. But it is. And our own long-time HSI panelist Dr. Makise is one of the key driving forces behind studying this herbal phenomenon, and bringing it directly to you—before anyone else in the United States has access to it.

This miraculous plant is so rare, there's only one place on the planet where it's found, a Pacific island made up mainly of coral rock... and that adds a unique twist to the healing powers of everything that grows there.

This powerhouse of cures is called shell ginger, and it may just be the next 'superfood' you hear about.

The underground herb that's (quietly) wiping out disease

So why hasn't anyone heard about the miraculous curative powers of shell ginger? Dr. Makise told me that scientists are too busy picking on single components to look at the plant as a whole—even though the whole works much more powerfully than the sum of its plentiful parts.

And while shell ginger may still be flying far under the radar, Dr. Makise has been prescribing it to patients, and seeing some pretty stunning effects.

Real people are seeing spectacular results

While there still aren't any completed formal clinical trials supporting shell ginger, there are plenty of case studies showing its value in fighting disease—even against advanced prostate cancer.

Jack R., a 50-year-old man riddled with prostate cancer, was about to go under the knife when a friend told him to call a natural doctor he knew. Jack made the call, and was excited about trying something—anything—other than surgery. He couldn't really afford a lot of treatment, but he did try one of the doctor's recommendations.

He felt the difference right away, especially when it came to urination. And within just two weeks of taking this miraculous natural remedy, Jack's doctor called off the surgery. Two weeks!

Rob M., a 51-year-old airline executive, had a small tumor on his left kidney. Doctors removed the kidney surgically and treated with interferon (a standard cancer therapy). But after all that, the cancer metastasized to his lungs.

Instead of suffering through more chemotherapy and surgery, or enduring radiation, Rob said no to mainstream cures. He began one therapy, then Dr. Makise added in shell ginger and lactoferrin. Rob began to get his energy back, and was able to work and live his life again—which would not have happened with chemo and radiation. And though scans show that he still has lung cancer, there has been no growth or change from the original scan—his cancer is under control.

And cancer isn't the only problem shell ginger has been instrumental in curing…

Overactive thyroid under control in just one month

Back in April 2009, Dr. Makise met with Irene S., a 45-year-old patient. She looked different than she had the month before, especially her eyes. Irene told him that she didn't feel anything much, but a few palpitations and maybe a little sweatier than usual. She'd suffered from hyperthyroidism (overactive thyroid) in the past, so Dr. Makise sent her straight to a specialist.

With a confirmed diagnosis, the specialist put Irene on Mercazole, a common synthetic thyroid drug used around the world. She'd been on that drug before, and it took more than a year to regulate her thyroid properly.

About a month later, Dr. Makise prescribed shell ginger… and her thyroid was under control within a month. The specialist was very surprised by the rapid improvement, and began to decrease her medication. Six months later, Irene was doing very well, even gaining back some weight.

Though scientists aren't sure which compound (or compounds) in shell ginger reduce thyroid hyperactivity, they have seen it work. In fact, they think it may also work to restore underactive thyroid (called hypothyroidism) as well, since plants in the ginger family often work as adaptogens, which work to balance systems in whichever way they need.

Erasing eczema quickly and easily

Dr. Makise has also treated hundreds of patients suffering from eczema (officially called atopic dermatitis), with stunning results. Rather than following the mainstream protocol of cortisone ointment—which lose power, and can cause unpleasant side effects—he takes the "inside out" approach, with a shell ginger twist.

For years he treated people with a focused mix of vitamins, minerals, and herbs, which was effective, "but not perfect." Then in June 2009, he started adding shell ginger into the regimen for more than one hundred patients—and he saw better results almost right away.

One reason for shell ginger's success here, believes Dr. Makise, is its detoxification effect. Many patients starting on shell ginger notice an immediate improvement in their bowel movements—and that's essential for detoxification.

"Be careful when you take the supplement of shell ginger," says Dr. Makise, "because 60 – 70 percent of the patients may suffer from some aggravation of symptoms temporarily. And some may suffer from diarrhea. This is due to the detoxification effect of shell ginger, and do not worry. Reduce the dose and gradually increase."

Jam-packed with healing substances for a wide range of healthy effects

Shell ginger is packed with dozens of healing components, all with unique curative effects on the body. No other plant contains this rare and abundant mix of more than fifty polyphenols and plenty of bioflavonoids—and that's why no other plant has such widespread curative capabilities.

Take a look at some of its most powerful compounds:

- Ferulic acid has powerful antioxidant properties with wide-ranging functions, from anti-aging support to improved cholesterol management to cancer prevention
- Kawain (which is the key polyphenol of Kava) enhances sleep, relaxation, and collagen production
- Kaempferol stifles production of two cytokines that cause allergic reactions, giving shell ginger an impressive anti-allergy effect
- Quercetin, a potent bioflavonoid, can fight tumors, lower blood pressure, prevent cataracts, and may even help prevent

Alzheimer's disease… among other things

- Epicatechin (best known as a component of green tea) shows promise in controlling blood sugar levels and preventing liver cancer

- Chlorogenic acid seems to prevent the cell mutations that cause cancer, and appears particularly beneficial in the fight against skin cancer

- Catechin helps prevent gastric ulcers, ward off viral infections, and seems to lower the risk of gastrointestinal cancers

Shell ginger is also known to increase body temperature, just like its cousins in the rest of the ginger family. Proper body temperature is critical to optimal enzyme function—they just can't get their jobs done if they aren't warm enough. And it turns out that, overall, the average body temperature has dropped at least one degree (celsius) over time, so we all need that warming factor.

Another huge benefit of mixed polyphenols is their ability to boost up your immune system and keep you in robust good health.

Can shell ginger stop Alzheimer's disease?

So far, there's no proof that shell ginger can help prevent or even reverse Alzheimer's disease, but scientists believe that it can have a very beneficial effect against this life-robbing condition.

Shell ginger contains key compounds that have been found useful in combating AD, which could mean that this supplement might be able to keep the decline from starting.

Two of its main components, known as DK and DDK, get converted in the body to a substance called hispidin. Hispidin appears to inhibit an enzyme called beta-secretase, which seems to be very involved in the onset of AD.

Shell ginger also contains ferulic acid, which has been studied as a cure for Alzheimer's disease. Ferulic acid can stop the destructive and toxic properites of amyloid-beta protein in their tracks—and amyloid-beta protein is widely known as a cause of mental decline.

Take shell ginger every day for optimum health

While shell ginger does grow in a few places in the world, the variety grown on the remote Japanese island of Okinawa is the only one Dr. Makise will work with. The soil of Okinawa is unique, as its made of weathered coral limestone which makes the pH level a weak alkaline—the most optimal level for good health.

Dr. Makise has made the only shell ginger supplement containing this special variety available in the United States for HSI Members. It's called JIPANG Ginger®, and in addition to shell ginger's plentiful and potent polyphenols, the formula also contains astaxanthin and Vitamin K2.

To support your immune system, you can take four to six tablets per day, about thirty minutes before going to bed. If you experience any stomach upset (like diarrhea), decrease the dose to one capsule daily for the first week, and increase the dose gradually by adding one capsule per week until you reach the full dose.

You can find ordering information for JIPANG-Ginger® in the Member Source Directory on page 529.

CHAPTER THIRTEEN

Just-discovered rare substance takes the sting out of menopause... and so much more

In a very small region in the heart of Brazil lies the secret to a virtually unnoticeable menopause... and quite possibly the solutions for oddly diverse health issues, from cancer to candida infections to gingivitis.

This extremely rare and unusual substance can turn menopause around, making dreaded night sweats and hot flashes a thing of the past. And when paired with a proprietary herbal blend, it smoothes out even more menopause symptoms—so you'll barely notice you're going through a change.

A life-changing encounter with a swarm of bees

This unlikely story begins with a businessman and a swarm of bees. The successful—but unhappy—Brazilian engineer was looking to change his life. Little did he know that the answer would come to him as an almost deafening buzz, as he and this distinct swarm of bees mysteriously crossed paths.

In no time at all, Alessandro Esteves gave up his old career, bought a farm, and dedicated his life to beekeeping. But these weren't just any bees. They held a secret that had caught the interest of researchers from across the globe—red propolis.

Now bee propolis is ridiculously common. It's a key component of every beehive in the world. But this propolis, Brazilian red propolis, is extremely rare—and its unique components give it distinctive healing powers.

Getting to the source

The research team just had to discover where the bees got that propolis, and Alessandro (with his intimate knowledge of the landscape) joined the expedition. And discovering the botanical origin (*dalbergia ecastophyllum*) brought them closer to learning its secrets.

The scientists were most interested in its red color and unique antioxidant and flavonoid activity, which was different than any other propolis they'd ever seen.

In fact, studies showed that these flavonoids were actually special isoflavones, something no other propolis in the world lays claim to. Not only that, but these isoflavones have a unique composition, making them more easily absorbable by the body than the standard variety. And therein lies their power to deliver a carefree menopause experience.

The aglycone difference

This Brazilian red bee propolis created by Alessandro's hives contains several isoflavones—some of which are still unidentified because they've never been seen before. But the key to their healing capabilities is well-known... the lack of a glucose ring, which is called *aglycone*.

This naturally aglycone isoflavone (called IsoFactor™) is much more efficiently absorbed by the body than isoflavones with the ring (which is virtually all others), including treated isoflavones. For example, aglycone soy isoflavones actually require a special fermentation process to remove that glucose ring—meaning they need to be treated like the ones naturally found in this red propolis.

And one study[1] found that aglycone isoflavones were absorbed substantially better than those with the glucose ring intact (called glucosides)—more than five times better (based on blood levels). What's more, those higher blood levels remained higher even four weeks later.

And its natural aglycone property gives IsoFactor™—the key ingredient in a revolutionary menopause formula called EaseFemin—a distinct advantage over other isoflavones.

Unique isoflavones balance hormones without damaging side effects

Isoflavones, like the ones in this Brazilian red bee propolis, are phytoestrogens—plant substances that are similar to human estrogen in their chemical structure, but are much weaker.

When these compounds mimic human estrogen in specific sites throughout the body, they bring on an abundance of health benefits. For one thing, they can directly relieve troubling menopause symptoms by creating a balancing effect for estrogen levels. You see, the cell receptors in your body are used to getting a steady supply of estrogen, and when that declines (as happens during menopause), unpleasant symptoms can set in.

Phytoestrogens gently balance that estrogen supply, boosting it enough to ease hot flashes and night sweats, without setting off a domino effect of negative effects (as is often seen when women use artificial hormone replacement therapy). On top of that, these isoflavones can also stop 'bad' estrogen (the form implicated in some forms of cancer) from causing harmful effects.

And that's not all! Isoflavones and other flavonoids found in this unique propolis are also highly powerful antioxidants. And that's especially true (but not at all surprising) here: Thanks to the very red resin of the *dalbergia ecastophyllum*, the antioxidant profile is quite unique and powerful. In fact, a DPPH test (a commonly used scientific test that measures free radical scavenging ability) showed 84.3 percent effectiveness of IsoFactor™ against free radicals—a very impressive score, especially for bee propolis.

As impressive as that is, it's only the beginning of the benefits propolis can offer—and has been offering for centuries.

The amazing protective powers of bee propolis— warding off infections, fighting cancer, and more

Did you know that bee propolis has been used for healing since ancient times? The Greeks, Romans, and Egyptians relied on this miraculous substances to cure any manner of ailment… and for good reason.

You see, propolis is what bees use to protect their hives from, well, everything. In fact, propolis is literally the hive's immune system, and it keeps the entire inner environment pure and sterile. That's an amazing feat, especially considering that the inside of the hive is very hot (around 90°), making it a prime breeding ground for bacteria, viruses, and other dangerous organisms. But thanks to propolis, the inner hive remains pristine.

That antimicrobial power works for us, too. When we consume propolis (or even rub it on wounds), it offers up anti-fungal, anti-viral, and anti-bacterial powers that can protect us against a wide variety of infections ranging from the common cold to candida (yeast infections) to gingivitis to salmonella.

And the latest research shows us that propolis also has cancer-fighting capabilities. In fact, Brazilian red propolis in particular was tested to see just how effective it could be against one of the deadliest diseases known to man: pancreatic cancer.

In the lab, a group of scientists studied the impact of key compounds in the red propolis against extremely hard to kill PANC-1 pancreatic cancer cells[2]. Now this particular type of cancer is known to be resistant to most chemotherapies, and even thrives when deprived of nutrients. But the PANC-1 cells met their match in red propolis extract, which 'displayed 100 percent cytotoxicity.' That means it was able to kill off *all* of the pancreatic cancer cells.

That's pretty amazing—especially when you consider that HRT, the old gold standard menopause treatment, is now believed to cause some forms of cancer.

Five synergistic ingredients heighten EaseFemin's effectiveness

While Brazilian red propolis is the star ingredient of EaseFemin, the formula also contains a carefully selected set of nutrients and a proprietary 'calming herbal blend.' Each of these ingredients was specifically chosen for its synergistic effect with the red propolis, and for its proven capabilities in easing menopause symptoms.

Because menopause is often associated with loss of bone density, EaseFemin includes calcium and high potency vitamin D to support bone health.

And while calcium is known primarily as a bone builder, it handles a lot of other tasks as well. One of those is as a mood soother—and we all know that mood dips can be caused by the hormonal changes brought on by menopause. Calcium deficiency plays a proven role in anxiety, depression, nervousness, and irritability... so a calcium boost can help lighten these darker moods.

The herbal blend contains three herbs well-known for their calming and healing properties: valerian, chamomile, and passionflower. This soothing trio helps take the edge off hormone-related mood dips, as well as easing insomnia and pains.

Valerian has a well-earned reputation as a sleep herb, mainly because of its extraordinary calming powers. It's a known stress-buster, as well as a natural antidepressant. And, of course, it helps you fall asleep and sleep better. What you may not know about valerian is that it's also been used traditionally to relieve painful menstruation and cramps—and that could translate into easing some of the pains associated with menopause.

Chamomile is another well-known calming herb. This medicinal plant has also been used for centuries to relieve insomnia, primarily because of its sedating effect on the central nervous system—a trick that also allows the herb to alleviate anxiety. Chamomile, like valerian, has some lesser known properties that can help women specifically—it's been used historically as a tonic for the uterus.

The final herb of this trio is *passionflower*, and it also combines menopause relief with good mood support. On the emotional side, passionflower may be used to ease anxiety, depression, and irritability. It's also sometimes used to level out mood swings, and may help you enjoy deeper sleep with fewer waking disturbances. On top of that, this herb has been often prescribed by herbalists in Europe as a remedy for the pains that can accompany menopause, possibly due to its antispasmodic properties.

The proof is in the happy customers

While there aren't yet any completed studies measuring the effectiveness of EaseFemin on menopause symptoms, J L Paes-Leme (Alessandro's business partner) told me that customers are coming back in droves. (And that they do want to run trials with the product in the near future—so stay tuned for more information about that.)

And while a 75 percent repeat sales rate sounds impressive, letters from satisfied customers offer a better picture.

W. Hargam wrote…

"I just wanted to express how pleased I am with your product. I have taken EaseFemin for almost 30 days now. I cannot believe how good I feel already! I never want to be without EaseFemin. It's wonderful! All post-menopause women need to be on your product. Thank you!"

P. Smillaw said…

"I have no hot flashes and no negative side effects from EaseFemin, and I feel confident that taking something natural is an advantage to my body. It has truly improved my health and quality of life! Thanks EaseFemin for a wonderful product!"

And Y. Lacer had this to say…

"I started this [EaseFemin] over a month ago and I ran out and have noticed an immediate difference in my perimenopause symptoms. I just purchased a 3 month supply so I don't run out again. It has truly made a difference and reduced my night sweats within just two weeks of taking the supplement."

Try EaseFemin for an unnoticeable menopause experience

Once you start taking EaseFemin, you'll probably notice a vast improvement in menopause symptoms in about six weeks (but for some women it may take ten to twelve weeks for the full effects of the remedy to kick in).

And, according to J L, it's best to take EaseFemin after dinner, before you go to bed.

The manufacturer recommends taking one capsule daily.

You'll find ordering information for EaseFemin in the Member Source Directory on page 529.

CHAPTER FOURTEEN

Unique protein supplement relieves Crohn's disease, eases chemotherapy side effects, heals open wounds... and more

I t's disgusting: Pre-digested hydrolyzed fish protein.

But it just might be the perfect solution to severe gastrointestinal ailments like Crohn's disease, ulcerative colitis, and 'leaky gut' syndrome... and a whole lot more.

Because the 'side effects' of this revolutionary supplement may improve your health in ways you'd never expect.

Pure protein goes to work instantly to nourish and heal your body

Pre-digested fish protein is actually not as gross as it sounds. All it means is that the nutrients in the fish have already been broken down by enzymes, so your body can absorb them easily and instantly.

How does that work? While it sort of sounds like someone else has chewed up the fish, it's really a highly sanitary process. The fish protein, which comes from fillets of deep-ocean white fish, is broken down by a unique process, and converted into pure components of protein: amino acids and peptides. And since that protein is already broken down, your body can use it right away—it sidesteps your body's digestion process completely.

Normally, your digestive system has to work extremely hard to break down large protein molecules—but it doesn't always work. And when your body doesn't completely break down proteins, you can't absorb all the individual nutrients.

But since the protein in this supplement is already broken down (pre-digested), your body doesn't have to do any work at all to reap all of its benefits. Some of the specific nutrients released by the process are small-chain peptides. Peptides are small compounds derived from protein, and are much more easily absorbed by your body. And with direct, instant access to these peptides, your body's digestive system gets stronger.

What's more, these powerful peptides seem to bring on healing in other areas of the body, too.

Crohn's disease symptoms eased in just three days

These healing peptides come to you in a supplement called Seacure—a perfect name for a pure fish protein that works to help your body cure itself.

There is plenty of science to back up Seacure's effectiveness when it comes to a wide range of GI diseases. But none of the studies—as impressive as they are—are nearly as persuasive as the stories of people whose lives have been forever changed by this deep sea supplement.

Kara M. from Texas said, "After a year of being very ill and struggling with chronic diarrhea, I was diagnosed with Crohn's. My doctor suggested that I take Seacure. In only three days I noticed a measurable reduction in activity in my gut. I was truly amazed at the results I personally experienced in only three days of taking Seacure."

Janet G. from Ohio used Seacure to combat chronic gastritis and acid reflux.

"Seacure has helped me tremendously! I have suffered from Gastritis and also acid reflux for the past 5 years. I was prescribed Prilosec and had been taking it longer than I felt was safe without long term side effects... Then I read about Seacure... I have to admit, I was a little skeptical at first, but ordered a bottle anyway. I have been taking Seacure a little over 3 months and have not had to take not even one antacid!

Seacure helps cancer patients thrive during chemotherapy

If you've ever seen someone suffer the ravages of chemotherapy, you know it can take as big a toll as cancer itself.

And since Seacure was developed to combat malnourishment—a very common side effect of mainstream cancer treatments—it follows that the supplement could help people struggling through chemotherapy. And based on anecdotal reports, it really does.

Dr. K. Jowerd of Hawaii sees Seacure help many people through devastating cancer treatments.

"I have used Seacure with many patients. Some of these patients were receiving chemotherapy for cancer and taking Seacure at the same time. Most of these individuals did very well during their chemotherapy. They experienced fewer side-effects from the chemotherapy, i.e. nausea, vomiting, diarrhea, lack of appetite and fatigue. I strongly recommend Seacure to anyone undergoing chemotherapy."

And Pamela T. of South Australia knows first-hand just how much Seacure can help someone through chemotherapy.

"After a mastectomy I began Chemotherapy treatment which lasted for four months. During the treatment, the Seacure enabled me to eat fairly normally and the nausea was largely diminished. I didn't lose weight either. The Seacure really did enable my stomach to work properly after the effects of the Chemo."

Open wounds heal faster with Seacure

How can a fish supplement help wounds heal? It's the power of pure protein, which helps your body jumpstart its own natural healing process. And based on reports from Seacure users, its wound healing properties are truly miraculous.

Perhaps the most amazing was the story of Benton Ludwig, a registered nurse from Arkansas who nearly lost his legs, and was saved by Seacure.

Benton had suffered from highly painful open-wound ulcers on both ankles, brought on by poor circulation. (I saw the pictures— they were truly horrifying.) He had undergone surgery at the Mayo Clinic, to no avail. The ulcers weren't healing, and the severe pain was constant.

He'd almost given up hope when he came across Seacure, and decided to give it a try.

Within four weeks of taking Seacure, his leg ulcers cleared up… and stayed that way.

Heal from the inside out with Seacure

Seacure's remarkable healing capabilities may just help you start feeling better right away—especially if you suffer from a debilitating GI condition like Crohn's or ulcerative colitis.

The recommended dosage is six capsules daily. For the best results, take your Seacure before meals.

A word on the fishy smell... Seacure capsules do smell fishy, and they're supposed to. If you can't get past the smell, put the capsules in your freezer. That will erase the smell (and won't smell up your freezer) without impacting Seacure's effectiveness.

You can find ordering information for Seacure in the Member Source Directory on page 529.

CHAPTER FIFTEEN

HSI Member's own kitchen concoction provides option to oral surgery

During a conversation with one of our members, Joe Lesky told me that back in 1997 his son Jim, 31 at the time, went for a regular dental checkup only to be told his gums were in such bad shape that his teeth either needed to be removed or they would fall out. This situation starts with gingivitis (inflammation of the gums), which is caused by plaque. If plaque isn't removed regularly, it grows and causes pockets between the teeth and gums. Healthy gums rest on the teeth without any gaps or pockets, but Jim's gums had pockets that measured 12 to 14 millimeters. Even half this measurement would have indicated a need for oral surgery. But Jim wasn't about to let the dentist pull any of his teeth. So he went for a second opinion—same diagnosis.

Still not ready to give up his teeth, Jim went for a third opinion, this time to a periodontist who diagnosed him with severe gum infection and periodontal disease. What disturbed Jim most was that he had no idea that he even had gum disease. And he's not alone: According to the American Dental Association, three out of four adults over age 35 have some form of gum disease-and most people don't even realize it until the first signs of gum tenderness or some blood on their toothbrush. It seems that even with the current tooth-whitening trend, many of us have been neglecting our smiles. Or maybe the treatments that have been available to us so far are not living up to the need.

The periodontist treated him with an antibiotic for the infection, but, even after the infection was treated, he was told he still needed surgery to reduce the depth of gum pockets. Jim was still hesitant about having such a major procedure, so he called his dad for advice and help.

Joe Lesky had treated himself with homemade remedies for years and has compiled an extensive file of information on herbs and other natural healers. So when Jim called him asking for advice, Joe pulled out his herbal references, and, as he told me in our phone conversation, "After much research, I combined several herbal extracts and essential oils, which were reported to be beneficial to gum health."

The result was a powerful herbal mouthwash that combines:

- Cayenne—fights infection, stimulates circulation and healing, and relieves pain.
- Bloodroot—prevents bacteria from forming plaque via natural antiseptic properties.
- Echinacea—boosts the immune system, relieves pain, and acts as an antiseptic and antibacterial agent
- Bayberry—tightens and stimulates gums. Also an astringent
- White oak bark—eases inflammation, has astringent and antiseptic qualities, tightens gums
- Tea tree oil—offers protection from harmful bacteria and behaves as a natural antiseptic and anti-inflammatory.
- Peppermint oil—stimulates circulation and freshens breath.

Joe instructed his son to mix the formula with water and rinse with it every morning and night. Jim was skeptical, but he figured he had nothing to lose and might save his teeth.

A few weeks later, he went back to the periodontist for a checkup and cleaning. The periodontist noted that Jim's gums looked healthier and the pockets in them had gone down a little, but he would still need surgery. Jim bargained with the periodontist and got him to agree to wait several more months to see if he could achieve even better results using his father's homemade mouthwash.

A few months later, the pockets had gone down more and his gums were pink and healthy. The periodontist was pleased with the progress and they both agreed to hold off on the surgery indefinitely. Today Jim's gums are still in good shape and he continues to use the solution regularly to keep them that way.

Even reverses oral bone loss

But even more amazing than Jim's return to gum health without surgery is that the bone loss associated with the severe infection had completely reversed. Many times, infections as severe as Jim's end up requiring bone grafts in order to replace lost bone. And that not only hurts your mouth-it also hurts your bank account. But Jim avoided this fate using the home made mouthwash, and he was able to reverse the deterioration altogether.

Sounds great, but we need more than one son's endorsement to cover a product in HSI. After all, this is just an herbal concoction that someone brewed up in his kitchen once, right? Well, as a matter of fact, Lesky wasn't just getting great results from his son—he was getting great results and feedback from a lot of his relatives, friends, and neighbors who had also tried his formula, and all wanted more. It seemed that the demand had outgrown his kitchen, so Lesky took the next step.

Coming to a store near you?

Lesky took the necessary steps of patenting his formula, designing and printing a label, and working with a manufacturer to produce 2,000 bottles of the product, which he named Peri-Gum. With that, the Lesky family hit the streets to get the word out locally. Joe, Jim, and Jim's wife Terri went around with cases to local health food stores telling of their successes with the formula. Joe even wrote an article for his local New Jersey paper.

Locally, Lesky received a phone call from a dentist detailing how a patient had brought in a copy of his article. It turned out that this dentist's wife and brother were both in need of oral surgery and were able to avoid it using Peri-Gum.

But getting the product out there on a national level didn't happen until a representative from a national natural product distributor heard about Peri-Gum. He also knew someone in need of oral surgery, and, once again, Peri-Gum offered that person effective healing without going under the knife. He was so impressed, he contacted Lesky and worked with him to bring Peri-Gum into health food stores nationwide.

Now Peri-Gum is available across the country. And it's even been the subject of several studies—all of which have confirmed that it works.

Most notably, one pilot study, completed at a prominent northeastern dental school, showed that volunteers' gum and oral health were significantly improved after just four weeks of using Peri-Gum. Researchers evaluated the subjects' progress by measuring the reduction of gingival health scores and reduction of plaque. Overall, they found a 20 percent reduction in the subjects' gingival health scores and a 16 percent reduction in plaque, And according to the study, Peri-Gum was found not to harm oral tissues.

Not what you'd expect from an ordinary mouthwash

The Peri-Gum concentrate formula is so powerful that when it's diluted with water according to the instructions, just one 1 oz. bottle makes up to 90 ounces of actual mouthwash. For use as a daily rinse, mix five drops of Peri-Gum with 1/2 oz. water and vigorously work the mouthwash between your teeth and gums for at least 30 seconds—the longer the better. Do not swallow.

Lesky recommends using Peri-Gum at least twice a day, especially at bedtime after you complete your normal dental hygiene routine (brushing teeth, etc.). He also suggests taking a very soft toothbrush, dipping it in the diluted Peri-Gum solution, and brushing with that instead of toothpaste.

I admit, my first reaction to a mouthwash containing cayenne was that it would burn—but I was game to at least try it. To my surprise, it didn't burn at all. But it did clean and refresh my mouth. In fact, it didn't just feel clean, it felt rejuvenated.

A leading developer and manufacturer of botanical extracts has picked up where Joe Lesky left off in his kitchen and has taken over the manufacturing of Peri-Gum, and now it's distributed across the country. You can purchase it in various health food stores or on-line directly through Lesky's company: Lesko Care, L.L.C. Contact information is listed in the Member Source Directory.

CHAPTER SIXTEEN

You could be just one bottle away from getting rid of your allergies for good

It all started when Jim English got a package from one of his contacts in China. In the box were several sample bottles of a new supplement, along with a note from the doctor that said "This is great allergy stuff." As CEO of a supplement company, English gets boxes of samples every day. So his first thought was "Oh great—<u>another</u> allergy remedy," and he promptly put it away up on the shelf. It wasn't until just over a year ago—when he needed it—that he thought of the samples again and got his first clue into AllerPhase's potential.

What prompted him to reach for the sample on the shelf was his son's friend Stephen. Twelve years old at the time, he had come over to their house to play when he started having an allergy attack. English remembered the sample of AllerPhase up on his shelf. He called Stephen's mother, explained what was in the product, and asked if it was okay to give it to her son. She told him to go ahead. So Stephen took the AllerPhase, and English sent the boys to sit quietly for a while, to give the formula a chance to work. Amazingly enough, about 30 minutes later, his son and his friend said they wanted to go out to the park.

English noticed that the swelling and redness from the allergic reaction had virtually disappeared from Stephen's face. He was shocked at how quickly the boy had recovered. English agreed to let them go and the kids were off—as though nothing had happened.

Seeing Stephen's results, he realized that the bottle that had just sat on his shelf for so long really might be "great allergy stuff."

Herbal teamwork wipes out symptoms

AllerPhase contains 10 traditional Chinese herbs specifically selected for their ability to quickly and safely relieve allergic symptoms while gently resolving the underlying immune system imbalance that triggers allergic reactions in the first place.

The first herb on this list, Gastrodia, is one I hadn't seen before in an allergy formula: It's commonly used in China to treat hypertension, improve circulation, and resolve headaches. But it appears exclusively as an allergy herb in AllerPhase and is largely responsible for the formula's ability to relieve brain fog—one of the main symptoms of allergies. Recent research suggests that Gastrodia aids in improving memory by promoting blood flow to the brain. But better blood flow also enhances the ability of other herbs to quickly reach brain tissue. This strategy works on allergy symptoms because allergic reactions don't just happen in your nose, your eyes, and your ears—they're also in your brain, since they affect your central nervous system (CNS), which is what causes the brain fog.

Two of the formula's other herbs are also rarely seen in allergy products: Paeonia sufruticosa and Pseudostellaria. English told me that these herbs actually help desensitize you from allergens so they become less and less of a problem over time.

AllerPhase's other ingredients— Centipeda, Xanthium, Angelica, Schizonepeta, Fritillaria, Platycodon, and licorice—work together in various groupings to target specific allergy symptoms.

- Centipeda, Xanthium, and Angelica work to clear nasal and sinus congestion

- Schizonepeta reduces inflammation responsible for itching eyes and irritated respiratory tissues

- Fritillaria, Angelica, Paeonia and Platycodon work together to reduce inflammation and tissue swelling

- Centipeda, Fritillaria, Platycodon and licorice all act to reduce fluids—running nose, watery eyes, etc.

Since many of these ingredients can be found in other allergy formulations, what makes this product different? Well, the answer to that goes back to the Chinese doctor who gave English the sample.

The allergy formula treated like a fine wine

First, let me tell you—this is one elusive man. Even when English and his partner offered him $10 million, then $15 million, to buy the exclusive rights to the AllerPhase formula outright, he turned them down. So they settled for exclusive distribution rights and worked with the doctor to build a $6 million pharmaceutical manufacturing facility in China that rivals anything in America.

The lab is used to manufacture other products as well, but when it's time to make AllerPhase, the lab director has to clear out the staff and turn the whole plant over for 10 days to the doctor, his sons, and the rest of his crew—all trained licensed doctors—so that the team can privately go through the traditional, step-by-step process for making this product.

It's similar to making a fine wine: They take the raw materials (grown in a region in China where the herbs have been cultivated for 5,000 years) and enzymatically ferment them. As each herb ferments, the manufacturing team captures the "released volatile oils" (the active part pf the herb), then reintroduces them into the product at a specific point in the formulation process.

This process is so rigorous that any slight deviation would result in a completely different product, as the doctor, his team, and Jim English learned firsthand.

One tiny change makes a huge difference—
and not for the better

One batch the doctor sent to English was darker than the usual color, so he decided to do a small trial on some people who had been using the original samples to see if it was just a variation in color—which does happen sometimes in herbal products—or if it was something more. English gave the darker samples to a few people, and just a few days later they each came back to him and asked what he'd given them. The darker sample hadn't worked.

When he asked what was different, they all replied that the quick relief they got before just wasn't there. English had no choice but to call up the doctor and send the whole batch back. And I'm not talking about a couple of bottles—I'm talking tens of thousands of dollars worth of supplements. English told them it simply wasn't what he ordered and explained the reactions he got in his small trial.

Turned out that one of the doctor's sons deviated from the usual process, and this tiny change ruined the formula. Once they knew what had happened, they returned to the original process and have worked diligently ever since to make sure it never deviates again.

One patient tosses her 3 inhalers in favor of AllerPhase

Typical allergy remedies have limited effectiveness because they tend to be more reactive than proactive: They react to the symptoms instead of preventing them, which usually doesn't do much for you in the long run. AllerPhase, on the other hand, actually goes where the mainstream allergy remedies don't—straight to your immune system. It has an immune-normalizing effect. English explains that, basically, AllerPhase reminds your immune system of what it's supposed to be doing and not doing. It actually re-trains your immune system to attack viruses and other harmful invaders—not the kinds of harmless substances that trigger allergy symptoms. This is why AllerPhase is getting such a positive response from the people who have gotten a chance to try it—people like Rose.

For a big part of her life, Rose had been suffering from allergic-induced asthma. She'd been using three different inhalers up to four times a day and had been using Flonase for about 15 years. It wasn't unusual for her to have such an extreme allergy attack that she would end up in the emergency room.

Over the years, she just couldn't find a reasonable amount of relief from any of the products she'd tried—and the cost was making it difficult for her as well. Last December she decided to stop using Flonase. Like a lot of people, Rose just wanted to feel better without the side effects. Shortly after she stopped taking the Flonase, she went to visit a friend who had cats—one of Rose's major allergens. It was no surprise that, once again, Rose ended up in the ER.

A couple of weeks later, she ran into a girl at her local pharmacy who had just started using AllerPhase and recommended it to Rose. Rose gave it a chance and began to feel better right away. Four days after she started taking AllerPhase, Rose was supposed to go back to her friend's house. Still feeling good when she arrived, she decided to put AllerPhase to the test. She did all the things she knew would provoke an attack: She drank alcohol, she ate dairy and almonds, and she didn't avoid the cat. Not only did Rose not have an attack, but she didn't even use her inhaler once. Obviously, Rose's experiment falls under the "Do Not Try This At Home" category. If you decide to try AllerPhase, be sure to work closely with your doctor and don't test your limits without consulting him first.

Word spreads—and so do the benefits

As impressive as Rose's story is, I wanted more firsthand information. So Rose introduced me to her roommate, Miranda. As you know, when a product works, people tell their friends about it—and that person tells a friend who then tells a neighbor, and the neighbor tells a relative, and so on. Well, in this case, Miranda saw such a miraculous change in the quality of Rose's life that she decided to try AllerPhase too.

Miranda has had chronic allergies since she was a young girl. She'd tried various remedies over the years with some success, but nothing had really come close to resolving all of her symptoms without any side effects. As she told me, her most irritating problems were migraine headaches and stuffed-up ears.

She started taking AllerPhase in mid-January, and the first clue that something was changing came a few days into treatment when she realized she was starting to get a migraine. But this time it went away in a matter of hours instead of days. Then, her hearing cleared up. She could actually hear her own voice, unmuffled. From there, word about AllerPhase spread to Miranda's mother, Anne.

Anne had also suffered from allergies since childhood. Because they had gotten so much worse over the years, she had also developed significant lung damage. When I spoke with her about her experience, she explained that she was plagued by maddening skin itching and terrible fatigue. She was dazed and had trouble walking even half a block, since her constant coughing drained her. At Miranda's urging, Anne tried AllerPhase. Just a few days later, she realized she wasn't itching anymore. And about three weeks later, she had a "huge leap in energy."

One bottle could be all it takes

From what I've found in my conversations with the people who have tried it, AllerPhase's effects are unique to each person.

But while AllerPhase has different results for different people, it does seem to help most people who try it. HSI panelist Hyla Cass, M.D., was one of the first clinicians to evaluate AllerPhase. She's given the formula to numerous patients over the past year. As she explains,

"Even in cases where patient's allergic symptoms were severe and unresponsive to traditional and alternative therapies, AllerPhase brought about almost immediate and profound relief within 30 to 40 minutes."

The recommended dose is two capsules as soon as your allergy symptoms start. Then take one or two capsules twice a day as needed until the symptoms stop.

English told me his own family started taking AllerPhase after his son's friend's experience and that they all swear by it. He also says that a lot of people who have tried it report back that they actually don't need to take any more after the first bottle—their symptoms just don't come back. For ordering information, see the Member Source Directory.

CHAPTER SEVENTEEN

Powerful antioxidant may save you from America's leading cause of blindness

O n the shoreline of Kona, Hawaii, an industrial-sized incubator is cultivating microscopic algae. Normally such algae would be nothing more than fish food. But this algae may yield one of the world's most potent safeguards against cancer, heart disease, and blindness.

More than 13 million Americans over the age of 40 suffer from age-related macular degeneration (ARMD). This gradual decay of the macula—a central area of the retina that provides our most acute vision—is caused by ultraviolet light, air pollution, genetics, drug use, and countless other factors that degrade eye cells. ARMD produces irreversible vision loss and ranks as the single leading cause of blindness.

Researchers at Aquasearch Inc. of Hawaii and the University of Illinois Urbana-Champaign, however, believe they've discovered a phytonutrient in the ocean that could prevent the onset of ARMD...as well as lower the risk of cancer, cardiovascular disease, and neurodegenerative diseases.

At HSI, we've been looking for something that addresses ARMD for a long time. This is the first promising discovery we've found, and we thought you should know about it.

Study concludes nutrient is 80 times more effective than vitamin E

Astaxanthin [as-ta-zan-thin] is a xanthophyll (a derivative of the pigment, carotene). It's found in certain varieties of algae and produces a pink tint in the flesh of fish that consume it (namely, salmon, shrimp, crawfish, crab, lobster, and trout).

Laboratory research has demonstrated that astaxanthin has exceptional capabilities as an antioxidant (an agent that prevents the oxidation or mutation of cells) and an anti-inflammatory.[1,2] In recent animal studies at the College of Human Ecology in Seoul, Korea, astaxanthin protected the liver from toxin damage and stimulated the body's own cellular antioxidant system.[3]

Japanese researchers at the National Institute of Health and Nutrition conducted a placebo-controlled study on human subjects and found that astaxanthin inhibits the accumulation of LDL ("bad") cholesterol.[4]

Additional studies compared astaxanthin to other carotenoids and concluded that it's twice as effective as beta-carotene and nearly 80 times more effective than vitamin E at preventing oxidation within a chemical solution.[5]

Those results convinced some researchers that astaxanthin could quite capably deliver the same benefit as other antioxidants, namely lower the risk of cancer, heart diesease, high cholesterol, neurodegenerative diseases, and other age-related ailments. Now, researchers also surmise that it may help you keep your sight.

Carotenoids cross blood-brain barrier to protect eyes

To give your eyes extra protection, you may already be taking eye-specific antioxidants like lutein and zeaxanthin. Known collectively as xanthophylls, these carotenoids are found most abundantly in corn, kiwi, red seedless grapes, orange-colored peppers, spinach, celery, Brussel sprouts, scallions, broccoli, and squash.[6] And many people include these foods or xanthophyll supplements in their diets to help prevent ARMD and cataracts. (Cataracts, which sometimes appear to be caused by light-induced oxidation of eye cells, currently afflict 14 percent of Americans over the age of 40.)

What makes xanthophylls special is their ability to affect the eyes. Not all antioxidants can do that, since not all are able to cross the blood-brain barrier (BBB). The BBB is a protective mechanism designed to prevent infectious organisms and chemicals from entering the nervous system. This is an effective way to prevent illness from spreading to areas that control life itself, such as the brain. Unfortunately, it also stops beneficial substances, like many antioxidants, from protecting those same organs. Very few antioxidants can penetrate the BBB. Lutein and zeaxanthin can. And so apparently can astaxanthin.

University of Illinois researchers Mark O.M. Tso, M.D., D.Sc., and Tim-Tak Lam, Ph.D., made this key discovery in tests on rats. In a successful petition to patent astaxanthin, they state, "The administration of astaxanthin also retards the progress of degenerative eye diseases and [benefits] the vision of the individuals suffering from degenerative eye diseases, such as age-related macular degeneration."[7]

Astaxanthin levels differ by 800 percent in wild and farmed fish

One simple way to benefit from astaxanthin is to include more fish containing this xanthophyll in your diet. Salmon is the richest source. However, not all salmon have the same chance to accumulate high levels of astaxanthin. Even though aquaculture operations supplement their fish food with astaxanthin, farmed salmon have dramatically less astaxanthin than do wild salmon. Different varieties of the fish raised in different stretches of ocean also contain different levels.

For example, farm-raised Atlantic salmon fed synthetic astaxanthin contain only 0.5 mg of the antioxidant in a 4-oz serving. Free-range sockeye salmon from the North Pacific that feed on wild microalgae containing natural astaxanthin, provide about 4.5 mg in a 4-oz serving.[8] By eating the right salmon variety, you could increase your astaxanthin intake by as much as 800 percent.

Patented incubator maximizes xanthophyll's production

A potent source of astaxanthin is a microalgae called *Haemotoccus pluvialis* (H. pluvialis) that grows in the rocky coastal areas around Hawaii. Scientists at Mera Pharmaceuticals, a local biotechnology company, have harvested samples of H. pluvialis, studied them, and created special cultivating techniques to maximize the microalgae's production of astaxanthin.

After building high levels of the antioxidant in the microalgae, Mera Pharmaceuticals subjects the plant to a special churning process to break open the cells and release the astaxanthin. Next, the algae are pasteurized and dried at a low temperature, and the astaxanthin is extracted and sealed in a softgel capsule. Mera Pharmaceuticals markets the formula under the name AstaFactor. For ordering information, refer to the Member Source Directory at the back of this book.

CHAPTER EIGHTEEN

Believe it when you see it: 3-nutrient eyedrop formula dissolves cataracts without surgery

If you're like me, you don't like putting anything in your eye. Even thinking about it makes me nervous. And the thought of eye surgery? Forget it. But develop cataracts, and it's either surgery or blindness, right? Not anymore.

Doctors in Europe have developed eyedrops with a natural ingredient that can safely and painlessly break up cataracts. These drops have been used successfully in Britain since they were introduced there several years ago, and now they're also available in the U.S.

TV show trial sparks interest in natural cataract solution

OcuPhase combines N-acetyl L-carnosine (a.k.a. NAC) with vitamins A and E and appears to have the ability to reverse the aging process of cells that lead to cataracts.

The formula was originally introduced in Europe by Professor Steven Charles Gallant, after his father's experience with cataracts led him to investigate NAC more closely. Gallant had been studying another carnosine derivative, L-carnosine, for many years. When his father developed cataracts and was reluctant to go under the knife, Gallant remembered that the NAC form of carnosine had been proven in previous studies to have positive effects on the condition.

"I tried to get some for him," Gallant explained, "but unfortunately, at the time, it wasn't easily obtainable. My father had to have the operation, which thankfully was successful. But that got me to thinking how great it would be if we were to develop, and make readily available, a product that could address this condition with a simple course of eye drops as opposed to invasive surgery."

After many years of research and development, Gallant came up with an eyedrop formula he called Bright Eyes, which is the basis for the OcuPhase formula available here in the U.S.

In Europe, it seems to have gained popularity after being featured on a U.K. television program called *The Richard & Judy TV Trials* show.[1]

The show conducted its own short experimental trial to see if the eye drops could live up to their claim of improving vision. The four people who tried it (including the hostess, Judy) did say they noticed their vision had improved.

After seeing the show, hundreds of other people tried the Bright Eyes formula. I'll fill you in on some of those testimonials in a minute, but right now let's talk a bit about the mechanics behind cataracts and what's wrong with conventional treatments for it.

Why you're not seeing clearly

The lens of the eye is made up mostly of protein and water that combine as a clear tissue that allows light to pass through and focus on the retina. Over time, the tissue can become damaged by free radicals that occur as a result of any number of reasons—diabetes, long-term use of corticosteriods, heredity, ultra- violet light, poor nutrition, smoking, high blood pressure, aging, etc.

One of the other major causes of damage to the eye is glycation. Glycation occurs when sugars combine with proteins to create a whole new type of compound called glycated proteins, which produce 50 times more free radicals than normal proteins. The end result is that the water-soluble structural proteins in the lens of the eye clump together, or become cross-linked. (They also become oversaturated with water, creating internal pressure in the eye.) This causes the characteristic clouding of the eye lens associated with cataracts. Think of it like cooking an egg white: It's clear and fluid as it hits the pan, but as it becomes stressed by the heat, it becomes opaque and rubbery.

The fix? We need to break down these protein cross-links, restore transparency, and reduce internal pressure—and that's precisely what OcuPhase eyedrops do. But before we talk about how OcuPhase clears the eye lens, let's talk about the most common treatment option for cataracts.

Surgery isn't always a one-time solution

During cataract surgery, the damaged lens is removed and replaced with a synthetic lens implant. Sounds simple, but it turns out that cataract surgery is a two-part ordeal.

The new lens implant is held in place inside the eye by a thin membrane called the posterior capsule, part of the original covering of the lens that is intentionally left behind for this purpose. The problem is, in up to 50 percent of patients who have this procedure, the lens capsule begins clouding up again within two years. This isn't quite the same thing as the cataract coming back, since the cloudy posterior capsule is much thinner than the original cataract, and it can be opened up with a laser beam.

The corrective procedure is considered a "follow-up visit" and can apparently be done in the opthalmologist's office. But to those of us who are squeamish about this sort of thing to begin with, having to do it twice is hardly a selling point—especially considering the other possible complications, like glaucoma, detached retinas, corneal edema, severely compromised corneas requiring corneal transplants, and internal eye infections, which can all potentially cause complete loss of vision.

Apparently, I'm not the only one who finds this option less than appealing. Our contacts at Pure Tango, Inc. also saw a need for more options, which is why they worked to develop OcuPhase: their own version of the highly effective and successful British Bright Eyes formula.

Nutrient drops work from the outside in

The Pure Tango OcuPhase formula contains NAC, vitamin A, and vitamin E. Vitamin A is essential for the health and function of epithelial cells, the cells in the top-most layer of tissues like those in the lens of the eye. When it's used topically in the eye, vitamin E can increase the survival time of corneal endothelial cells, decrease inflammation, speed up healing of eye tissues, regenerate gluta-thione in the eye (which naturally decreases with age), and even prevent cataracts in some animal studies.[2-7] Add the power of NAC, which seems to act synergistically with vitamin E, and the vitamin combination is suddenly supercharged.[8] But what exactly makes NAC so effective?

The NAC in OcuPhase acts as a time-release version of L-carnosine. It's important to understand that OcuPhase isn't "just" L-carnosine in eyedrop form. Apparently, the results from NAC are achieved safely because of its time-release action: It breaks down and transforms into L-carnosine gradually. To speed up the process could ultimately cause more damage to the eye.

What's amazing is that even though our eyes and lenses are very impermeable, NAC is able to slowly permeate the lens structure. It's able to do this because unlike straight carnosine, NAC is soluble in lipids as well as in water.[9] The eyes contain both.

So after it enters the lipid components of the eye, NAC transforms into L-carnosine. This small molecule performs a remarkable variety of functions—most notably anti-oxidation and anti-glycation.

L-carnosine actually restores the lens by removing those cross-linked protein groups we talked about earlier. A 1999 Chinese study demonstrated that carnosine has a 100 percent success rate on early-stage senile cataracts and an 80 percent success rate on more advanced cases.[10]

Vision improves in 90 percent of study participants

I found that most of the recent research on N-acetyl carnosine has been carried out in Russia—all with encouraging results.[11-13]

In a 2001 study, Russian scientists conducted two randomized, double-blind, placebo-controlled trials—one for six months, one for 24 months—using an NAC eyedrop formula. A total of 49 patients (average age 65) with cataracts ranging in severity from minimal to advanced (but not to the point of requiring surgery) were treated with two drops of the NAC solution per day. The team monitored the condition of the cataracts, visual acuity, and glare sensitivity.

They found that the eyes treated with NAC were substantially improved in six months— transmissivity (the amount of light penetrating the lens of the eye) increased in 42 percent; glare sensitivity improved in 89 percent; and overall vision improved in 90 percent of the study participants. Even more good news: These improvements held up for the entire 24-month duration of the trial. And there was no worsening in any of the NAC-treated eyes, whereas visual acuity dropped in 89 percent of the controls after 24 months.[14]

British customers back up eyedrops' benefits

As I mentioned earlier, the OcuPhase formula has just become available in the U.S., so there isn't much feedback on it yet. But the very similar Bright Eyes formula has been available in Britain for some time. The following letters were written to the British distributor of

Bright Eyes after it was featured in several articles and on the *Richard & Judy* TV show.

"I want to tell you about my experiences with the special eye-drops. At first I didn't think there were any real differences, but I persisted in using the drops twice a day in the affected eye. Now after about three months I believe that there are significant changes to my vision. It's been a fairly gradual thing, which may explain why I didn't appreciate any changes early on, but now it's obvious to me that my eyesight has improved. The changes are slower than I anticipated, but I for one am sold on the drops!"

—C.B.S.

"Some 10 years ago I was told I was developing cataracts from the outside of my eyes to the inside. Five years ago I was told I must not drive: having never learnt I was not too upset. But two years ago I was warned that the cataracts were just about fully formed and I needed check-ups every six months... I have now been using carnosine eye drops for six months. I recently went to the optician and was told I only had a bit of a cataract. Also I do not need to see an optician for two years. I could not believe it... So very, very many thanks. My husband went to the optician last week, and he is just starting to form a cataract in his right eye. Needless to say he will be using carnosine eye drops."

—J.C.

"In October 2002, I was diagnosed with a small cataract in my left eye. Shortly afterwards a work colleague told me about the eye drops as seen on channel 4 'Richard & Judy.' I started using them. In April 2004, I had an in-depth eye test: NO SIGN OF THE CATARACT."

—M.S.

See for yourself

As a preventive, the suggested use of OcuPhase is one or two drops in each eye every day. Those with any kind of eye problem may want to apply one or two drops several times a day. Most people report that they start noticing positive results over a three to six month period. Early intervention allows OcuPhase to work even better, since the lens is more permeable in the early stages.

Keep in mind that even though this treatment can be done in the comfort of your own home, it's always a good idea to work with your healthcare provider to assure safety and to monitor your progress.

CHAPTER NINETEEN

Keep your bladder healthy naturally with this exclusive herb & mineral blend

There's a strange irony in modern society in that the most hushed topics are often the ones that need the most discussion. And bladder health is typically on that list of taboo subjects. So let's open it up and talk about what you can do now to keep your bladder strong and toned for the long haul, starting with a formula available from NorthStar Nutritionals called UroConfidence.™ UroConfidence was specifically designed to help support bladder tone and function. The bladder is, after all, a muscle. And just as the other muscles in your body need nourishment, so does your bladder.

Define "normal"

So just what is "normal" bladder function? Typically, people empty their bladders about every three to four hours during the day. And it's not unusual to get up once during the night to use the bathroom. Keep in mind as well that some bladder issues—like urgency and frequency—can be indications of larger problems. These problems can only be determined during an examination. So, as always, if you develop any of these symptoms or any other serious health conditions, or if you are currently taking any medications or supplements, you should consult with your health-care provider.

Power-packed plants

The natural ingredients in UroConfidence work together to improve the tone of the bladder wall and the surrounding area—supporting the bladder's ability to correctly and efficiently fill and empty. The two signature ingredients are the herbs Crateva nurvala and Equisetum arvense. Crateva comes from a small tree (commonly known as the three-leaf caper) often found along riverbanks and cultivated throughout India, where it's traditionally used to maintain bladder health.

Preliminary studies (one on dogs and one on 30 human subjects) involving traditional Ayurvedic therapies show that Crateva helps support bladder tone and function. The Crateva used in UroConfidence is actually a special, high-potency extract called Cratevox.™ Cratevox ensures the strength and absorbability of each capsule thanks to a specialized extraction method.

Equisetum arvense (more commonly known as horsetail) acts as a mild diuretic, which is soothing to the urinary tract. Its toning and astringent properties make it useful for maintaining healthy urinary function. It also has antispasmodic effects, which support the bladder sphincter.

A noticeable difference
in just a few weeks

While research is preliminary, it does offer some insight into the product's potential. A pilot study showed improvements for over 80 percent of subjects in bladder frequency, leakage, urgency and bladder discomfort. A larger scale placebo-controlled trial also showed improved bladder symptoms of incontinence, frequency, nocturia, urgency and bladder discomfort for 85 percent of participants. The results suggested that the preparation was suitable and effective for both men and women. According to the manufacturer, UroConfidence has

The Bladder-Strengthening Exercise
You Can Do Anytime, Anywhere

You also may want to consider adding your bladder to your exercise routine. Kegel exercises help strengthen the muscles that control the bladders of both men and women. They can be done anytime, anywhere (and without anyone else knowing).

Kegel Exercises:

• To locate the right muscles, try stopping or slowing your urine flow.

• Squeeze your muscles. Hold for a count of 10. Relax for a count of 10.

• Repeat this movement 20 times.

• Repeat the above steps three to four times a day.

You may need to start slower, perhaps squeezing and relaxing your muscles for four seconds each and doing this 10 times, three or four times a day. Work your way up from there. It will take about three to six months before you'll see any improvement, so don't get discouraged.

no recorded side effects and is not known to interfere with any prescription drugs or supplements. Of course, you should always consult with your healthcare practitioner for advice on any interactions. Although very unlikely, there is some evidence to indicate that Equisetum may enhance the effects of diuretic blood pressure drugs.

The suggested dosage as a dietary supplement is two capsules in the morning and two capsules at night with meals for the first two to three months.

About 50 percent of people notice an effect within three weeks, but give it some time. UroConfidence's herbal ingredients need a couple of months to build up in your system. Optimal effects are usually achieved in two to three months. At that point, you may be able to lower your dosage by half for maintenance.

Please note: HSI doesn't accept fees from outside companies for editorial coverage. However, NorthStar Nutritionals is one of HSI's dietary supplement affiliate companies. Even though we would never recommend any product we don't believe in, you should know about that relationship when deciding whether to try their products.

Member Source Directory

Açaí, Sambazon Global Headquarters. 1160 Calle Cordillera, San Clemente, CA 92673. Tel: (877)726-2296; www.sambazon.com; (see website for retail availability at Whole Foods markets.)

AdvaCal Calcium Supplement, LaneLabs. Tel: (800)510-2010; www.lanelabs.com. AdvaCal costs US$28.95 per bottle, but HSI Members get special pricing with coupon code HSIB2G1A. Buy 2 bottles of AdvaCal and you'll receive a bonus bottle FREE.

AllerPhase, Tango Advanced Nutrition. Tel: (866)778-2646; www.puretango.com. A 30-capsule bottle costs US$39.95 plus shipping.

AMAS Cancer Test, Oncolab, Inc. Tel: (800)922-8378; www.oncolabinc.com.

Ambrotose and **Ambrotose AO,** Mannatech, Inc. 600 S. Royal Lane, Suite 200, Coppell, TX 75019. Tel: (800)281-4469; www.mannatech.com.

Amyloban 3399, Mushroom Wisdom, Inc. Tel: (800)747-7418; www.MushroomWisdom.com. Amyloban 3399 normally costs US$89.95, but HSI members will get a 15% discount by using code HSI-AML (both online and phone orders).

Arjuna, Himalaya Herbal Healthcare. 1101 Gillingham Lane, Sugar Land, TX 77478. Tel: (800)869-4640 or (713)863-1622; www.himalayausa.com. A 60-caplet bottle costs US$17.95 plus shipping.

ArthriPhase, Tango Advanced Nutrition. Tel: (866)778-2646 or (805)504-9563, ext. 1; www.puretango.com. One bottle of 60 capsules costs US$39.95 plus shipping.

Astafactor, Mera Pharmaceuticals, Inc. 73-4460 Queen Ka'ahumanu Hwy., Suite 110, Kailua Kona, HI 96740; Tel: (800)480-6515 or (808)326-9301; www.astafactor.com.

AvéULTRA (Avemar fermented wheat germ extract), The Harmony Company. P.O. Box 567, Valley Cottage, NY 10989. Tel: (800)521-0543; www.theharmonycompany.com. A box of 30 single-serving packets costs US$199.95 plus shipping.

Botanical Vitality 200+, Great Life Labs. Tel: (800)526-4240; www.greatlife.com. A bottle of 60 capsules (a 30-day supply) is US$36.00 plus shipping.

Brain Protex, The Herbs Place. 27 Fleetwood Dr, Palmyra, VA 22963; Tel: (434)591-1249; www.theherbsplace.com. A 60-capsule bottle of Brain Protex is normally US$25.15.

Breast-Mate™, Mushroom Wisdom, Inc. Tel: (800)747-7418; www.mushroomwisdom.com. One bottle normally costs US$59.95 plus shipping, but HSI Members can save 15 percent by mentioning code HS-BM (both online and phone orders).

C-Statin, Aidan Products. Tel: (800)529-0269; www.aidanproducts.com. A bottle of C-Statin is US$98.00.

Cat's Claw (contains TOA), Rainforest Natural Products, Inc. Tel: (305)235-9880; www.rainpharm.com.

Cat's Claw—TOA-free (Prima Una De Gato), NutriCology. 2300 North Loop Rd., Alameda, CA 94502. Tel: (800)545-9960; www.nutricology.com. A 90-caplet bottle of Cat's Claw is US$110.78.

Cesium Chloride, The Wolfe Clinic. Tel: 1-877-359-6950; www.shopthewolfeclinic.com. Call the clinic for more information and pricing.

Citrus Bergamot, Herbal Powers. Tel: (877)903-9657; www.herbal-powers.com. Citrus Bergamot costs US$34.95 per bottle.

Cognizin, Healthy Origins. Tel: (888)228-6650; www.healthyorigins.com. You can buy Cognizin at a discount by mentioning HSI (no code is needed on the website): A 30-count bottle of Cognizin normally costs US$19.99.

Concentrated Flax Hull Lignans, Flax Lignan Health. Tel: (817)710-6918; www.FlaxLignanHealth.com. One tub of FHL Concentrated Flax Hull Lignans (a one-month supply) costs US$36.00. You can also Buy 2 and Get 1 Free for the price of $72.00, but HSI members will receive an additional $5 off when using the Buy 2 Get 1 Free offer. Simply use code VAULT5.

Corvalen M, Douglas Labs. Tel: (800)245-4440; www.douglaslabs.com. A 12-oz. jar of powder costs US$60.

CSI Anti-Aging Fruit Stem Cell Serum, Vitacost.com. Tel: (800)381-0759; www.vitacost.com. One bottle costs US$20.00 plus shipping.

Del-Immune V, Pure Research Products. 6107 Chelsea Manor Court, Boulder, Colorado, 80301. Tel: (888)466-8635; www.delimmune.com. A 30-capsule bottle costs US$19.50 plus shipping. Discounts offered when ordering in bulk.

Digest RC, CX Research, Inc. Tel: (855)773-7755; www.cxresearch.net. A 30-tablet pack costs US$17.95, plus shipping.

EaseFemin, Natura Nectar. Tel: (800)609-7794; www.naturanectar.com. EaseFemin costs US$30.99 per box, but HSI Members will get a 15% discount plus free shipping when they mention code BESTALERT.

Eczema Rescue, Peaceful Mountain. Tel: (888)303-3388; www.peaceful mountain.com. A 1-oz. tube of Eczema Rescue is US$15.95 plus shipping.

EpiCor®, Embria Health Sciences. Tel: (877)362-7421; www.epicorimmune.com.

Farabloc, Farabloc Development Corp.; www.farabloc.com.

Femmenessence MacaHarmony, Natural Health International. Tel: (415)243-9991; www.naturalhi.com. One box is US$34.99.

GalantaMind (Galantamine), Life Enhancement Products, Inc. P.O. Box 751390, Petaluma, CA 94975-1390; Tel: (800)543-3873 or (775)783-1600; www.life-enhancement.com.

Glabrinex, Vitamin Research Products. Tel: (800)877-2447; www.vrp.com. A bottle of 90 capsules is US$64.95 plus shipping.

GlucoComplete, Real Advantage Nutrients. Tel: (800)913-2602 or (443)353-4306; www.RealAdvantageNutrients.com. GlucoComplete normally costs US$49.95, but HSI Members are entitled to a special 20% discount. Simply use code G655M602 when you order.

Glucotor v.2, Baseline Nutritionals. Tel: (800)440-3120; www.baselinenutritionals.com. A 180-capsule bottle costs US$49.95 plus shipping.

Healthy Prostate & Ovary, Nutricology. Tel: (800)545-9960; www.nutricology.com. A 180-tablet bottle costs US$59.03 plus shipping.

Homocysteine Formula, Vitacost. Tel: (800)381-0759; www.vitacost.com. A 60-capsule bottle costs US$9.59 plus shipping.

Huanarpo Macho, Rainforest Natural Products, Inc. Tel: (305)235-9880; www.rainpharm.com. A 2 oz. bottle costs $25 plus shipping.

ImmPower (AHCC), Harmony Company. P.O. Box 567, Valley Cottage, NY 10989. Tel: (800)521-0543; www.theharmonycompany.com. US$54.95 (30 capsules 500mg) plus US$9.95 for shipping.

JIPANG Ginger, Makise Lifeup International. Tel: (808)537-2050; www.makiselifeupusa.com. JIPANG Ginger costs US$50 for a 60-capsule bottle.

KGP Flush, Baseline Nutritionals. Tel: (800)440-3120; www.baselinenutritionals.com. One 4 oz bottle costs US$49.95 plus shipping. HSI members are entitled to exclusive savings: Buy one bottle and get a second bottle for 25% off. Simply use coupon code HSIKGP9 when you order. You can also purchase the tincture as part of Baseline's Liver Detox Kit (including Liver Tea, Liver Tincture, Blood Support, and Colon Corrective) for $170.00.

Kold Kare, Kare N Herbs. Tel: 1-800-774-9444; www.karenherbs.com. A pack of 40 tablets is $15.95, plus shipping.

L-Tryptophan, Vitamin Research Products. Tel: (888)362-1699; www.vrp.com. A 90-capsule bottle of L-Tryptophan is $39.00 plus shipping.

Lactoferrin Caps, Life Extension Foundation. Tel: (800)544-4440; www.lef.com. A 60-capsule bottle of Lactoferrin Caps costs US$52.

Lyprinol, LyprinolUSA, LLC. 2215-B Renaissance Drive, Las Vegas, NV 89119. Tel: (888)433-6223 or (480)829-0154; www.lyprinolusa.com. A 60-capsule bottle of Lyprinol costs $49.95 plus $9.95 shipping.

MigraSpray, Nature Well, Inc., 110 West C Street, Suite 1300, San Diego, CA 92101. Tel: (800)454-6790; www.migraspray.com. 1 bottle costs US$39.95 plus US$7.95 for shipping.

MindCare, Himalaya Herbal Healthcare. 1101 Gillingham Lane, Sugar Land, TX 77478. Tel: (800)869-4640 or (713)863-1622; Fax: (713)863-1686; www.himalayausa.com. A 60-capsule bottle of MindCare costs US$20.95, and a 120-capsule bottle costs $35.95.

Mitochondria Ignite (with NT Factor), ProHealth. 2040 Alameda Padre Serra, Santa Barbara, CA 93103. Tel: (800)366-6056; www.prohealth.com; One bottle of 90 tablets costs US$51.49 plus shipping.

Modifilan (Fucoidan), Fucoidan Sales. Tel: (877)516-5433; Fax: (913)856-0212; www.Fucoidan.net. 1 bottle of 90 capsules costs US$29.00 plus shipping.

Mucolyxir, NutriCology. Tel: (800)545-9960 or (510)263-2000; Fax: (800)688-7426; www.nutricology.com. 12 ml liquid is US$41.57 plus shipping.

NattoZyme (Nattokinase), NutriCology. Tel: (800)545-9960, www.nutricology.com. A 90-capsule bottle of NattoZyme costs US$53.56 plus shipping.

NEO40 Daily lozenges and test strips, Neogenis Labs, Tel: (855)NEO-4040 [855-636-4040]; www.neogenis.com. One box of NEO40 Daily lozenges costs US$59.95, and one package of Neogenis Test Strips costs US$21.95. Products are available only in the US.

NGF, Vitamin Research Products. Tel: (888)362-1699 or (817)785-4652; www.vrp.com. One bottle of 120 capsules costs US$59.95 plus shipping.

N-Tense, Rainforest Natural Products, Inc. Tel. (305)235-9880; www.rainpharm.com.

OcuPhase Eyedrops, Tango Advanced Nutrition. Tel: (866)778-2646 or (805)504-9563; www.puretango.com. A box of 2x5 ml vials costs US$39.95, but HSI Members will receive 10% off their order when they use coupon code OCU2.

Olive Leaf Extract, Seagate. Tel: (888)505-4283; www.seagateproducts.com. One bottle of 90 capsules is US$29.95. One 1 oz bottle of nasal spray is US$9.99.

Osteoking, Crystal Natural Pharmaceutical Corp. www.osteoking.com. A one-month supply (15 bottles) costs US$118 plus shipping (free shipping to USA).

Osteophase, Tango Advanced Nutrition. Tel: (866)778-2646 or (805)504-9563; www.puretango.com. A 60-capsule bottle costs US$39.95 plus shipping.

Ostera, Metagenics. Tel: (800)921-4271; www.thenaturalonline.com. A bottle of 60 tablets is US$53.95.

Ostinol™, ZyCal Bioceuticals, Inc., Tel: (888)779-9225; www.zycalbio.com. A 30-capsule bottle costs US$79 with 350mg capsules and US$109 with 450mg capsules.

Padma Basic, Econugenics. Tel: (800)308-5518; www.econugenics.com. A 180-tablet bottle is US$99.95 plus shipping and handling.

PectaSol-C, Econugenics. Tel: (800)308-5518; www.econugenics.com. PectaSol-C costs $34.95 per bottle of 90 capsules. HSI members can get one bottle free when they buy three, or two bottles free when they buy five. Simply mention HSI when ordering to take advantage of this special deal.

Peri-Gum, Lesko Care, L.L.C. Tel: (908)272-3081; www.peri-gum.com. A 1 oz. bottle of concentrate is US$21.00 plus $4.95 shipping and handling. Online orders only, using PayPal. Website also offers individual state listings of retailers carrying Peri-Gum or by mail at Lesko Care, LLC 18 Connecticut Street, Cranford, NJ 07016.

Phytocort, NutriCology. Tel: (800)545-9960; www.nutricology.com. One bottle of 120 capsules costs US$47.70.

Policosanol, Life Extension Foundation. Tel: (954)766-8144; www.lef.org. One bottle (60 tablets) is US$20.00 plus shipping.

Prelief®, DSE Healthcare, LLC. Tel: (800)338-8079; www.prelief.com. One bottle of Prelief® (120 tablets) is US$13.00 plus shipping and handling.

ProstaCaid, Econugenics. Tel: (800)308-5518; www.prostacaid.org. ProstaCaid normally costs $99.95 per 120-capsule bottle, but HSI Members can get one bottle free when they buy three, or two bottles free when they buy five. Simply mention HSI when ordering to take advantage of these special deals.

Raphacholin C®, QLIFE Inc. Fax: (973)633-8410; www.qlife.mybigcommerce.com. A pack of 30 tablets costs US$10.00, plus shipping.

RegeneCell, NorthStar Nutritionals. Tel: (800)913-2592 or (443)353-4354; www.northstarnutritionals.com. A 30-day supply is $399.95 plus shipping, but HSI Members will receive 20% off their RegeneCell purchase when using coupon code WNSNS2AA.

Resprin, Resprin, Inc. Tel: (877)473-7774; Email: customerservice@resprin.com; www.resprin.com. A bottle of 90 capsules is US$26.99 plus shipping.

Samento, Vitamin Research Products. Tel: (800)877-2447; www.vrp.com. One bottle of Samento costs US$44.95.

Seacure, Proper Nutrition, Inc. Tel: (800)555-8868 or (610)939-0414; www.propernutrition.com. Seacure costs US$48.49 for 180 capsules.

Seditol, Pure Encapsulations. Tel: (800)753-2277; www.pureencapsulations.com. A bottle of 60 capsules costs $54.00.

Seratonin, NutriCology. Tel: (800)545-9960; www.nutricology.com. One bottle of 90 capsules costs US$56.24 plus shipping.

Serrapeptase, The Green Willow Tree. Tel: (828)254-3220; Fax: (208)330-2445; www.greenwillowtree.com. A bottle of Serrapeptase is US$42.98, plus shipping.

Sleep Apnea Relief, Nature's Rite. Tel: (888)465-4404; www.mynaturesrite.com. One bottle costs US$45.99, but if you buy three or more bottles, you will save 10 percent.

Soothanol X2, NorthStar Nutritionals. Tel: (800)913-2592, www.northstarnutritionals.com. A 1 oz bottle is US$49.95 plus $6.95 shipping and handling ($14.95 outside the USA. Cannot fulfill orders to Australia, Germany, Austria or New Zealand). HSI Members will receive 20% off their Soothanol X2 purchase when using coupon code WNSNS2BB.

StemEnhance, E3Live. Tel: (888)800-7070; www.E3Live.com. A bottle of 60 capsules (a one-month supply) is US$70.95 plus shipping.

SUGARSolve, Harmony Company. P.O. Box 567, Valley Cottage, NY 10989; Tel: (800)521-0543; www.theharmonyco.com. A bottle of SUGARSolve costs US$29.95 for 60 softgels.

Super Royal Agaricus, Agaricus Blazei Murill Extract (ABM), Mushroom Wisdom, Inc. Tel: (800)747-7418; www.mushroomwisdom.com. A bottle of Super Royal Agaricus costs US$34.95 plus shipping.

SynerFlex, NorthStar Nutritionals. Tel: (800)913-2592 or (443)353-4354; www.northstarnutritionals.com. A 30 day supply is US$39.95 plus US$6.95 shipping and handling (US$14.95 outside the USA. Additional duties and fees may apply upon delivery. Not available in Australia, Austria, or Germany). HSI Members will receive 20% off their Synerflex purchase when using coupon code WNSNS2CC.

Syntra5, Syntratech. Tel: (888) 447-4898; www.BloodSugarHealth.com. A one month supply (180 count bottle) normally costs US$69.87, but HSI members pay only US$59.87, an exclusive 15% discount on a single bottle, or HSI members can buy two 180-count bottles at the discount price AND get one free. Product only available in the U.S., Canada, Australia, and the United Kingdom.

Taurox 6X (COBAT), NutriCology. Tel: (800)545-9960 or (510)263-2000; Fax: (510)263-2100; www.nutricology.com. A 13.5 ml bottle of Taurox 6X costs US$49.47 plus shipping.

Toki Collagen Drink, LaneLabs. Tel: (800)510-2010; Fax: (201)236-0090; www.lanelabs.com. Toki costs US$175.00 per box, but HSI members get special pricing: Buy 2 boxes and save $100 with coupon code HSI100T.

Ultra H-3, Uni Key Health Systems, Inc., 181 West Commerce Drive, Hayden Lake, ID 83835 Tel: (800)888-4353; www.unikeyhealth.com. A bottle of Ultra H-3 costs US$34.50 plus shipping.

UroConfidence, NorthStar Nutritionals. Tel: (800)913-2592; www.northstarnutritionals.com. A one-month supply (60-capsules) is US$49.95 plus $6.95 shipping ($14.95 shipping outside the USA. Cannot fulfill orders to Australia, Germany, Austria or New Zealand). HSI Members will receive 20% off their UroConfidence purchase when using coupon code WNSNS2DD.

Vasotensin, Center for Natural Medicine Dispensary. 1330 S.E. 39th Avenue, Portland, OR 97214. Tel: (888)305-4288 or (503)232-1100; www.mmilner.metagenics.com. A 120-tablet bottle of Vasotensin costs US$57.25.

Vital Cell, Tango Advanced Nutrition. Tel: (866)778-2646; www.puretango.com. A 180-capsule bottle costs US$39.95 plus shipping.

Wound Honey, Eras Natural Sciences. Tel: (800)308-6284; www.woundhoney.com. One 80-g tube is US$19.95.

*Please note: HSI verifies all product information when reports are written; however, pricing and availability can change by the time reports are delivered. We regret that not all products and services are available in all locations worldwide.

The above statements have not been evaluated by the U.S. Food and Drug Administration. These products are not intended to diagnose, treat, cure or prevent any disease.

References

Part I: Pain

Ancient herb meets modern science to slash rheumatoid arthritis symptoms in half

[1] Wurm M, Kacani L et al "Pentacyclic oxindole alkaloids from uncaria tomentosa induce human endothelial cells" *Planta Med* 1998 Dec;64(8):701-704

[2] Keplinger K, Laus G et al "Uncaria tomentosa (Willd.) DC.—ethnomedicinal use and new pharmacological, toxicological and botanical results" *J Ethnopharmacol* 1999 Jan;64(1):23-34

[3] Reinhard KH "Uncaria tomentosa (Willd.) DC:cat's claw, una de gato, or saventaro" *J Altern Complement Med* 1999 Apr;5(2):143-151

[4] ibid

[5] Somova LO et al "Cardiovascular, antihyperlipidemic and antioxidant effects of oleanolic and ursolic acids in experimental hypertension" *Phytomedicine* 2003 Mar;10(2-3):115-21

Breakthrough Chinese formula sends drug-resistant joint pain packing

[1] Newman NM, Ling RS. "Acetabular bone destruction related to non-steroidal anti-inflammatory drugs." *Lancet.* 1985 Jul 6'2(8845):11-4.

Eliminate excruciating kidney pain for good with this all-in-one stone-crushing cure

[1] Barros, ME, et. al. "Effects of an aqueous extract from Phyllanthus niruri on calcium oxalate crystallization in vitro." *Urol. Res.* 2003; 30(6): 374-9.

[2] Campos, AH, et. al. "Phyllanthus niruri inhibits calcium oxalate endocytosis by renal tubular cells: its role in urolithiasis." *Nephron.* 1999;81(4):393-97.

[3] Nakagiri R, Hashizume E, Kayahashi S, et. al. "Suppression by Hydrageae Dulcis Folium of D-galactosamine-induced liver injury in vitro and in vivo." *Biosci Biotechnol Biochem.* 2003 Dec;67(12):2641-3.

Your glucosamine supplement could be useless… Uncover the secret source of your joint discomfort

[1] Blanco. (2005). "Study of the differences between the Hyal-Joint and hyaluronic acid ex fermentation on synovial fluid." *Bioiberica.*

[2] Kalman, Douglas, et al. (2008). Effect of a natural extract of chicken combs with a high content of hyaluronic acid (Hyal-Joint) on pain relief and quality of life in subjects with knee osteoarthritis: a pilot random-

ized double blond placebo-controlled trial. *Nutrition Journal* 7(3).

[3] DeLuca, Hector. (2002) Calcium fructoborate (Fruitex B) increases bone density in vitamin D depleted rats. Department of Biochemistry, University of Wisconsin.

[4] Miljkovic, Natasa. (2002) Osteoarthritis and calcium fructoborate supplementation: An open-label pilot study. Department of Orthopedic Medicine, University of Novi Sad, Novi Sad, Yugoslavia.

Soothe your pain on contact

[1] *Lancet* 2000;355(9199): 233-34

[2] Reuters Health Information, April 23, 2000

Want relief from migraine headaches? A few drops under the tongue may be all you need...

[1] Murphy JJ, Heptistall S, Mitchell JR "Randomized double-blind placebo-controlled trial of feverfew in migraine preparations" *Lancet* 1988 Jul;2(8604):189-192

[2] Johnson ES, Kadam NP, et al "Efficacy of feverfew as prophylactic treatment of migraine" *Br Med J* (Clin Res Ed) 1985 Aug;291(6495):569-573

[3] www.migraspray.com

[4] Hoffman D Herbal Materia Medica http://www.healthy.net

[5] Felter HW, Lloyd JU King's American Dispensatory http://www.ibilio.org/herbmed

[6] Blum JM, Marshall P, "Herbal someopathic support for the treatment of migraine-type headache symptoms" Executive Summary, NatureWell Inc. LaJolla CA Aug 29, 2001

[7] Miller LG "Herbal medicinals: selected clinical considerations focusing on known or potential drug-herb interactions." *Arch Intern Med* 1998 Nov;158(20):2200-2211

[8] ibid

Tibetan medicine relieves chronic leg pain

[1] MCP Hahnemann University Libraries, Health Reviews on the Internet, "A Meta-analysis of the Treatment of Intermittent Claudication," Richard Neil, M.D.

[2] Schweizerische Medizinische Wochenschrift 1985;115(22): 752-56

[3] *Angiology* 1998;44(11): 863-67

[4] *Journal of Vascular Investigation* 1998;4: 129-36

[5] *The Express*, March 31, 1999

[6] *Annales Academiae Medicae Stetinensis* 1991;37: 191-202

Raw bar favorite offers arthritis relief

[1] *Practioner* 1980; 224: 955-60
[2] *Gazette Medicale* 1986; 93(38): 111-16
[3] *Inflammopharmacology* 1997;5 : 237-46
[4] *Allergie et Immunologie* 2000; 32(7): 272-78

Part II: Cancer

The Lactoferrin miracle

[1] *Japanese Journal of Cancer Research* 1997;88: 184-190
[2] *Cancer Research* 1994;54(9): 2310-2312
[3] *Advances in Experimental Medicine and Biology* 1994;357: 143-156
[4] *Journal of Ocular Pharmacology and Therapeutics* 1998;14(2): 99-107
[5] *Medical Microbiology and Immunology* 1993;182(2): 97-105
[6] *Antiviral Research* 2001;52(3): 225-39

Discover the cancer-fighting potential of Brazil's "Mushroom of God"

[1] *Agricultural and Biological Chemistry* 1990;54(11): 2897-2906
[2] *Bioscience, Biotechnology, and Biochemistry* 1998;62(3): 434
[3] *Cell Structure and Function* 2001;26(2): 103-8
[4] *Journal of Nutrition* 2001;131(5): 1409-13
[5] *Japanese Journal of Pharmacology* 1994;66(2): 265-71
[6] *Biotherapy* 1998;11(4): 259-65

This overlooked 'waste product' may be the cancer-fighting breakthrough of the century

[1] Chen, J; Stavro, PM; Thompson, LU. Dietary flaxseed inhibits human breast cancer growth and metastasis and downregulates expression of insulin-like growth factor and epidermal growth factor receptor. *Nutr Cancer.* 2002;43(2):187-92.
[2] Thompson, LU; Chen, GM; Li, T; Strasser-Weippi, K; Goss, PE. Dietary flaxseed alters tumor biological markers in postmenopausal breast cancer. *Cancer Res.* 2005 May 15;11(10):3828-35.
[3] Li, D; Yee, JA; Thompson, LU; Yan, L. Dietary supplementation with secoisolariciresinol diglycoside (SDG) reduces experimental metastasis of melanoma cells in mice. *Cancer Lett.* 1999 July 19; 142(1):91-6.
[4] Horn-Ross, Pamela L.; John, Esther M.; Canchola, Alison J.; Stewart, Susan L.; Lee, Marion M. Phytoestrogen Intake and Endometrial Cancer Risk. *J Natl Cancer Inst.* 2003;95:1158-1164.
[5] Cotterchio, Michelle; Boucher, Beatrice A.; Manno, Michael; Gallinger,

Steven; Okey, Allan; Harper, Patricia. Dietary phytoestrogen intake is associated with reduced colorectal cancer risk. *Journal of Nutrition.* December 2006;136:3046-3053.

[6] Rossi, Marta; Negri, Eva; Talamini, Renato; et al. Flavonoids and colorectal cancer in Italy. *Cancer Epidemiology Biomarkers and Prevention.* August 2006;15:1555-1558.

[7] Obermeyer W, et al (US Food and Drug Administration, Center for Food Safety and Applied Nutrition, Div. Contaminants Chem., Natural Products Branch), Meeting of the Federation of American Societies for Experimental Biology March/April 1993, Faseb J (Fed Am Soc Exp Biol), A863, 1993.

[8] Vanharanta, M; Voutilainen, S; Rissanen, TH; Adlercreutz, H; Salonen, JT. Risk of cardiovascular disease-related and all-cause death according to serum concentrations of enterolactone: Kuopio Ischaemic Heart Disease Risk Factor Study. Arch Intern Med. 2003;163(9):1099-1104.

[9] Prasad, K. Hypocholesterolemic and antiatherosclerotic effect of flax lignan complex isolated from flaxseed. *Atherosclerosis.* 2005 April;179(2):269-275.

[10] Patade, A; Devareddy, L; Lucas, EA; Korlagunta, K; Daggy, BP; Arjmandi, BH. Flaxseed reduces total and LDL cholesterol concentrations in Native American postmenopausal women. *Womens Health.* 2008 March 8. [Epub ahead of print].

[11] "Flax Lignan Ingredient May Reduce Prostate Size." Flax Lignan Information Bureau. 2005 May. http://www.flaxlignaninfo.com.

[12] Demark-Wahnefried, W; Price, DT; Polascik, TJ; Robertson, CN; Anderson, EE; Paulson, DF; Walther, PJ; Gannon, M; Vollmer, RT. Pilot study of dietary fat restriction and flaxseed supplementation in men with prostate cancer before surgery: exploring the effects on hormonal levels, prostate-specific antigen, and histopathologic features. *Urology.* 2001;58:47–52.

[13] AIDS Research Assistance Institute

The metal that shrinks tumors within weeks—your blood will actually REPEL cancer

[1] Brewer, A. Keith. (1984) The high pH therapy for cancer, tests on mice and humans. Pharmacology, Biochemistry, and Behavior 12(supp. 1): 1-5.

[2] "Cesium chloride: Alternative cancer treatment." Alternative Cancer Treatments: Comparison and Testing. http://alternativecancer.us.

[3] "Liquid Cesium Chloride / DMSO - Directly Targets and Kills Cancer Cells and Stops Pain." Alternative Cancer Treatment. Puna Wai Ora Mind-Body Center. http://www.alternative-cancer-care.com.

[4] Howenstine, James. (2004) Use of cesium chloride to cure malignancies. Newswithviews.com.

"Choking" weed starves tumors by cutting off blood supply

[1] Oudhia P., and Tripathi R.S. (1998) Medicinal weeds of kharif crops in the plains of Chhattisgarh. Bhartiya Krishi Anusandhan Patrika 13(1/2):33-38.

[2] Meng, X.L., et al. (2002) Effects of a high molecular mass Convolvulus arvensis extract on tumor growth and angiogenesis. *P R Health Sci J* 21(4):323-8.

[3] Riordan, N.H., et al. (2000) Anti-angiogenic, anti-tumor, and immunostimulatory effects of a non-toxic plant extract (PGM). Presented at Comprehensive Cancer Care 2000, Arlington, VA.

The magic mushroom formula that can conquer breast cancer

[1] D. Sliva, et al. Phellinus linteus suppresses growth, angiogenesis and invasive behaviour of cancer cells through the inhibition of AKT signalling. *British Journal of Cancer* (2008)

[2] T. Sasaki, et al. Antitumor polysaccharides from some Polyporaceae, Ganoderma applanatum (PERS.) PAT[1]) and Phellinus linteus (BERK. et CURT) AOSHIMA[2]). *Chem. Pharm. Bull.* (1971)

[3] T. Lu, et al. Hispolon from Phellinus linteus has antiproliferative effects via MDM2-recruited ERK1/2 activity in breast and bladder cancer cells. *Food and Chemical Toxicology* (2009)

[4] Kumar KMP, Dharmalingham M. Evaluation of clinical efficacy of Diabecon with reference to insulin-levels in diabetic patients. *Medicine Update* (2002)

[5] Preuss, H., et al. Enhanced insulin-hypoglycemic activity in rats consuming a specific glycoprotein extracted from maitake mushroom. *Molecular and Cellular Biochemistry* (2007)

[6] I. Wolf, et al. Diabetes mellitus and breast cancer. *Lancet Oncology* (2005)

[7] G.C. Kabat, et al. A longitudinal study of the metabolic syndrome and risk of postmenopausal breast cancer. *Cancer Epidemiology, Biomarkers & Prevention* (2009)

[8] P. Pasanisi, et al. Metabolic syndrome as a prognostic factor for breast cancer recurrences. *International Journal of Cancer* (2006)

[9] Bradlow, H.L., et al. Indole-3-carbinol. A novel approach to breast cancer prevention. *Annals of the New York Academy of Sciences* (1995)

[10] Cover, C. M., et al. Indole-3-carbinol and tamoxifen cooperate to arrest the cell cycle of MCF-7 human breast cancer cells. *Cancer Research* (1999)

[11] Chatterji, U., et al. Indole-3-carbinol stimulates transcription of the

interferon gamma receptor 1 gene and augments interferon responsiveness in human breast cancer cells. *Carcinogenesis* (2004)

[12] Nakachi, K., et al. Influence of drinking green tea on breast cancer malignancy among Japanese patients. *Japanese Journal of Cancer Research* (1998)

[13] Chen, Z. P., et al. Green tea epigallocatechin gallate shows a pronounced growth inhibitor effect on cancerous cells but not on their normal counterparts. *Cancer Letters* (1998)

[14] Liao, S., et al. Growth inhibition and regression of human prostate and breast tumors in athymic mice by tea epigallocatechin gallate. *Cancer Letters* (1995)

[15] Shrubsole, et al. Dietary folate intake and breast cancer risk: results from the Shanghai Breast Cancer Study. *Cancer Research.* (2001)

Defeat even advanced prostate cancer with "killer" herbs

[1] Guess, B.W., et al. Modified citrus pectin (MCP) increases the prostate-specific antigen doubling time in men with prostate cancer: a phase II pilot study. *Prostate Cancer and Prostatic Diseases* (2003) 6, 301–304.

[2] Azemar, M, et al. Clinical benefit in patients with advanced solid tumors treated with modified citrus pectin: a prospective pilot study. *Clinical Medicine: Oncology.* 2007:1, 73-80.

[3] Yan, J. and A. Katz. PectaSol-C Modified Citrus Pectin Induces Apoptosis and Inhibition of Proliferation in Human and Mouse Androgen-Dependent and–Independent Prostate Cancer Cells. *Integrative Cancer Therapies.* 9(2) 197-203, 2010.

[4] Yan, J. and A. Katz. ProstaCaid Induces G2/M Cell Cycle Arrest and Apoptosis in Human and Mouse Androgen-Dependent and–Independent Prostate Cancer Cells. *Integrative Cancer Therapies.* 9(2) 186-196, 2010.

[5] Nachshon-Kedmi, M., et al. Induction of apoptosis in human prostate cancer cell line, PC3, by 3,3'-diindolylmethane through the mitochondrial pathway. *Br J Cancer.* 91(7):1358-1363, 2004.

[6] Garikapaty, V. P., et al. 3,3'-Diindolylmethane downregulates pro-survival pathway in hormone independent prostate cancer. *Biochem Biophys Res Commun.* 340(2):718-725, 2006.

[7] Nachshon-Kedmi, M., et al. Therapeutic activity of 3,3'-diindolylmethane on prostate cancer in an in vivo model. *Prostate.* 61(2):153-160, 2004.

[8] Durak, I., et al. Aqueous extract of urtica dioica makes significant inhibition on adenosine deaminase activity in prostate tissue from patients with prostate cancer. *Cancer Biol Ther.* 3(9), 2004.

[9] Konrad, L., et al. Antiproliferative effect on human prostate cancer cells by a stinging nettle root (Urtica dioica) extract. *Planta Medica.* 66(1):44-47, 2000.

[10] Chen, S., et al. Effects of the flavonoid baicalin and its metabolite baicalein on androgen receptor expression, cell cycle progression and apoptosis of prostate cancer cell lines. *Cell Prolif.* 34(5):293-304, 2001.

[11] Zhang, D. Y., et al. Inhibition of cancer cell proliferation and prostaglandin E2 synthesis by Scutellaria baicalensis. *Cancer Res.* 63(14):4037-4043, 2003.

[12] Mantena, S. K., et al. Berberine, a natural product, induces G1-phase cell cycle arrest and caspase-3-dependent apoptosis in human prostate carcinoma cells. *Mol Cancer Ther.* 5(2):296-308, 2006.

[13] Pantuck, A. J., et al. American Urological Association Annual Meeting. San Antonio, USA. May 21-26, 2005.

[14] Albrecht, M., et al. Pomegranate extracts potently suppress proliferation, xenograft growth, and invasion of human prostate cancer cells. *J Med Food.* 7(3):274-283, 2004.

[15] Malik, A., et al. Prostate cancer prevention through pomegranate fruit. *Cell Cycle.* 5(4), 2006.

[16] Malik, A., et al. Pomegranate fruit juice for chemoprevention and chemotherapy of prostate cancer. *Proc Natl Acad Sci U S A.* 102(41):14813-14818, 2005.

[17] Jiang, J., et al. Ganoderma lucidum inhibits proliferation and induces apoptosis in human prostate cancer cells PC-3. *Int J Oncol.* 24(5):1093-1099, 2004.

[18] Johnston, N. Medicinal mushroom cuts off prostate cancer cells' blood supply. *Drug Discov Today.* 10(23-24):1584, 2005.

[19] Stanley, G., et al. Ganoderma lucidum suppresses angiogenesis through the inhibition of secretion of VEGF and TGF-beta1 from prostate cancer cells. *Biochem Biophys Res Commun.* 330(1):46-52, 2005.

[20] Sliva, D., et al. Ganoderma lucidum suppresses motility of highly invasive breast and prostate cancer cells. *Biochem Biophys Res Commun.* 298(4):603-612, 2002.

[21] Dufoour, B., et al. Controlled study of the effects of Pygeum africanum extract on the functional symptoms of prostatic adenoma. *J Ann Urol* (Paris), 18(3):193-195, 1984.

[22] Santa Maria Margalef, A., et al. [Antimitogenic effect of Pygeum africanum extracts on human prostatic cancer cell lines and explants from benign prostatic hyperplasia]. *Arch Esp Urol.* 56(4):369-378, 2003.

[23] Wojnowski, R., et al. Modified citrus pectin enhances the effect of novel dietary supplement formulas inhibition of invasiveness of breast and prostate cancer cells by down-regulation of urokinase plasminogen activator (uPA) secretion. Indiana University. 2010.

Vietnamese medicinal herb shows promise in healing prostate and ovarian disease

[1] Zvetkova E, Wirleitner B, Tram NT, Schennach H, Fuchs D Aqueous extracts of Crinum latifolium (L.) and Camellia sinensis show immuno-modulatory properties in human peripheral blood mononuclear cells. *Int Immunopharmacol.* 2001 Nov;1(12):2143-50

Is it really from heaven above?
The cancer miracle that leaves healthy cells healthy

[1] "A medical nutrient has supportive value in the treatment of colorectal cancer." *British Journal of Cancer Aug* 4; 89(3): 465-9

[2] "Antimetastatic effect of Avemar in high-risk melanoma patients." 18th UICC International Cancer Congress, Oslo, Norway, 30 June—5 July, 2002. *International Journal of Cancer* 2002; 100(S13): 408.

[3] "A medical nutriment study has supportive effect in oral cancer." (un-published, Márta Ujpál et al) see re

[4] "Wheat germ extract glucose uptake and RNA ribose formation but increases fatty acid synthesis in MIA pancreatic adenocarcinoma cells." Pancreas 2001; 23:141-147

"Metabolic profiling of cell growth and death in cancer: applications in drug discovery." *Drug Discovery Today* 2002; 7(6): 18-26

[5] "Fermented wheat germ extract inhibits glycolysis/pentose cycle enzymes and induces apoptosis through poly(ADP-ribose) polymerase activation in Jurkat T-cell leukemia tumor cells." *Journal of Biological Chemistry* 2002; 277: 46,408-46,414.

"Fermented wheat germ extract induces apoptosis and downregulation of major complex class I proteins in tumor T and B cell lines." *International Journal of Oncology* 2002; 20: 563-570

[5] "Fermented wheat germ extract induces apoptosis and downregula-tion of major complex class I proteins in tumor T and B cell lines." *International Journal of Oncology* 2002; 20: 563-570

"Avemar triggers apoptosis and downregulation of cell surface MHC 1 proteins in lymphoid tumor cells." Scientific meeting of the Albert Szent-Gyorgyi Medical and Pharmaceutical Center of the Szeged University. Szeged, Hungary, 2000.

[7] "Studies for the effect of Avemar on tumor necrosis induced cytotoxic-ity and on TNF production of immune cells." Institute of Biochemistry, Biological Research Center of the Hungarian Academy of Science. Szeged, 1999.

"Effects of Avemar on the early events of the immune response." Insti-tute of Genetics, Biological Research Center of the Hungarian Academy

of Sceince. Szeged, 1999.
"Effect of Avemar on macrophages and microvascular endothelial cells."
Scientific meeting of the Albert Szent-Györgyi Medical and Pharmaceutical Center of the Szeged University. Szeged, Hungary, 2000.
[8] Letter from James Heimbach, Ph.D. of Jheimbach LLC, 10/28/05
[9] Avemar Published Research, (www.avemarresearch.com)

Part III: Heart

Prevent heart attack and stroke with enzyme that dissolves blood clots in hours

[1] "Interview with Doctor of Medicine Hiroyuki Sumi," Japan Bio Science Laboratory Co. Ltd.
[2] *Acta Haematologica* 1990;84: 139-43
[3] *Biological & Pharmaceutical Bulletin* 1995;18(10): 1,387-91
[4] *Acta Haematologica* 1990;84: 139-43
[5] *Plant Foods for Human Nutrition* 1995;47(1): 39-47
[6] JTTAS 1995
[7] JTTAS 1995

Reverse Metabolic Syndrome—high blood sugar, high cholesterol, high triglycerides!—with this rare Italian fruit

[1] Jung, U. J., et al. Naringin supplementation lowers plasma lipids and enhances erythrocyte antioxidant enzyme activities in hypercholester-olemic subjects. *Clinical Nutrition.* 22(6):561-568, 2003.
[2] Jung, U. J., et al. The hypoglycemic effects of hesperidin and naringin are partly mediated by hepatic glucose-regulating enzymes in C57BL/KsJ-db/db mice. *Journal of Nutrition.* 134(10):2499-2503, 2004.
[3] Bok, S. H., et al. Plasma and hepatic cholesterol and hepatic activities of 3-hydroxy-3-methyl-glutaryl-CoA reductase and acyl CoA: cholesterol transferase are lower in rats fed citrus peel extract or a mixture of citrus bioflavonoids. *Journal of Nutrition.* 129(6):1182-1185, 1999.
[4] Choia, K. M. D., et al. Effect of naringin supplementation on cholesterol metabolism and antioxidant status in rats fed high cholesterol with different levels of vitamin E. *Annals of Nutrition & Metabolism.* 45(5):193-201, 2001.
[5] Mollace, V., et al. Potent hypolipemic and hypoglycemic effect of bergamot-derived poliphenolic fraction: role in 3-hydroxy-3-methyl glutaryl CoA reductase inhibition. (ahead of publication)

Sugar cane extract rivals popular cholesterol-lowering drugs, without the dangerous side effects

[1] *Arch Med Res*, 29(1):21-4, 1998
[2] *Rev Med Chil*, 127(3):286-94, 1999
[3] *Int J Clin Pharmacol Res*, 19(4):117-27, 1999
[4] *Gynecol Endocrinol*, 14(3):187-95, 2000
[5] *Angiology*, 52(2):115-25, 2001
[6] www.ahaf.org/alzdis/research/awards_body.htm

The link between homocysteine and heart disease

[1] *New England Journal of Medicine* 1974;291: 537-43
[2] Research Communications in Molecular Pathology and Pharmacology 1995; 89(2): 208-20
[3] *American Journal of Clinical Nutrition* 1998;68(5): 1104-10

The single-ingredient formula rivaling a major class of blood pressure drugs

[1] *What Your Doctor May Not Tell You About(TM): Hypertension : The Revolutionary Nutrition and Lifestyle Program to Help Fight High Blood Pressure*, New York: Warner Books, 2003
[2] Fujita H, Yamagami T, Ohshima K. "Effect of an ace-inhibitory agent, katuobishi oligopeptide, in the spontaneously hypertensive rat and in borderline and mildly hypertensive subjects." Nutr Res 2001; 21: 1,149-1,158
[3] "LKPNM: a prodrug-type ACE-inhibitory peptide derived from fish protein." Immunopharmacology 1999; 44: 123

The silkworm's secret: Ease inflammation and respiratory illness with this enzyme

[1] *J Int Med Res* 1990; 18(5): 379-88
[2] *Pharmatherapeutica* 1984: 3(8): 526-30
[3] *J Int Med Res* 1990; 18(5): 379-88
[4] *J Assoc Physicians India* 1999 Dec; 47(12): 1,170-2
[5] *Minerva Cardioangiol* 1996 Oct; 44(10): 515-24

Ayurvedic herb fights angina, heart disease, atherosclerosis, and more

[1] *Journal of the Association of Physicians of India* 2001;49: 231-35
[2] *Journal of Ethnopharmacology* 1997;55(3): 165-69
[3] *Journal of Ethnopharmacology* 1997;55(3): 165-69
[4] *Journal of the Association of Physicians of India* 1994;42(4): 287-89
[5] *International Journal of Cardiology* 1995;49(3): 191-99
[6] *International Journal of Cardiology* 1995;49(3): 191-99
[7] *Indian Journal of Physiology and Pharmacology* 1998;42(1): 101-06

[8] *International Journal of Cardiology* 1998;67(2): 119-24
[9] *Journal of Ethnopharmacology* 1998;62(2): 173-82
[10] *Indian Journal of Experimental Biology* 1997;35(5): 478-82
[11] *Journal of the Association of Physicians of India* 1994;42(4): 287-89
[12] *Journal of Ethnopharmacology* 1997;55(3): 165-69
[13] *Journal of Environmental Pathology, Toxicology and Oncology* 2001;20(1): 9-14
[14] *In Vitro Cellular & Developmental Biology: Animal* 2000;36(8): 544-47

One miracle molecule can stop heart attack, stroke...even pull you back from the brink of death

[1] Bryan, N., et al. All-natural nitrite and nitrate containing dietary supplement promotes nitric oxide production and reduces triglycerides in humans. *Nutrition Research*. 31(2011) 262-269.

[2] Petkov, V. Plants with hypotensive, antiatheromatous and coronary dilating action. *American Journal of Chinese Medicine*. 7:197-236, 1979.

[3] Wegrowski, J., et al. The effect of procyanidolic oligomers on the composition of normal and hypercholesterolemic rabbit aortas. *Biochem Pharm*. 33(21):3491-3497, 1984.

[4] Taskov, M. On the coronary and cardiotonic action of Crataemon. *Acta Physiol Pharm*. 3:53-7, 1977.

[5] Tauchert, M., et al. Effectiveness of hawthorne extract LI 132 compared with the ACE inhibitor Captopril: multicenter double blind study with 132 NYHA Stage II. *Muench Med Wochenschr*. 136(Supplement):S27-S33, 1994.

[6] Jayalakshmi, R., et al. Cardioprotective effect of tincture of Crataegus on isoproterenol-induced myocardial infarction in rats. *J Pharm Pharmacol*. 56(7):921-926, 2004.

[7] Bobek, P., et al. The effect of red beet (Beta vulgaris var. rubra) fiber on alimentary hypercholesterolemia and chemically induced colon carcinogenesis in rats. *Nahrung*. 44(3):184-187, 2000.

[8] Webb, A. J., et al. Acute blood pressure lowering, vasoprotective, and antiplatelet properties of dietary nitrate via bioconversion to nitrite. *Hypertension*. 51(3):784-790, 2008.

[9] Maier, J. A., et al. High concentrations of magnesium modulate vascular endothelial cell behaviour in vitro. *Biochim Biophys Acta*. 1689(1):6-12, 2004.

[10] Bartlett, M. K., et al. Vitamin C and wound healing. II. Ascorbic acid content and tensile strength of healing wounds in human beings. *New England Journal of Medicine*. 226:474-481, 1942.

[11] Hayashi, T., et al. l-Citrulline and l-arginine supplementation retards the progression of high-cholesterol-diet-induced atherosclerosis in rabbits. *Proc Natl Acad Sci U S A*. 102(38):13681-13686, 2005.

[12] Bryan, N., et al. Effects of hemodialysis on the nitric oxide congeners nitrite and nitrate: Implications for cardiovascular health in dialysis patients. (submitted for publication, but not yet published).

Part IV: Asthma and COPD

Stamp out even the worst asthma: A breakthrough approach to easy breathing without devastating side effects

[1] Wen M, Wei C, Hu Z, et al. "Efficacy and tolerability of antiasthma herbal medicine intervention in adult patients with moderate-severe allergic asthma." *J Allergy Clin Immun* 2005 517-524.
[2] Hoang B, Shaw D, Levine S, et al. "New approach in asthma treatment using excitatory modulator." Publication pending.
[3] ibid.

Part V: Anti-Aging, Energy, and Weight Loss

The secret energy-boosting weapon trusted by pro athletes

[1] Seidman MD, Khan MJ et al "Influence of lecithin on mitochondrial DNA and age-related hearing loss" *Otolaryngol Head Neck Surg* 2002;127(3):138-144
[2] Agadjanyan M, Vasilevko V et al "Nutritional Supplement (NT Factor) Restore Mitochondrial Function and Reduces Moderately Severe Fatigue in Aged Subjects" *J Chronic Fatigue Syndr* 2003;11(4)
[3] Ellithorpe R, Settineri R, Nicholson G "Pilot Study: Reduction of Fatigue by Use of Dietary Supplement Containing Glycophospholipids" *JANA* 2003;6(1):23-28
[4] Colodny L, Lynch K et al "Results of a Study to Evaluate the Use of Propox to Reduce Adverse Effects of Chemotherapy" *JAMA* 2000;3(2)

Anti-aging therapy so easy you can do it in your sleep

[1] Vgontzas A., Bixler E. et al: Chronic insomnia is associated with nyctohemeral activation of the hypothalamic-pituitary-adrenal axis: clinical implications. *J Clin Endrocinol Metab* 86: 3787-3794,2001
[2] Wurtman RJ, Hefti F, Melamed E. Precursor control of neurotransmitter synthesis. *Pharmacol Rev* 1981;32:315-35.
[3] *The Journal of the American Medical Association* August 16, 2000;284:861-868, 880-881.

Single formula unlocks the 4 strongest secret weapons of a life-extending diet

[1] Gronbaek M., et al. "Type of alcohol consumed and mortality from all causes, coronary heart disease, and cancer." *Annals of Internal Medicine* 2000 Sep 19;133(6):411-9.

[2] Frankel EN, et al. "Inhibition of human LDL oxidation by resveratrol." *Lancet* 1993 Apr 24;341(8852):1103-4.

[3] Bowers JL, et al. "Resveratrol acts as a mixed agonist/antagonist for estrogen receptors alpha and beta." *Endocrinology* 2000 Oct;141(10):3657-67.

[4] Subbaramaiah K, et al. "Resveratrol inhibits cyclooxygenase-2 transcription in human mammary epithelial cells." *Ann NY Acad Sci* 2000;889:214-223.

[5] Howitz KT, et al. "Small molecule activators of sirtuins extend Saccharomyces cerevisiae lifespan." Nature 2003 Sep 11; 425 (6954):191-6. Epub 2003 Aug 24 (http://webweekly.hms.harvard.edu/archive/2003/8_25/inprint.html).

[6] ibid.

[7] Rice-Evans CA. "The relative antioxidant activities of plant-derived polyphenolic flavonoids." *Free Radical Res* 1995 Apr; 22(4): 3785-93.

[8] Mian E, et al. "Anthocyanosides and the walls of the microvessels: further aspects of the mechanism of action of their protective effect in syndromes due to abnormal capillary fragility" *Minerva Med* 1977 Oct 31; 68(52): 3565-81.

[9] Wang H, et al. "Antioxidant and anti-inflammatory activities of anthocyanins and their aglycon, cyanidin, from tart cherries." *J Nat Prod.* 1999 Feb;62 (2):294-6.

[10] Gil Mi, et al. "Antioxidant activity of pomegranate juice and its relationship to phenolic composition and processing." *J Agric Food Chem.* 2000 Oct; 48 (10): 4581-9.

[11] Aviram M and Dornefeld, L. "Pomegranate juice consumption inhibits serum angiotensin converting enzyme activity and reduces systolic blood pressure." *Atherosclerosis.* Volume 158, Issue 1, September 2001, 195 –198

[12] Aviram M, et al. "Pomegranate juice consumption for 3 years by patients with carotid artery stenosis reduces common carotoid intima-media thickness, blood pressure and LDL oxidation." *Clin Nutr* 2004 Jun; 23(3): 423-33

[13] Barch DH, et al. "Structure-function relationships of the dietary anticarcinogen ellagic acid." *Carcinogenesis* 1996,17/2(265-269).

[14] Losso JN, et al. "In vitro anti-proliferative activities of ellagic acid." *J Nutr Biochem.* 2004 Nov;15(11): 672-8.

[15] Aviram M, et al. "Pomegranate juice flavonoids inhibit low density lipoprotein oxidation and cardiovascular diseases: studies in atheroscle-

rotic mice and in humans." *Drugs Exp Clin Res.* 2002; 28(2-3): 49-62.

[16] Miodini P, et al. "The two phyto-oestrogens genistein and querce-tin exert different effects on oestrogen receptor function." *Br J Cancer* 1999;80:1150-5.

[17] Zeisel, SH. "Choline: needed for normal development of memory." *Journal of American College of Nutrition* 2000. 19:528S-531S.

[18] Free Radical Biology Medicine, Volume 8, 1990; *Journal Biological Chemistry*, August 25, 1987.

Shrinking that spare tire has never been easier

[1] Cukierman-Yaffe T, et al. (2009) Relationship between baseline glyce-mic control and cognitive function in individuals with type 2 diabetes and other cardiovascular risk factors: the action to control cardiovas-cular risk in diabetes—memory in diabetes (ACCORD-MIND) trial. *Diabetes Care* 32:221-226.

[2] Kamisoyama H, et al. (2008) Investigation of the anti-obesity action of licorice flavonoid oil in diet-induced obese rats. *Biosci Biotechnol Biochem* 72(12):3225-31.

[3] Nakagawa K, et al. (2004) Licorice flavonoids suppress abdominal fat accumulation and increase in blood glucose level in obese diabetic KK-A(y) mice. *Biol Pharm Bull* 27(11):1775-8.

[4] Aoki F, et al. (2007) Suppression buy licorice flavonoids of abdominal fat accumulation and body weight gain in high-fat diet-induced obese C57BL/6J mice. *Biosci Biotechnol Biochem* 71(1):206-14.

[5] Tominaga Y, et al. (2006) Licorice flavonoid oil effects body weight loss by reduction of body fat mass in overweight subjects. *Journal of Health Science* 52(6):672-683.

[6] Aoki F, et al. (2007). Clinical safety of licorice flavonoid oil (LFO) and pharmacokinetics of glabridin in healthy humans. *Journ Amer Col of Nutr* 26(3):209-218.

An anti-aging breakthrough that will change the way you think about taking supplements forever!

[1] Willcox, J. K., S. L. Ash, et al. (2004). "Antioxidants and prevention of chronicdisease." *Crit Rev Food Sci Nutr* 44(4): 275-95.

[2] Frei, B., L. England, et al. (1989). "Ascorbate is an outstanding antioxi-dant in human blood plasma." *Proc Natl Acad Sci U S A* 86(16): 6377-81.

[3] Balch, J. F. and P. A. Balch (1997). Minerals. Prescription for Nutri-tional Healing. Garden City Park, Avery Publishing Group: 22-29.

[4] Emara, A. M. and H. El-Bahrawy (2008). "Green tea attenuates benze-neinduced oxidative stress in pump workers." *J Immunotoxicol* 5(1): 69-80.

[5] Murray, M. T. and J. E. Pizzorno, Jr. (1999). Chapter 80: Curcuma

longa(turmeric). Textbook of Natural Medicine. J. E. Pizzorno, Jr. and M. T. Murray. New York, Churchill Livingstone. 1: 689-693.

[6] Kandere-Grzybowska, K., D. Kempuraj, et al. (2006). "Regulation of IL-1-induced selective IL-6 release from human mast cells and inhibition by quercetin." *Br J Pharmacol* 148(2): 208-15.

[7] Viuda-Martos, M., Y. Ruiz-Navajas, et al. (2008). "Functional properties of honey, propolis, and royal jelly." *J Food Sci* 73(9): R117-24.

[8] Ajmani, R. S. and J. M. Rifkind. (1998). "Hemorheological changes during human aging." *Gerontology* 44:111-120.

[9] Fujita, M., K. Hong, et al. (1995). "Thrombolytic effect of nattokinase on a chemically induced thrombosis model in rat." *Biol Pharm Bull* 18(10):1387-91.

[10] Suzuki, H., T. Ohyama, et al. (2002). "Effect of oral administration of nattokinase extract on blood mobility." 25(4): 333-338.

[11] Richter, C., J. W. Park, et al. (1988). "Normal oxidative damage to mitochondrial and nuclear DNA is extensive." *Proc Natl Acad Sci U S A.* 85(17):6465-7.

[12] Trifunovic, A., A Hannson, et al. (2005). "Somatic mtDNA mutations cause aging phenotypes without affecting reactive oxygen species production." *Proc Natl Acad Sci U S A.* 102(50):17993-8.

[13] Pauly, D. F. and C. J. Pepine (2000). "D-Ribose as a supplement for cardiac energy metabolism." *J Cardiovasc Pharmacol Ther* 5(4): 249-58.

[14] McDaniel, M. A., S. F. Maier, et al. (2003). "Brain-specific" nutrients: a memory cure?" *Nutrition* 19(11-12): 957-75.

[15] Chapuy, M. C., R. Pamphile, et al. (2002). "Combined calcium and vitamin D3 supplementation in elderly women: confirmation of reversal of secondary hyperparathyroidism and hip fracture risk: the Decalyos II study." *Osteoporos Int* 13(3): 257-64.

[16] Flynn, C. A. (2004). "Calcium supplementation in postmenopausal women." *American Family Physician* 69(12): 2822-2823.

[17] Higdon, J. and V. J. Drake (2007). Vitamin B12, The Linus Pauling Institute (Micronutrient Information Center).

[18] Penland, J. G. (1998). "The importance of boron nutrition for brain and psychological function." *Biol Trace Elem Res* 66(1-3): 299-317.

[19] Pettegrew, J. W., J. Levine, et al. (2000). "Acetyl-L-carnitine physical chemical, metabolic, and therapeutic properties: relevance for its mode of action in Alzheimer's disease and geriatric depression." *Molecular Psychiatry* 5(6): 616-632.

[20] Passeri, M., D. Cucinotta, et al. (1990). "Acetyl-L-carnitine in the treatment of mildly demented elderly patients." *International Journal of Clinical Pharmaceutical Research* 10(1-2): 75-79.

[21] Suarez, F., M. D. Levitt, et al. (1999). "Pancreatic supplements reduce

symptomatic response of healthy subjects to a high fat meal." *Dig Dis Sci* 44(7): 1317-21.

Replenish your body's supply of this natural moisturizer and say good-bye to wrinkles and joint pain

[1] *The Journal of Rheumatology*, 1998; (25)11: p. 2,203-12
[2] Research report of MDS Panlabs Pharmacology Services, Taiwan
[3] Quality assurance report from StillMeadow Inc., March 2000

Erase debilitating pain and fatigue by recharging your cell batteries

[1] Gebhart B, Jorgenson JA. "Benefit of Ribose in a Patient with Fibromyalgia." *Pharmacotherapy* 2004; 24(11): 1,646-1,648
[2] Bengtsson A, Henriksson KG "Reduced high-energy phosphate levels in the painful muscles of patients with primary fibromyalgia." *Arthritis Rheum* 1986; 29: 817-821

Turn back the clock with nature's new fountain of youth

[1] *Science* 2000;287: 2486-92
[2] www.smart-drugs.com/ias-info/gh3-prevention.htm

Part VI: Osteoporosis

Build bone density and heal fractures in half the time with the Chinese tradeshow secret

[1] Zhao Hong Bin ZH, et al. "Experimental Research on The Treatment of Hormonal Necrosis of the Femoral Head." The 1st Affiliated Hospital of Kunming Medical College Department of Orthopedics, 12/15/02
[2] Shu Ye. "Pharmacodynamic Research on OSTEOKING." Kunming Medical College, Kunming, China. 12/28/98.
[3] Maoming X, Yuanshan W, Minquan Z, et al. "Observation of the effect of OSTEOKING on traumatic fractures." 59th Central Hospital of PLA, Kunming City, China, 6/00
[4] Hong BZ, Bing W, Xueling Z, et al. "Long Term Observation of 76 cases of ischemic necrosis of femoral head treated with OSTEOKING." 1st Affiliated Hospital of Kunming Medical College/Kunming Huaxi Traditional Medicine Research Institute in Western China/The 1st People's Hospital of Kunming City, 12/03

Addressing bone density is not enough… Breakthrough reverses osteoporosis by actually rebuilding bone

[1] (2009) Effect of a novel combination of RIAA, berberine, and vitamins D and K on bone remodeling in postmenopausal women with low estrogen. Functional Medicine Research Center.

Part VII: Diabetes

Blood sugar buster THREE TIMES more effective than top-selling diabetes drugs

[1] Montgomery, M, et al. (2007) Human clinical trial evaluating the safety and efficacy of Diatroxal: a randomized, double-blind placebo controlled study. Fenestra Research Labs.

[2] Tully, Lisa. (2007) Peer review of clinical research on Diatroxal by Fenestra Research.

[3] Preuss, HG, et al. (2004) An overview of the safety and efficacy of a novel, natural(-)-hydroxycitric acid extract (HCA-SX) for weight management. *J Med* 35(1-6):33-48.

[4] Preuss, HG, et al. (2004) Effects of a natural extract of (-)-hydroxycitric acid (HCA-SX) and a combination of HCA-SX plus niacin-bound chromium and Gymnema sylvestre extract on weight loss. *Diabetes Obes Metab* 6(3):171-80.

Forget willpower: Overcome sugar addiction in 21 days with a natural herb

[1] *Rat studies show evidence of "sugar dependence,"* Reuters Health News, June 18, 2001

[2] *Trends in Neurosciences*, 24(8):443, 2001

[3] *Eur J Biochem*, 264(2):525-33, 1999

[4] *Am J Physiol Regul Intergr Comp Physiol*, 278(6):R1513-7, 2000

[5] *Eur J Biochem*, 264(2):525-33, 1999

[6] *Eur J Biochem*, 264(2):525-33, 1999

Cutting-edge sugar research may revolutionize your health

[1] Endo T, Toda T "Glycosylation in congenital muscular dystrophies" *Biol Pharm Bull* 2003; 26(12):1641-1647

[2] Sasisekharan R, Myette JR "The Sweet Science of Glycobiology" *American Scientist* 2003; 91(5)

[3] ibid

[4] Endo T, Toda T "Glycosylation in congenital muscular dystrophies" *Biol Pharm Bull* 2003; 26(12):1641-1647

[5] Kuroda Y, Nakata N et al "Structural studies on IgG oligosaccharides of patients with primary Sjogren's syndrome" *Glycoconjugate Journal*

2002;19:23-31

[6] Haston JL, FitzGerald O et al "Preliminary observations on the influence of rheumatoid alpha-1-acid glycoprotein on collagen fibril formation" *Biomed Chromatogr* 2002;16(5):332-342

[7] Backlund J, Treschow A et al "Glycosylation of type II collagen is of major importance for T cell tolerance and pathology in collagen-induced arthritis" *Eur J Immunol* 2002;32(12):3776-3784

[8] Seelen MA, Trouw LA et al "Autoantibodies against mannose-binding lectin in systemic lupus erythematosus" *Clin Exp Immunol* 2003;134(2):335-343

[9] Gupta JK, Ingegno AP et al "Multiple sclerosis and malabsorption" *Am J Gastroenterol* 1977;68(6):560-565

[10] See DM, Cimoch P et al "The in vitro immunomodulatory effects of glyconutrients on peripheral blood mononuclear cells of patients with chronic fatigue syndrome" *Integr Physiol Behav Sci* 1998;33(3):280-287

[11] Lefkowitz DL, Stuart R et al "Effects of a glyconutrient on macrophage functions" *Int J Immunopharmacol* 2000;22(4):299-308

The Battle is Won: Maintain healthy blood sugar, once and for all

[1] Loew, D. Pharmacokinetics of thiamine derivatives especially of benfotiamine. *Int J Clin Pharmacol Ther.* 34(2):47-50, 1996.

[2] Hammes, H. P., et al. Benfotiamine blocks three major pathways of hyperglycemic damage and prevents experimental diabetic retinopathy. *Nature Medicine.* 9(3):294-299, 2003.

[3] Hammes, H. P., et al. Benfotiamine blocks three major pathways of hyperglycemic damage and prevents experimental diabetic retinopathy. *Nature Medicine.* 9(3):294-299, 2003.

[4] Balakumar P, Rohilla A, et al. The multifaceted therapeutic potential of benfotiamine. *Pharmacol Res* 2010;61(6):482-488.

[5] Beltramo E, Berrone E, et al. Effects of thiamine and benfotiamine on intracellular glucose metabolism and relevance in the prevention of diabetic complications. *Acta Diabetol* 2008;45(3):131-141.

[6] Marchetti V, Menghini R, et al Benfotiamine couteracts glucose toxicity effects on endothelial progenitor cell differentiation via Akt/FoxO signaling. *Diabetes* 2006;55:2231-2237.

[7] Beltramo E, Berrone E, et al. Thiamine and benfotiamine prevent increased apoptosis in endothelial cells and pericytes cultured in high glucose. *Diabetes Metab Res Rev* 2004;20(4):330-336.

[8] Beltramo E, Nizheradze K, et al. Thiamine and benfotiamine prevent apoptosis induced by high glucose-conditioned extracellular matrix in human retinal pericytes. *Diabetes Metab Res Rev* 2009;25(7):647-656.

[9] Hammes, H. P., et al. Benfotiamine blocks three major pathways of

hyperglycemic damage and prevents experimental diabetic retinopathy. *Nature Medicine.* 9(3):294-299, 2003.

[10] Schmid U, Stopper H, et al. Benfotiamine exhibits direct antioxidative capacity and prevents induction of DNA damage in vitro. *Diabetes Metab Res Rev* 2008;24(5):371-377.

[11] Katare RG, Caporali A, et al. Vitamin b1 analog benfotiamine prevents diabetes induced diastolic dysfunction and heart failure through akt/pim-1- mediated survival pathway. *Circ Heart Fail* 2010;3(2):294-305.

[12] Katare RG, Caporali A, et al. Vitamin b1 analog benfotiamine prevents diabetes induced diastolic dysfunction and heart failure through akt/pim-1- mediated survival pathway. *Circ Heart Fail* 2010;3(2):294-305.

[13] Ceylan-Isik AF, Wu, S, et al. Vitamin B1 analog benfotiamine prevents diabetes induced diastolic dysfunction and heart failure through Akt/Pim-1- mediated survival pathway. *J Appl Phyiol* 2006;100:150-156.

[14] Anderson RA, Broadhurst CL, et al. Isolation and characterization of polyphenol type-a polymers from cinnamon with insulin-like biological activity. *J Agric Food Chem* 2004;52(1):65-70.

[15] Qin B, Nagasaki M, et al. Cinnamon extract (traditional herb) potentiates in vivo insulin-regulated glucose utilization via enhancing insulin signaling in rats. *Diabetes Res Clin Pract* 2003;62(3):139-148.

[16] Khan A, Safdar M, et al. Cinnamon improves glucose and lipids of people with type 2 diabetes. *Diabetes Care* 2003;26(12):3215-3218.

[17] Ziegenfuss TN, Hofheins JE, et al. Effects of a water-soluble cinnamon extract on body composition and features of the metabolic syndrome in pre-diabetic men and women. *J Int Soc Sports Nutr* 2006;345-53.

[18] Anderson RA. Chromium, glucose intolerance and diabetes. *J Am Coll Nutr* 1998;17(6):548-555.

[19] Cefalu WT, Rood J, et al. Characterization of the metabolic and physiologic response to chromium supplementation in subjects with type 2 diabetes. *Met Clin Exp* 2010;59:755-762.

[20] Anderson RA. Chromium, glucose intolerance and diabetes. *J Am Coll Nutr* 1998;17(6):548-555.

[21] Mita, Y., et al. Supplementation with chromium picolinate recovers renal Cr concentration and improves carbohydrate metabolism and renal function in type 2 diabetic mice. *Biol Trace Elem Res.* 105(1-3):229-248, 2005.

[22] Anderson, R. A., et al. Elevated intakes of supplemental chromium improve glucose and insulin variables in individuals with type 2 diabetes. *Diabetes.* 46:1786-1791, 1997

Dodge the sugar bullet—and double your chances of beating this leading killer

[1] *Eur J Clin Nutr* 1990; 44(4): 301-6
[2] *Prostaglandins Leukot Essent Fatty Acids* 1997; 56 (5): 379-384
[3] *Plant Foods Hum Nutr* 1999; 53(4): 359-365
[4] *J Biochem* (Tokyo) 1992; 111(1): 109-112
[5] *J. Endocrinol* 1999; 163 (2): 207-212
[6] *J Ethnopharmacol* 1990; 30: 281-294
[7] *J. Ethnopharmacol* 1990; 30(3): 295-300
[8] *Bio Environ Sci* 1990 Jun; 3(2): 123-131
[9] *Diabetes Care* 2000; 23(1): 9-14
[10] *Diabetes Care* 1999; 22(6): 913-919
[11] *Int J Obes* 1984; 8(4): 289-293
[12] *Diabetes Care* 1999; 22(6): 1-7
[13] "Medical Implications of Prickly Pear Cactus," Texas A&M University (www.tamuk.edu)
[14] *Gac Med Mex* 1992; 128(4): 431-436
[15] Anderson R, et al. "Isolation and characterization of polyphenol type-A polymers from cinnamon with insulin-like biological activity." *J Agric Food Chem* 2004; 52(1): 65-702 ibid
[16] Cheng N, Anderson RA, et al. FASEB J 2002 Mar 20;16(4):A647) Cheng N et al. "Hypoglycemic effects of cinnamon, heshouwu & mushroom extracts in Type II diabetes mellitus." *FASEB J* 2002: 16(4): A647
[17] Khan A, et al. "Cinnamon improves glucose and lipids of people with type 2 diabetes." *Diabetes Care* 2003; 26(12): 3,215-3,218

Part VIII: Memory

Focus your mind, sharpen your memory with Ayurvedic medicine

[1] *Psychopharmacology* 2001;156(4): 481-84
[2] *Angiology* 2001;52 Suppl 2:S9-13
[3] *Journal of Alternative & Complementary Medicine* 1995;1(3): 249-55
[4] *Phytotherapy Research* 2001;15(6): 544-48
[5] *Phytotherapy Research* 2001;15(6): 524-48
[6] *Arzneimittel-Forschung* 1978;28(1): 7-13
[7] *Journal of Ethnopharmacology* 1996;54(2-3): 119-24
[8] *Probe* 1998;37(3): 179-81
[9] *Fitoterapia* 1995;66(3): 216-22
[10] *Indian Journal of Experimental Biology* 1994;32(1): 37-43
[11] *Mentat [MindCare] Product Monograph*, pages 131-32

Memory-boosting breakthrough proves 'science' wrong by regrowing

dead brain cells

[1] Tagliatatela G, Angelucci L, Ramacci MT, Werrbach-Perez K, et al. Acetyl-L-carnitine enhances the response of PC-12 cells to nerve growth factor. *Brain Res Dev Brain Res.* 1991 Apr 24;59(2):221-30.

[2] Taglialatela, G, Navarra D, Olivi A, Ramacci MT, Werrbach-Perez K, et al. Neurite outgrowth in PC12 cells stimulated by acetyl-L- carnitine arginine amide. *Neurochem Res.* 1995 Jan;20(1):1-9.

[3] Westlund KN, Lu Y, Werrbach-Perez K, Hulsebosch CE, Mrgan B, et al. Effects of nerve growth factor and acetyl-L-carnitine arginyl amide on the human neuronal line HCN-1A. *Int J Dev Neurosci.* 1992 Oct;10(5):361-73.

[4] Scorziello A, Meucci O, Calvani M, Schettini G. Acetyl-L-carnitine arginine amide prevents beta 25-35-induced neurotoxicity in cerebellar granule cells. *Neurochem Res.* 1997 Mar;22(3);257-65.

[5] Sima AA, Calvani M, Mehta M, Amato A. Acetyl-L-carnitine Study Group. Acetyl-l-carnitine improves pain, nerve regeneration, and vibratory perception in patients with chronic diabetic neuropathy: an analysis of two randomized placebo-controlled trials. *Diabetes Care.* 2005 Jan;28(1):89-94.

[6] Montgomery SA, Thal LJ, Amrein R. Meta-analysis of double-blind randomized controlled clinical trials of acetyl-L-carnitine versus place-bo in the treatment of mild cognitive impairment and mild Alzheimer's disease. *Int Clin Psychopharmacol.* 2003 Mar;18(2): 61-71.

[7] Vermeulen RC, Scholte HR. Exploratory open label, randomized study of acetyl and propionylcarnitine in chronic fatigue syndrome. *Psychosom Med.* 2004 Nar-Apr;66(2):276-82.

[8] Tomassini V, Pozzilli C, Onesti E, Pasqualetti P, Marinelli F, Pisani A, et al. Comparison of the effects of acetyl-L-carnitine and aman-tadine for the treatment of fatigue in multiple sclerosis: results of a pilot, randomized, double-blind, crossover trial. *J. Neurol Sci.* 2004 Mar 15;218(1-2):103-8.

[9] Wang, L, Pooler AM, Albrecht MA, Wurtman, RJ. Dietary uridine-5'-monophosphate supplementation increases potassium-evoked do-pamine release and promotes neurite outgrowth in aged rats. *J Mol Neurosci.* 2005;27(1):137-45.

[10] Dawson DM. Enzymatic conversion of uridine nucleotide to cytidine nucleotide by rat brain. *J Neurochem.* 1968 Jan;15(1):31-4.

[11] Silei V, Politi V, Lauro GM. Uridine induces differentiation in human neuroblastoma cells via protein kinase C epsilon. *J Neurosci Res.* 2000 Jul 15;61(2):206-11.

[12] Pooler AM, Guez DH, Benedictus R, Wurtman RJ. Uridine enhances

neurite outgrowth in nerve growth factor-differentiated PC 12 (corrected). *Neuroscience.* 2005;134(1):207-14.

[13] Rao SB, Chetana M, Uma Devi P. Centella asiatica treatment during postnatal period enhances learning and memory in mice. *Physiol Behav.* 2005 Nov 15;86(4):449-57.

[14] Soumyanath A, Zhong YP, Gold SA, Yu X, Koop DR, Bourdette D, Gold BG. Centella asiatica accelerates nerve regeneration upon oral administration and contains multiple fractions increasing neurite elongation in-vitro. *J Pharm Pharmacol.* 2005 Sept;57(9):1221-9.

[15] Garcia-Alloza M, Dodwell SA, Meyer-Luehmann M, Hyman BT, Bacskai BJ. Plaque-derived oxidative stress mediates distorted neurite trajectories in the Alzheimer mouse model. *J Neuropathol Exp Neurol.* 2006 Nov;65(11):1082-9.

Flower power keeps your brain alive

[1] *Behavioral* Brain Research 2000;113(1-2): 11-19
[2] The Newsletter of the Memory Disorders Project at Rutgers-Newark, Winter 2001
[3] *Dementia and Geriatric Cognitive Disorders* 2000;11(Suppl 1): 11-18
[4] *Drugs* 2000;60(5): 1095-1122
[5] *Dementia and Geriatric Cognitive Disorders* 2000;11(Suppl 1): 19-27
[6] *Neurology* 2000; 54(12): 2269-76
[7] National Institute on Aging
[8] *Dementia and Geriatric Cognitive Disorders* 2001;12: 69-77
[9] *Behavioral Brain Research* 2000;113(1-2): 11-19

Regrow brain cells, fight off toxic proteins, and reverse the signs of Alzheimer's and dementia

[1] Kasahara, K., et al. The benefits of lion's mane for aged-disabled. *Gunma Medical Supplementary* issue. 77-81, 2001.
[2] Mori, K., et al. Improving Effects of the Mushroom Yamabushitake (hericium erinaceus) on Mild Cognitive Impairment: A Double-blind Placebo-controlled Clinical Trial. *Phytotherapy Research.* 23, 367-72, 2009.
[3] Kawagishi, H. The inducer of the synthesis of nerve growth factor from lion's mane (Hericium erinaceus). *Explore.* 11(4), 2002.
[4] Nagai, K., et al. Dilinoleoyl-phosphatidylethanolamine from Hericium erinaceum protects against ER stress-dependent Neuro2a cell death via protein kinase C pathway. *Journal of Nutritional Biochemistry.* 17(2006) 525-530.
[5] Case study conducted by Dr. K. Inanaga, submitted for publication January 2008.
[6] Jiang, ZZ and Zhang, LY. New Drug Screening Center, China Pharma-

ceutical University, Unpublished Data

Part IX: Immune System

The Scandinavian secret to cutting colds by 50 percent

[1] *J Nat Prod*, 56(7):995-9, 1993
[2] *Indian J Exp Biol*, 39(1):41-6, 2001
[3] *Phytomedicine*, 4(2):101-4, 1997
[4] ibid. 6(4):217-23, 1999
[5] *Phytomedicine*, 7(5):341-50, 2000
[6] ibid. 7(5):351-64, 2000
[7] www.altcancer.com/andcan.htm (Chinese Herbal Med, 13(9):33-6, 1982)
[8] *J Tongi Med Univ*, 16(4):193-7, 1996
[9] *Clin Exp Pharmacol Physiol*, 27(5-6):358-63, 2000
[10] ibid. 23(8):675-8, 1996
[11] *Planta Med*, 58(2):146-9, 1992
[12] *Phytomedicine*, 6(1):27-31, 1999

Protect yourself from a flesh-eating hospital horror with this natural life-saver

[1] Wikipedia contributors. Methicillin-resistant Staphylococcus aureus. Wikipedia, The Free Encyclopedia. August 4, 2008, 05:25 UTC.
[2] Natural remedies for MRSA. Regenerativenutrition.com. 2008.
[3] Associated Content. Can MRSA be counteracted naturally? AssociatedContent.com. 15 November 2007.
[4] Olive Leaf Extract. Regenerativenutrition.com. 2008.
[5] Wikipedia contributors. Olive leaf. Wikipedia, The Free Encyclopedia. August 1, 2008, 04:03 UTC.
[6] Bisignano, G, et al. On the in-vitro antimicrobial activity of oleuropein and hydroxytyrosol. *J Pharm Parmacol.* 1999 Aug;51(8):971-4.

Scientists rediscover 3,000-year-old wound-healing marvel

[1] Zumla, A, Lulat, A. Honey - a remedy rediscovered. *J R Soc Med.* 1989;82:384-385.
[2] Molan, P.C. Honey as an antimicrobial agent. In: Mizrahi, A. and Lensky, Y. (eds.) Bee Products: Properties, Applications and Apitherapy Plenum Press, New York. 1997: 27-37.
[3] Molan, P.C. Manuka honey as a medicine. University of Waikato. 2001.
[4] Molan, P.C. Honey as a topical antibacterial agent for treatment of infected wounds. *World Wide Wounds.* 2001.
[5] Molan, P.C. What's special about active manuka honey? University of

Waikato. 2001.

Secret germ antidote knocks out Flu in 8 hours

[1] "Attenuation of influenza-like symptomatology and improvement of cell-mediated immunity with long-term N-acetylcysteine treatment," *Eur Respir J.* 1997; 10(7):1,535-1,541

Part X: Vital Health Secrets

Nature's perfect food: Discover the amazing health benefits of the fruit from the Amazon's "tree of life"

[1] Zenebe W, Pechanova O "Effects of red wine polyphenolic compounds on the cardiovascular system" Bratisl Lek Listy 2002;103(4-5):159-165
[2] Rosenkrantz S, Knirel D, Dietrich H et al "Inhibitiion of the PDGF receptor by red wine flavoinoids" FASEB J 2002 Dec;16(14):1958-1960
[3] ibid
[4] Hou DX "Potential mechanisms of cancer chemoprevention by anthocyanins" *Curr Mol Med* 2003 Mar;3(2):149-159
[5] Funari SS, Barcelo F, Escriba PV "Effects of oleic acid and its congeners, elaidic and stearic acids" *J Lipid Res* 2003 Mar;44(3):567-575
[6] Moghadasian MH "Pharmacological properties of plant sterols in vivo and in vitro observations" *Life Sci* 2000 Jun 30;67(6):605-615

Learn what may be causing your bladder control problems—and what you can do about it

[1] Whitmore K, Bologna R et al "Survey of the effect of Prelief on food-related exacerbation of interstitial cystitis symptoms" unpublished; 1998-1999
[2] Tu LM, Polansky M, Cordon DA et al "A retrospective analysis of calcium glycerophosphate (Prelief) in the treatment of food-sensitive interstitial cystitis patients" Quebec Urological Association, 1998

The Polish mothers' secret indigestion remedy

[1] Sipos P, Hagymasi K et al "Effects of black radish root (Raphanus sativus L. var niger) on the colon mucosa in rats fed a fat rich diet" *Phytother Res.* 2002 Nov;16(7):677-9.
[2] Esanu V, Prahoveanu E "The effect of an aqueous horse-radish extract, applied as such or in association with caffeine, on experimental influenza in mice" *Virologie.* 1985 Apr-Jun;36(2):95-8
[3] Speroni E, Cervellati R et al "Efficacy of different Cynara scolymus preparations on liver complaints" *J Ethnopharmacol.* 2003 Jun;86(2-3):203-11

[4] Saenz Rodriguez T, Garcia Gimenez D, de la Puerta Vazquez R "Choleretic activity and biliary elimination of lipids and bile acids induced by an artichoke leaf extract in rats" *Phytomedicine*. 2002 Dec;9(8):687-93

[5] Hiki N, Kurosaka H et al "Peppermint oil reduces gastric spasm during upper endoscopy: a randomized, double-blind, double-dummy controlled trial" *Gastrointest Endosc*. 2003 Apr;57(4):475-82

The key to good health is hiding in your bone marrow: Wake up your stem cells without stirring up controversy

[1] Wade, Nicholas. "Regrow Your Own." *The New York Times* 11 Apr. 2006 <www.nytimes.com>.

[2] Drapeau, Christian, MSc. "Triple-Blind Randomized Placebo-Controlled Study of the Effect of StemEnhance on Bone Marrow Stem Cell Mobilization." Summary available online <www.stemtechhealth.com>.

Steam up your sex life with this native secret from south of the equator

[1] Stanislavov R, Nikolova V. "Treatment of erectile dysfunction with pycnogenol and L-arginine." *J Sex Marital Ther*. 2003 May-Jun;29(3):207-13.

[2] Roseff SJ. "Improvement in sperm quality and function with French maritime pine bark extract." *J Reprod Med*. 2002 Oct;47(10):821-4.

[3] Benavides A, et.al. "Catechin derivatives in Jatropha macrantha stems: characterization and LC/ESI/MS/MS quail-quantitative analysis." *J. Pharm. Biomed. Anal*. 2006 Feb 24; 40(3): 639-47.

[4] Richard T, Verge S, Berke B, et.al. "NMR and stimulated annealing investigations of bradykinin in the presence of polyphenols." *J Biomol Struct Dyn*. 2001 Feb;18(4):627-37.

[5] Becker AJ, Uckert S, Stief CG, et.al. "Possible role of bradykinin and angiotensisn II in the regulation of penile erection and detumenscence." *Urology*. 2001 Jan;57(1):193-8.

Beat depression, migraines—and everything in between—with this single serotonin-boosting breakthrough

[1] Healy D, Herxheimer A, Menkes DB. "Antidepressants and violence: problems at the interface of medicine and law." *PloS Med*. 2006 Sep;3(9):e372

Forget dangerous HRT… You can balance your hormones safely and naturally—without adding a single hormone to your body

[1] Hudson, Tori. (2008/2009) Maca: New insights on an ancient plant. Integrative Medicine 7(6): 54-57.

[2] "Femmenessence (Maca-GO) balances hormonal fluctuation for menopause sufferers with all-natural alternative to HRT." Medical News

Today. 16 January 2008.

[3] Carter, Ronald. (2008) Clinical effects of a proprietary, standardized, concentrated, organic Lepidium peruvianum formulation (Maca-GO) as an alternative to HRT. Natural Health International.

[4] Meissner, H.O. (2005) Hormone-balancing and pharmacological effects of therapeutic doses of Lepidium peruvianum (Maca-GO) in postmenopausal women. Menopause 12(6).

[5] Meissner, H.O. (2006) Therapeutic effects of Lepidium peruvianum chacon (pre-gelatinized maca) used as a non-hormonal alternative to HRT in perimenopausal women – clinical pilot study. IJBS 2(2).

"Nothing—and I mean nothing—has ever had such a wonderful healing effect on my eczema"

[1] McNamara, M, et al. Clinical evaluation of an herbal, topical cream in the treatment of eczema: A double-blind, randomized, placebo controlled study. Klearson Corporation.

[2] McNamara, M, et al. Study of the Safety of PM Eczema Rescue for cases of eczema: A double-blind, randomized, placebo controlled study. Klearson Corporation.

[3] Widrig R, Suter A, Saller R, Melzer J (2007). "Choosing between NSAID and arnica for topical treatment of hand osteoarthritis in a randomised, double-blind study". Rheumatol. Int. 27 (6): 585–91.

Astonishing nutrient turns the tide on Alzheimer's disease, dementia, even strokes!

[1] Serra, F., et al. Effect of CDP-choline on senile mental deterioration. Multicenter experience on 237 cases. Minerva Med. 81:465-470, 1990.

[2] Adibhatla, R. M., et al. Cytidine 5′-diphosphocholine (CDP-choline) in stroke and other CNS disorders. Neurochem Res. 30(1):15-23, 2005.

[3] Silveri, MM, et al. Citicoline enhances frontal lobe bioenergetics as measured by phosphorous magnetic resonance spectroscopy. NMR Biomed. Nov 2008;21(10):1066-75

The government tried to keep this life-changing supplement from you… but HSI is giving you direct access

[1] Fujita, T., et al. Aging and Calcium Paradox. Increase of Red Cell Calcium Content with Age and its Reversal by Calcium Supplementation. Women and Aging: New Research. 2009

[2] Fujita, T. et al. Effect of Calcium Supplementation on Bone Density and Parathyroid Function in Elderly Subjects. Miner Electrolyte Metab. 21:229-231, 1995.

[3] Fujita, T., et al. A three-year comparative trial in osteoporosis treat-

ment: Effect of combined alfacalcidol and elcatonin. Journal of Bone and Mineral Metabolism. 15:223-226, 1997.

[4] Fujita, T. et al. Peripheral computed tomography (pQCT) detected short-term effect of AAACa (heated oyster shell with heated algal ingredient HAI): a double-blind comparison with CaCO3 and placebo. Journal of Bone and Mineral Metabolism. 18:212-215, 2000.

[5] Fujita, T. et al. Overnight suppression of parathyroid hormone and bone resorption markers by active absorbable algae calcium. A double-blind crossover study. Calcif Tissue Int. 60:506-512, 1997.

[6] Fujita, T., et al. Reappraisal of Katsuragi Calcium study, a prospective, double-blind, placebo-controlled study of the effect of active absorbable algal calcium (AAACa) on vertebral deformity and fracture. J Bone Miner Metab. 22:32-38, 2004.

[7] Ohgitani, S. and Fujita, T. Heated oyster shell with algal ingredient (AAACa) decreases urinary oxalate excretion.
J Bone Miner Metab. 18:283-286, 2003

[8] Fujita, T., et al. Exaggerated evening fall of serum calcium in Alzheimer's disease as a possible factor in sundown syndrome and its correction by active absorbable algae calcium (AAACa). Fifth International Conference on Alzheimer's disease and related disorders. July 1996.

Just-discovered rare substance takes the sting out of menopause… and so much more

[1] Izumi, T., et al. Soy Isoflavone Aglycones Are Absorbed Faster and in Higher Amounts than Their Glucosides in Humans. *Journal of Nutrition.* 1000;130:1695-1699.

[2] Awale, S., et al. Constituents of Brazilian red propolis and their preferential cytotoxic activity against human pancreatic PANC-1 cancer cell line in nutrient-deprived condition. *Bioorganic & Medicinal Chemistry.* 16 (2008) 181-189.

Powerful antioxidant may save you from America's leading cause of blindness

[1] *Lipids* 1989;24(7): 659-61

[2] *Physiological Chemistry and Physics and Medical NMR* 1990;22(1): 27-38

[3] *Methods and Findings in Experimental and Clinical Pharmacology* 2001;23(2): 79-84

[4] *Journal of Atherosclerosis and Thrombosis* 2000;7(4): 216-22

[5] www.astaxanthin.org

[6] *The British Journal of Ophthalmology* 1998;82(8): 907-10

[7] United States Patent No. 5,527,533;Tso, Mark O.M. and Lam, Tim-Tak; October 27, 1994

[8] *Journal of AOAC International* 1997;80(3): 622-32

Believe it when you see it: 3-nutrient eyedrop formula
dissolves cataracts without surgery

[1] http://www.ethos.ag/video/randj-update-1.wmv (video clip of Richard & Judy TV Trials Show)

[2] *Ophthalmologica* 2001; 215(3): 192-6

[3] *Aust N Z J Ophthalmol* 1987;15(4): 309-14

[4] *J Ocul Pharmacol Ther* 1999; 15(4): 345-350

[5] *Exp Eye Res* 1999; 68(6): 747-755

[6] *Ann Nutr Metab* 1999; 43(5): 286-289

[7] *Klin Oczna* 1998; 100(2): 85-88

[8] *Age and Ageing* 2000; 29: 207-210

[9] *Photochemistry and Photobiology* 2000; 71(5): 559-566

[10] Wang AM, et al. "Use of carnosine as a natural anti-senescence drug for human beings." Department of Biochemistry and Department of Neurobiology, Harbin Medical University, China, 1999

[11] Babizhayev MA, Deyev A. "Free radical oxidation of lipid and thiol groups in genesis of cataract." *Biophysics* (biofizika) 1986; 31: 119-125

[12] Babizhayev MA, Deyev AI, Linberg LF. "Lipid peroxidation as a possible cause of cataract." Mech Ageing Dev 1988; 44: 69-89

[13] Babizhayev MA. "Antioxidant activity of L-carnosine, a natural histidine-containing di-peptide in crystalline lens." *Biochem Biophys Acta* 1989; 1,004: 363-371

[14] Babizhayev MA, Deyev AI, Yermakova VN, et al. "N-Acetylcarnosine, a natural histidine-containing dipeptide, as a potent ophthalmic drug in treatment of human cataracts." *Peptides* 2001; 22: 979-994